Ultrasound in Critical Care

Ultrasound in Critical Care

Editor: Jonathan Hodges

AMERICAN
MEDICAL PUBLISHERS
www.americanmedicalpublishers.com

AMERICAN
MEDICAL PUBLISHERS
www.americanmedicalpublishers.com

Cataloging-in-Publication Data

Ultrasound in critical care / edited by Jonathan Hodges.
p. cm.
Includes bibliographical references and index.
ISBN 979-8-88740-543-8
1. Ultrasonic imaging. 2. Diagnostic ultrasonic imaging. 3. Critical care medicine.
4. Diagnostic imaging. 5. Ultrasonics in medicine. I. Hodges, Jonathan.
RC78.7.U4 U48 2023
616.075 43--dc23

American Medical Publishers,
41 Flatbush Avenue,
1st Floor, New York,
NY 11217, USA

ISBN 979-8-88740-543-8 (Hardback)

Contents

Preface

Every book is initially just a concept; it takes months of research and hard work to give it the final shape in which the readers receive it. In its early stages, this book also went through rigorous reviewing. The notable contributions made by experts from across the globe were first molded into patterned chapters and then arranged in a sensibly sequential manner to bring out the best results.

Ultrasound is a diagnostic method that uses high-intensity sound waves to produce the images of structures within the body. It serves as a valuable source of information for several purposes, including diagnosis of various diseases and monitoring the course of pregnancy. Ultrasound can also be used as an image guidance tool during certain medical procedures. The images generated by an ultrasound are known as sonogram. Ultrasound can be categorized into three main types, which includes pregnancy or prenatal ultrasound, diagnostic ultrasound, and ultrasound guidance for procedures. There are several procedures that need ultrasound guidance, such as guiding needle placement to sample fluid or tissue from joints, tendons, muscles, transplant organs, etc. Lesion localization procedures, embryo transfer for in vitro fertilization and nerve blocks are some other medical procedures that make the use of ultrasound guidance. Ultrasound is also used for the management of patients undergoing critical care. The diagnosis and assessment of various medical conditions such as pulmonary edema, pneumothorax and deep vein thrombosis can be done in a rapid manner through ultrasound. This book unravels the recent studies on ultrasound imaging. It strives to provide a fair idea about its applications in critical care. This book is appropriate for students seeking detailed information in this area as well as for experts.

It has been my immense pleasure to be a part of this project and to contribute my years of learning in such a meaningful form. I would like to take this opportunity to thank all the people who have been associated with the completion of this book at any step.

Editor

1

Common pitfalls in point-of-care ultrasound: a practical guide for emergency and critical care physicians

Pablo Blanco[1,2*] and Giovanni Volpicelli[3]

Abstract

Background: Point-of-care ultrasonography (POCUS) is a widely used tool in emergency and critical care settings, useful in the decision-making process as well as in interventional guidance. While having an impressive diagnostic accuracy in the hands of highly skilled operators, inexperienced practitioners must be aware of some common misinterpretations that may lead to wrong decisions at the bedside.

Objectives: This article provides a revision list of common POCUS misdiagnoses usually found in practice and offers useful tips to recognize and avoid them.

Discussion: The following aspects were selected and reviewed: pericardial effusion vs. pleural vs. ascites vs. epicardial fat; right ventricle dilation in acute pulmonary embolism and inferior vena cava for volume status assessment in cardiac ultrasound; lung point and lung pulse misinterpretations and mirror artifacts vs. lung consolidations in lung ultrasound; peritoneal fluid vs. the stomach and a critical appraisal of gallbladder signs of acute cholecystitis in abdominal ultrasound; the rouleaux phenomenon vs. deep vein thrombosis or acute right strain in vascular ultrasound.

Conclusions: Following some rules in technique and interpretation, and always integrating POCUS findings into the broader clinical context, most POCUS misdiagnosis can be avoided, and thus patients' safety can be enhanced. Being aware of a list of common pitfalls may help to avoid misdiagnoses.

Keywords: Ultrasonography, Point-of-care, Injuries, Critical care

Introduction

Point-of-care ultrasonography (POCUS) is living a gold era in emergency and critical care medicine, because it is now widely recognized its usefulness in complementing the physical examination and serving as a safe interventional guidance at the bedside [1, 2]. Moreover, an ultrasonography-supported paradigm is gradually becoming a routine approach when caring for critically ill patients [3, 4]. However, it is important to highlight some rising concerns regarding provoked patients' injuries that can result when POCUS is used inappropriately by novice or inexperienced practitioners. POCUS misdiagnoses due to inexperience may lead to errors in the treatment that may worsen patients' outcomes or even be fatal. It is important to remind that before taking any action and being independent in the decision-making process, practitioners must be properly trained and well prepared to the possibility of misinterpretations. Nowadays, POCUS competences are covered in many curricula [1, 5–8] and included in most hands-on training programs, which represent the best way to teach properly POCUS and train new operators. Here, we report a revision of some common POCUS misdiagnoses that may be encountered in the common clinical practice. We will highlight the potential impact of these mistakes on patient outcome,

*Correspondence: ohtusabes@gmail.com
[1] Intensive Care Unit, Hospital Dr. Emilio Ferreyra, 4801, 59 St., 7630 Necochea, Argentina
Full list of author information is available at the end of the article

and finally we will list several tips that may be of help for a correct interpretation of POCUS imaging.

Cardiac ultrasound

Pericardial effusion versus other diagnosis

Pericardial effusion (PEF) is often found in critically ill patients and is defined by transthoracic echocardiography (TTE) as a diastolic fluid-filled space located within the two layers of the pericardium. Pericardial fluid is usually anechoic but sometimes can show a complex echotexture as, for instance, when it contains clots, pus or fibrin. PEF can be circumferential or regional. Even when circumferential, PEF not always is easy to visualize because it may distribute irregularly, and thus several TTE views are needed to demonstrate its presence and real amount. Magnitude and short time of collection are the two main characteristics that influence the possibility of tamponade. The most important tips to recall regarding PEF recognition at POCUS are:

- Tracking anterior to descending aorta in parasternal long axis and apical 4-chamber views (Fig. 1a, b) [9, 10].
- PEF is always present in dependent segments (posterior wall, lateral wall, inferior wall).
- Checking diastolic collapse of cardiac chambers that is a sign of hemodynamically significant PEF: characteristically, the right ventricle outflow tract and the right atrium (RA) are the first parts of the cardiac chambers that collapse under the external pressure of PEF, followed next by the right ventricle (RV) with further increase in the pericardial pressure; diastolic collapse of the left atrium (LA) and left ventricle (LV) can be observed only in the most extreme cases [9, 10]. Right chambers will be fairly resistant to collapse in severe pulmonary hypertension, when abnormal high intracavitary pressure is opposed to the high intra-pericardial pressure [11]. Of note, diastolic collapse of both atriums in significant PEF occurs in ventricular systole (i.e., atrial diastole), and thus one can determine its presence when the atrioventricular valves are closed. This allow for distinction between diastolic collapses in PEF from the normal atrial systole which occurs when the atrioventricular valves are opened.
- Checking dilated (more than 2 cm diameter in long axis) and reduced or absent collapsibility (less than 20% collapse) of the inferior vena cava (tamponade) in spontaneously breathing patients [9, 10].

In case of hypovolemic patients with small, under-filled cardiac chambers, even a mild PEF may be overestimated because the hyper contractile heart could simulate a diastolic collapse of the right chambers. In these cases, the observation of a depleted inferior vena cava (more than 50% or complete collapse during respiration) is a key finding, allowing to rule out a significant role of PEF in the hemodynamic instability.

The most common problematic differential diagnosis of PEF are represented by pleural effusion, peritoneal free-fluid (ascites) and epicardial and/or mediastinal fat. In addition, a large hiatal hernia, pericardial or other mediastinal cysts or left ventricle pseudoaneurysm may sometimes be hardly differentiated but more rarely.

Pleural effusion is defined as a fluid-filled space located within the pleural space. When not directly investigated by lung ultrasound but incidentally detected during TTE, pleural effusion is usually present in a significant amount. Characteristically, left sided pleural effusion appears posterior and lateral to the descending aorta in parasternal long axis and apical 4-chamber views (Fig. 1b, c) [9, 10]. In subcostal views, a right pleural effusion can also be visualized besides the right cardiac chambers, extending over the bare area of the liver (Fig. 1d). When observed in detail, a mobile and consolidated lung is visualized into the pleural fluid (Fig. 1b–d). Additionally, lung ultrasound in coronal views will also show this effusion.

Ascites appears invariably in subcostal views, anterior to the right cardiac chambers. In these cases, the falciform ligament is observed within the fluid, which in addition with the visible diaphragmatic movement, allows to confirm the diagnosis (Fig. 2a) [12]. Moreover, extending the examination to the rest of the abdomen will easily demonstrate the presence of ascites to complete the diagnosis.

Epicardial fat is the adipose tissue accumulated between the visceral pericardium and the myocardium (i.e., epicardial region) [13, 14]. It is slightly isoechoic and is best observed in systole (obliterates completely in diastole) and exclusively in anterior regions. Thus, it is commonly visualized in parasternal long and short axis views (Fig. 2b) as well as in the subcostal 4-chamber view [13]. Mediastinal fat is located anterior to the pericardium and is best observed also in parasternal views (short and long axis) during systole (Fig. 2b) [13].

Error implication An erroneously diagnosed PEF in the unstable patient may lead to undue pericardiocentesis with the strong possibility of cardiac chamber perforation, pericardial tamponade, and eventually, death.

How to avoid this error It is essential to integrate the US findings in the clinical context and consider all the infor-

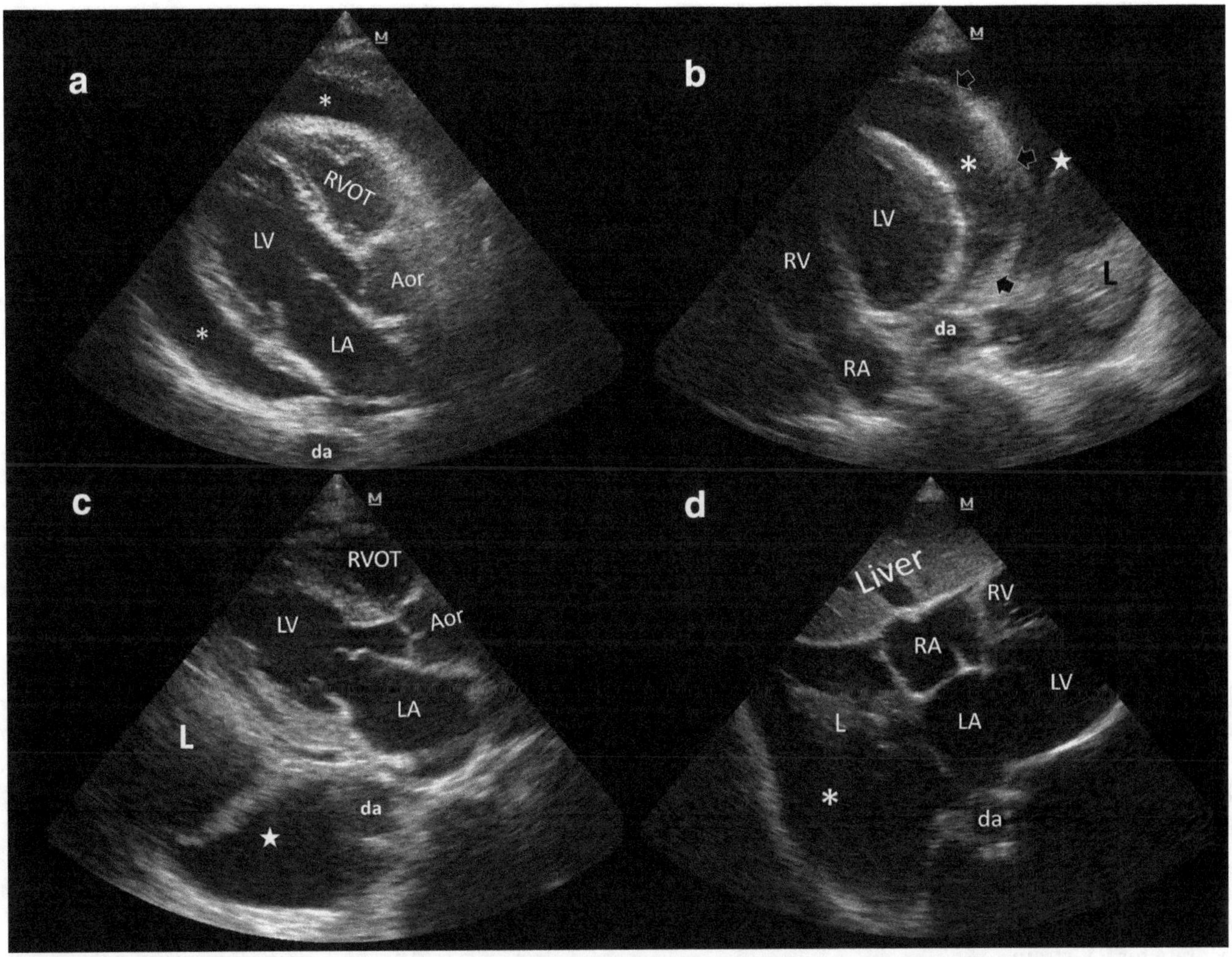

Fig. 1 Pericardial versus pleural effusion. **a** Parasternal long axis view. Pericardial effusion (*asterisks*) tracks anterior to the descending aorta (da); *LV* left ventricle, *LA* left atrium, *RVOT* right ventricle outflow tract, *Aor* aortic root. **b** Apical 4-chamber view. Pericardial effusion (*asterisk*) tracks anterior to the descending aorta (da); pleural effusion (*white star*) tracks posterior and lateral to the da. *Arrows* pericardial delineation, *L* lung consolidation, *LV* left ventricle, *RV* right ventricle, *RA* right atrium. **c** Pleural effusion (*white star*) tracks posterior and lateral to the da; *L* lung consolidation, *LV* left ventricle, *LA* left atrium, *RVOT* right ventricle outflow tract, *Aor* aortic root. **d** Right pleural effusion (*asterisk*) extending into the bare area of the liver, besides the heart in subcostal 4-chamber view; *L* lung consolidation, *RA* right atrium, *RV* right ventricle, *LA* left atrium, *LV* left ventricle, *da* descending aorta

mation on the patient condition, signs and symptoms; tamponade is a clinical diagnosis, which is supported by a compatible POCUS scan. Eventually, in doubtful cases it may be considered draining other effusions if these are well demonstrated and reevaluate thereafter the magnitude of a PEF. If PEF is still present but is not large and shows no hemodynamic consequences on the motility of the right cardiac chambers, drainage should be avoided unless an infectious PEF is suspected. In case of unusual regional location of PEF with intuitive difficulties in the procedure for draining, as it may be a posterior PEF, a surgical consult should be considered. In difficult cases, eventually, the correlation with other imaging methods (e.g., CT) is required.

Right ventricle dilation and acute pulmonary embolism

The diagnosis of right ventricle dilation is of paramount importance in the bedside diagnosis of pulmonary embolism in emergency situations and unstable patients. However, not always the dilation is clearly visible and many possibilities of error should be considered. The diagnosis of dilation basically relies on a comparison between the end-diastolic diameters of the RV and LV. A wrong and incomplete visualization of the cardiac chambers may lead to misdiagnosis. Moreover, the possibility of a chronic dilation not linked to acute right overload may induce further errors. This possibility may be encountered in case of evaluation of patients with chronic volume overload status (e.g., chronic significant

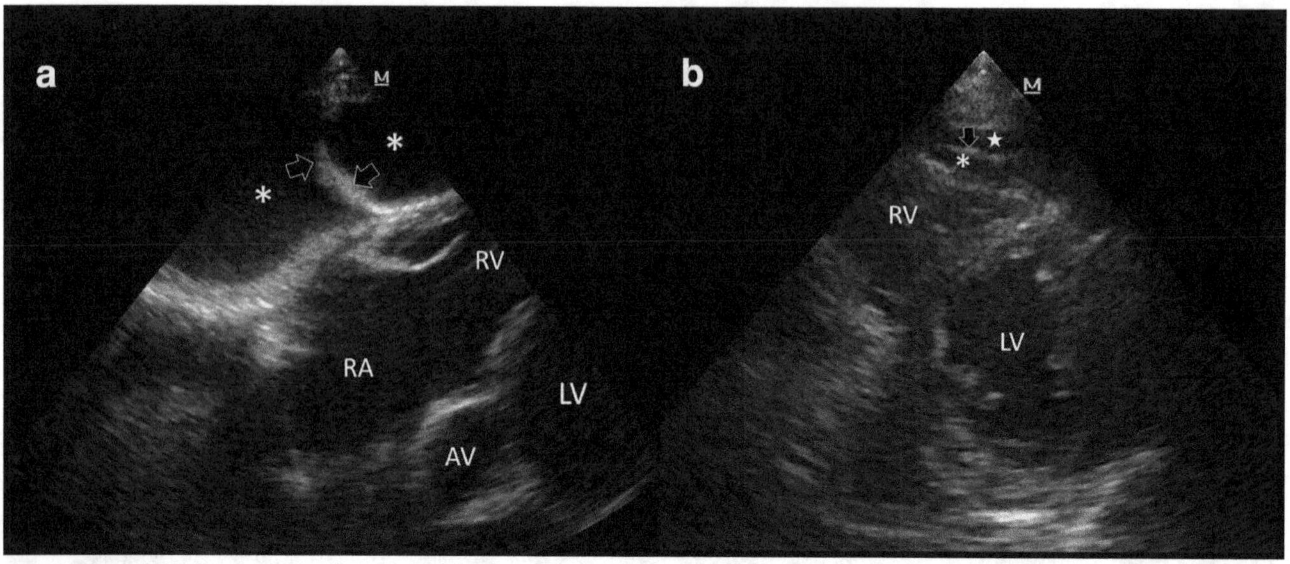

Fig. 2 **a** Pericardial effusion versus ascites. Ascites (*asterisks*) is shown anterior to the heart in subcostal 4-chamber view. The falciform ligament (*arrows*) is depicted, confirming this effusion. *LV* left ventricle, *AV* aortic valve, *RV* right ventricle, *RA* right atrium. **b** Epicardial (*asterisk*) and mediastinal fat (*white star*), demonstrated in parasternal short-axis view, in systole; *LV* left ventricle, *RV* right ventricle, *arrow* pericardium

tricuspid or pulmonary regurgitation) and chronic pressure overload conditions (e.g., chronic pulmonary hypertension) [15]. RV infarction is another condition coursing with RV dilation and impairment of RV function and sometimes hardly to differentiate from pulmonary embolism. In patients with cardiac arrest from any cause, ventricular chambers tend to equalize in short time, and thus applying RV dilation criteria may not be accurate for RV strain.

Error implication A wrong diagnosis of RV dilation in the extreme emergency may lead to the erroneous conclusion of a state of acute right pressure overload (massive pulmonary embolism) that may induce undue thrombolysis or more invasive treatments (e.g., thrombectomy). On the other hand, missing the visualization of real RV dilation from an acute status may delay proper treatment and be harmful for the patient.

How to avoid this error To diagnose correctly RV dilation, the two ventricles should be clearly and fully visualized, preferably in the apical 4-chamber view, and the two end-diastolic diameters taken beside at the level of the atrioventricular valve plane. When this view is not fully demonstrative, a conclusion should never be drawn. A ratio of at least 0.9 is indicative of dilated RV [16–19]. When other views are chosen for difficulty in obtaining a clear apical 4-chamber, different cut-offs should be applied (Table 1). Along with RV dilation, other signs of RV pressure overload may be considered, such as systolic interventricular septal flattening with systolic D-shaped RV (observed in short-axis views), impairment of RV systolic function (e.g., low TAPSE, RV free wall and RV inferior wall hypokinesia) as well as a RV-RA peak pressure gradient higher than 30 mmHg [15, 16, 19]. However, these additional signs are more laborious and need an advanced skill to be evaluated. Moreover, they are not sufficiently sensitive and specific when considered alone [15–17]. Finally, in cases of dilated RV, adjunctive signs of chronic dilation should be considered, like the thickness of the RV wall (superior to 5 mm), LV status, regional impairments, together with clinical history when available.

Table 1 Criteria for diagnosing right ventricle dilation at point-of-care bedside echocardiography (Adapted from [16]–[19])

Echocardiography view	Criteria for right ventricle dilation
4-Chamber apical view	Right/left ventricular end-diastolic diameter ratio >0.9
Parasternal long axis view	Right ventricular end-diastolic diameter >30 mm
Subcostal view	Right/left ventricular end-diastolic diameter ratio >0.7 or 0.9

For the evaluation of the dimension of the right ventricle the preferred view should be the apical 4-chamber. The other views should be used as second choice in case of doubtful measure or impossibility to obtain a clear image

RA thrombus in transit and thrombus located between both atriums in the foramen ovale are specific signs of pulmonary embolism, and thus should always be considered.

Inferior vena cava and fluid status

The inferior vena cava (IVC) is responsible for lower body systemic blood returning towards the heart. Thus, it is a common practice to consider that volemic status and/or fluid responsiveness may be in someway related to ultrasound measurement of the IVC diameter and its dynamics during the respiratory cycles, which allows a rough estimation of the right atrial pressure. While a depleted IVC is often observed in hypovolemic patients, typically the IVC is dilated in a hypervolemic condition with a less pronounced or null respiratory collapse [20]. However, some gray-zone conditions that alter this supposed linear relationship between the size of the vein and the actual volume status can be easily encountered and observed in practice. For instance, patients with high left ventricle filling pressures and normal IVC [21], potentially fluid responsive patients with physiologically dilated IVC [22], cases of acute right ventricular infarction, pericardial tamponade, acute massive pulmonary embolism, intraabdominal hypertension, asthma/COPD exacerbations and mechanically ventilated patients with positive pressures, all represent conditions where the IVC measurement may fail in indicating reliably the volume status. In addition, acute or chronic cor pulmonale, severe tricuspid regurgitation and pericardial constriction may show highly variable IVC dynamics, independent from the real volume status of the patient [23]. A further possibility of misinterpretation of the ultrasound study of the IVC may happen when the technique is not correctly applied. For a correct measure, the IVC should be visualized in long axis and the inner walls clearly imaged. In M-mode, the movement of the vessel under the probe may erroneously give the impression of a respiratory collapse that is not real. This must be checked observing simultaneously the M-mode with two dimensional imaging (Additional file 1: Video S1, Additional file 2: Video S2, Additional file 3: Video S3). Other phenomena observed is the inspiratory lateral translation of the IVC, producing a misalignment between the IVC and the US scanning plane, and thus simulating an inspiratory collapse [23]. These are common pitfalls that may trick even expert operators.

Error implications These misinterpretations may lead to avoid fluid treatment and even using undue diuretics in patients who are volume depleted and potentially fluid responsive (e.g., in cases of patients mechanically ventilated, or in some emergencies like myocardial infarction of the right ventricle and obstructive causes of shock). On the other hand, errors in the IVC ultrasound may lead to erroneous administration of fluid challenges in patients with high left sided cardiac pressures or conditions of non-responsiveness to volume load, sometimes inducing pulmonary congestion, worsening hemodynamic status and even delaying proper administration of vasopressors and inotropes.

How to avoid this error It is essential to integrate the IVC analysis with a comprehensive multi-organ ultrasound approach that should include a basic focused evaluation of the dimensions, ratio and function of the right and left cardiac chambers, a basic evaluation of the pulmonary congestion by assessing lung ultrasound for B lines, and of course, a full consideration of all the available clinical information. A correct interpretation of the volume status through the IVC assessment should always combine the respiratory variation of the IVC with its absolute size. In mechanically ventilated patients without inspiratory efforts and tidal volume >8 ml/kg (predicted body weight), IVC variation (distensibility index) distinguished fairly accurately the fluid responsive from non-responsive patients [23–25]. In patients with non-invasive ventilation, the interplay between the active respiratory efforts of the patient (negative pressure inducing an inspiratory flattening of the IVC) and the machine (positive pressure inducing an inspiratory engorgement of the IVC) has unpredictable effects on the inferior vena cava [23]. In spontaneously breathing patients with hypovolemia, a IVC collapsibility >42% may predict fluid responsiveness with high specificity (97%) [26]; however, normovolemic patients with large respiratory efforts may simulate this IVC dynamics [23]. Patients with shallow respiratory efforts may induce the opposite changes in the IVC collapsibility.

Other conditions affecting the transmural pressures between the thorax and the abdomen (e.g., asthma/COPD exacerbations, active expiratory efforts, patients with invasive mechanical ventilation and inspiratory efforts) may preclude the use of the IVC for volume assessment, as well as other situations that can induce high RA pressures (e.g., RV infarction, tamponade).

Lung ultrasound

Lung sliding, lung point, B lines and lung pulse in the diagnosis of pneumothorax

The lung point is a fundamental ultrasonographic sign highly specific for confirming pneumothorax [27]. Two other equivalent signs are also highly specific for diagnosing pneumothorax [27]: the hydro-point [28] and the heart-point sign [29]. However, some normal physiological conditions can be misdiagnosed for false lung points [30, 31]. The requirement necessary to define the real lung point is an absent lung sliding with absent subpleural parenchymal ultrasound signals (B-lines or consolidations) and the lung point as the contact between the aforementioned region and the sliding lung (or pleural fluid as in hydro-pneumothorax) [32]. Indeed, some similar ultrasound patterns representing the interphases between the expanding lung and the diaphragm (Additional file 4: Video S4) and between the expanding lung and the heart (Additional file 5: Video S5), may be misdiagnosed for false lung points, especially when observed with high frequency probes, sometimes inducing the operator to wrong conclusions.

A complex situation can also be encountered in patients with pulmonary peripheral blebs. These patients commonly have structural lung parenchymal alterations that sometimes are at risk to develop a secondary pneumothorax in a background of chronic obstructive pulmonary disease [33]. Thus, differential diagnosis with pneumothorax may be crucial. In these cases, sometimes a regular lung sliding can be demonstrated in large peripheral blebs even if with some difficulty [34]. However, very often, the presence of pleural adhesions precludes the visualization of the respiratory movement of the lung and may induce erroneous interpretation. In stable patients absence of sliding should never be considered enough to finalize the diagnosis of pneumothorax. Especially, in patients with complex pulmonary disorders (large blebs and adhesions), a more detailed chest CT study may be required.

Pneumomediastinum may mimic a left sided pneumothorax, producing air artifacts during the chest ultrasound examination and even obscuring a regular parasternal and apical echocardiographic views. Correlation with chest X-ray or CT is usually required to confirm the diagnosis and exclude a pneumothorax [35].

While a false pattern of absence of sliding may contribute to misdiagnose pneumothorax, sometimes a respiratory or cardiac movement of the lung image at ultrasound may be misinterpreted for a false lung sliding (Additional file 6: Video S6). Even the beat of an intercostal artery or the thoracic internal artery in parasternal region may simulate a false lung pulse (Additional file 7: Video S7), thus inducing the operator to misdiagnose the absence of pneumothorax. Similarly, in complex cases of recurrence of pneumothorax after abrasion pleurodesis, the visualization of B lines due to multiple septa still connecting the lung to the chest wall may induce to erroneously rule out the condition (Additional file 8: Video S8) [36].

Error implications The misdiagnosis of the absence of sliding or a false lung point may lead to an unnecessary pleural drainage. Furthermore, in doubtful cases, higher costs and irradiation exposure may arise if other unnecessary diagnostic imaging methods are ordered. In case of false sliding, false pulse or multiple septa, the diagnosis of pneumothorax may be dangerously delayed or even missed.

How to avoid these errors Use a set of criteria to define pneumothorax by combining the four basic signs: abolished lung sliding, absent parenchymal signs (B lines and consolidations), absent lung pulse and look for the lung point for final confirmation in stable patients. Eventually, rule in a pneumothorax by chest CT if the patient is stable or correlate the ultrasound pattern with previous images, when available, in case of history of blebs or previous abrasion pleurodesis. In complicated cases, like secondary pneumothorax, recurrences, post-procedural pneumothorax, and trauma, a complex pattern should always be considered a strong possibility and induce the caring physician to carefully scan the whole chest to improve the accuracy of lung ultrasound.

Mirror artifact vs. lung consolidation

Mirror artifacts consist in the repetition of a false image resulting from the ultrasound beam hitting against a highly reflective surface [37], such as the diaphragm. Most frequent in the right side, this artifact can simulate a lung consolidation by the repetition of the liver tissue pattern above the diaphragm (Fig. 3a).

Error implications This misdiagnosis may lead to higher costs and adverse effects derived from indications of antibiotics as well as unneeded chest X-ray or CT.

How to avoid this error Along with integration into the clinical picture, observing the same tissue pattern of the liver or spleen is usually enough to rule in this artifact. The presence of pleural effusion that invariably accompanies lung consolidations and sonographic air or fluid bronchograms (Fig. 3b) is never observed in mirror image artifacts, and thus may aid in differentiating real lung diseases.

Abdominal ultrasound

Peritoneal fluid versus the stomach

Peritoneal fluid recognition is recommended during the first evaluation of trauma patients [38] as well as in patients presenting with several abdominal complaints and shock [39, 40]. When the abdomen is evaluated in left coronal views, a full stomach appearing below the diaphragm may mimic a condition of peritoneal fluid

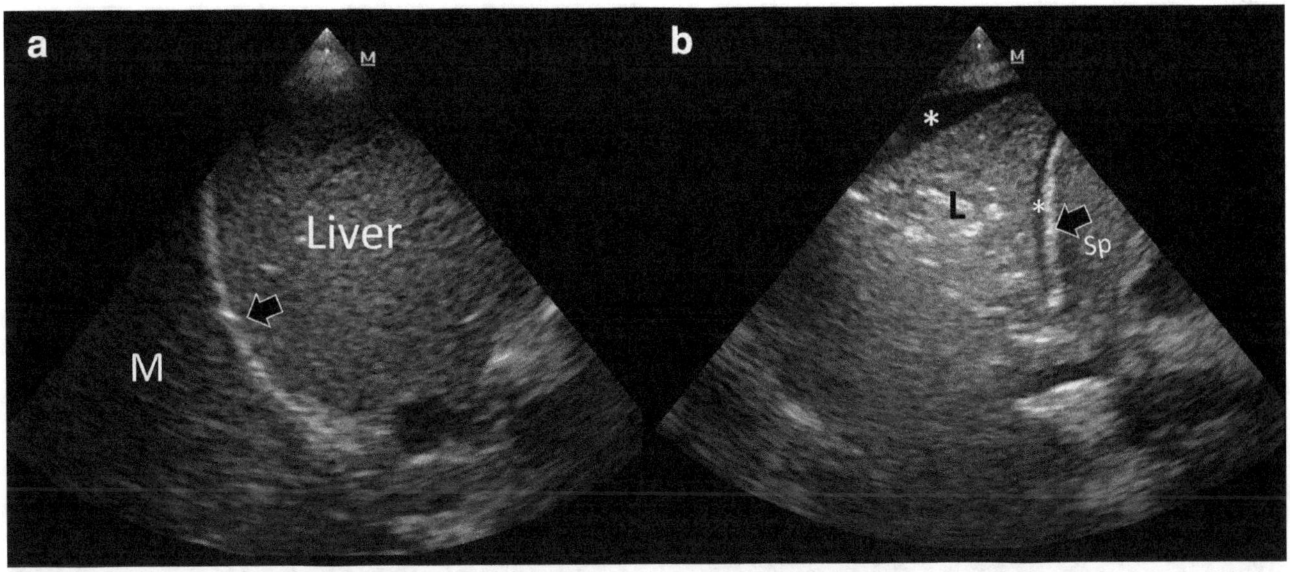

Fig. 3 **a** Mirror image artifact (M), showing a similar tissue-like pattern in comparison with the liver; *arrow*: diaphragm. **b** Lung consolidation (L). Distinctively, it is shown a tissue-like pattern, sonographic air bronchogram and pleural fluid (*asterisks*); *arrow* diaphragm, *Sp* spleen

(Fig. 4a). In other situations, the stomach may even appear in epigastric subcostal views and may simulate a fluid abdominal collection (Fig. 4b). Depending on gastric contents (fluid, air, food), the appearance of the stomach may vary, ranging from simple anechoic fluid up to a heterogeneous ultrasound pattern.

Error implications A misdiagnosis of false peritoneal fluid may lead to undue ultrasound-guided puncture and subsequent intraabdominal organ damage (i.e., spleen, diaphragm and stomach perforation), and eventually involving the pleural space causing pneumothorax. Furthermore, higher costs and undue irradiation may arise from confirmatory CT studies. Eventually, this misinterpretation may lead to laparotomy, and thus adjunctive surgical risks.

How to avoid this error First, it is important to consider the possibility of a full stomach since it is visible in most non-fasted patients as well as in patients with delayed gastrointestinal emptying, which is a common condition in the critically ill. In doubtful cases and when the patients are able to take oral fluids, a possibility for differential diagnosis consists in observing bubbles appearing after having asked to the patient to drink some water. In unconscious patients or in extreme emergency situations, such as in postoperative abdominal patients with sepsis of unknown origin or in trauma patients, the opposite may be done by using the nasogastric or orogastric tube and evaluating if the image persists after gastric drainage. Moreover, the gastric tube can be also visualized by ultrasound coming down to the stomach during the maneuver, confirming the location of the organ (Fig. 4c).

Distended gallbladder, thickened gallbladder walls and acute cholecystitis

Along with a compatible clinical picture, ultrasonographic criteria of acute cholecystitis are a distended gallbladder, thickened walls, biliary sludge and lithiasis (calculus type), pericholecystic fluid and sonographic Murphy's sign [41, 42].

Gallbladder distension and wall thickening, although important signs, are not specific for acute cholecystitis when considered alone (Tables 2, 3). For example, thickened gallbladder walls are commonly observed in patients coursing with generalized edemas such as those with cardiac failure (Fig. 5a, b), pre-eclampsia or renal failure. In non-fasted patients, the gallbladder is physiologically contracted, and thus may show thickened walls. In the presence of thickened walls, pericholecystic fluid and biliary sludge but the absence of clearly visible gallstones, acute cholecystitis during septic shock can be misdiagnosed [43].

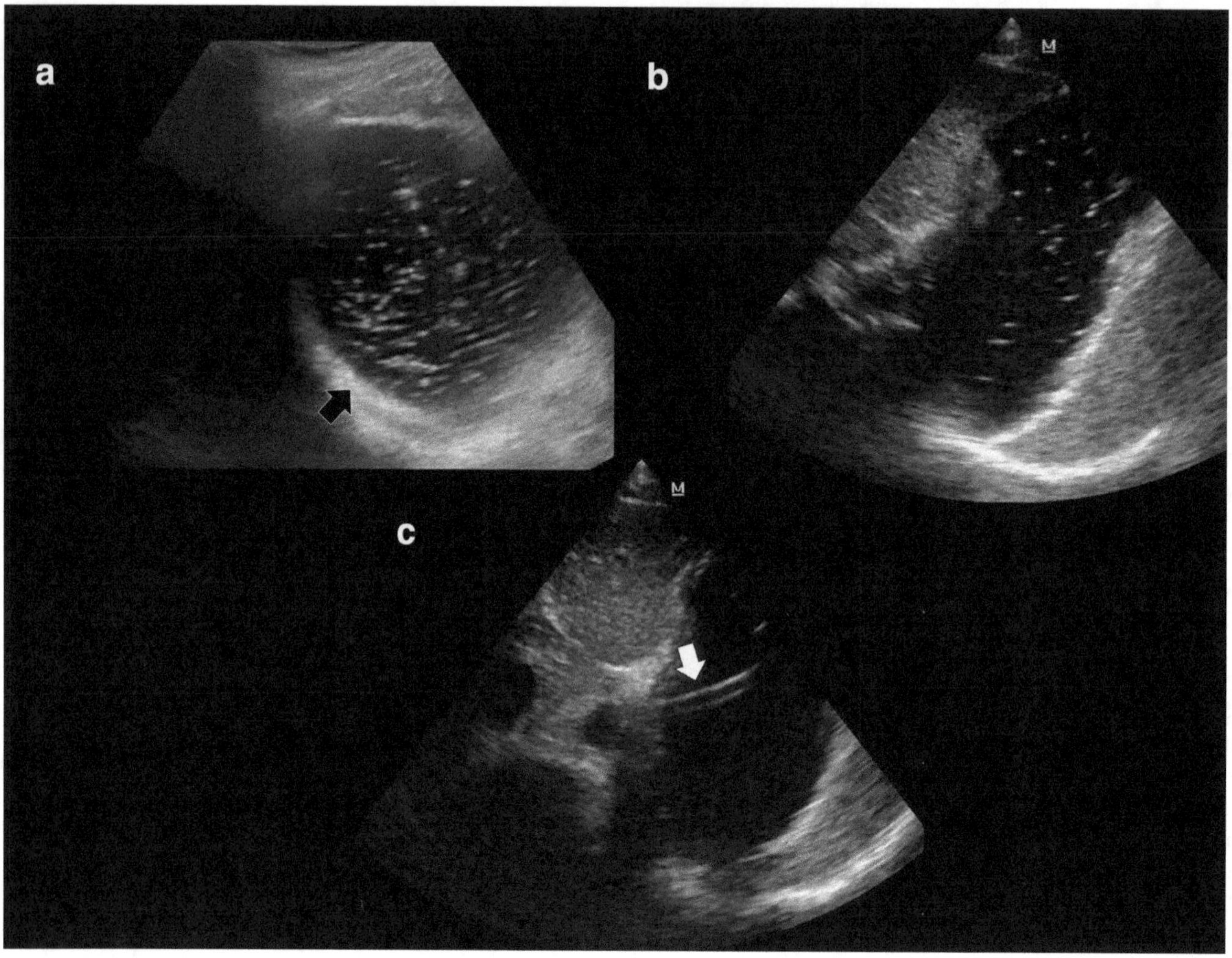

Fig. 4 **a** Stomach observed from the left coronal view. Note the fluid content and the echoes inside (air bubbles); *arrow* diaphragm. **b** Stomach observed from an epigastric view simulating a collection. **c** A gastric tube is observed confirming that it is the stomach (*white arrow*)

Table 2 Causes of gallbladder wall thickening (Modified from [39])

Generalized edematous states	Inflammatory conditions	Miscellaneous	Neoplastic	Physiological
Congestive heart failure	Acute and chronic cholecystitis	Adenomyomatosis	Gallbladder adenocarcinoma	Non-fasting patient (contracted gallbladder)
End-stage cirrhosis	Cholangitis	Cystic vein varices	Metastases	
Renal failure	Acute hepatitis	Malabsorption		
Hypoalbuminemia	Pancreatitis			
Pre-eclampsia	Perforated duodenal ulcer			

Table 3 Causes of gallbladder distension

Physiological	Obstruction
Fasting	Cystic duct (e.g., lithiasis) Common bile duct Pancreas

Error implications This misdiagnosis may lead to higher costs and adverse effects derived from the indications of antibiotics, and eventually, to cholecystectomy or cholecystotomy, and thus unnecessary surgery risks.

How to avoid this error It is essential to integrate ultrasound findings into the patient clinical context, always

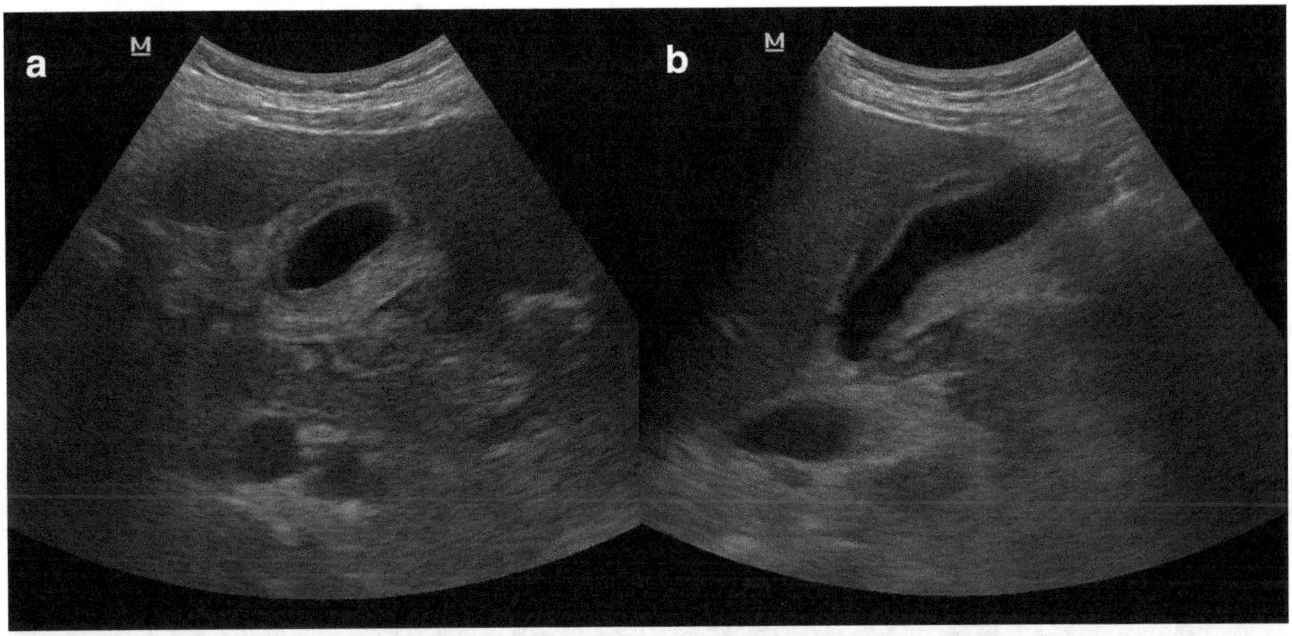

Fig. 5 Gallbladder wall thickening in short (**a**) and long (**b**) axis in a patient with severe heart failure, hepatomegaly and ascites

considering common underlying diseases resulting in morphological alterations of the gallbladder (e.g., cardiac failure). In the absence of clearly visible gallstones, the diagnosis of cholecystitis should always be confirmed by other methods [43].

Vascular ultrasound

Rouleaux vs. deep vein thrombosis

Most cases of deep vein thrombosis (DVT) are found in lower limbs, exposing patients to the risk of pulmonary embolism. A common differential diagnosis of DVT is the presence of "rouleaux formation" that is an accumulation of erythrocytes lying over the venous valves represented by spontaneously echogenic blood flow inside the vessel [44] (Fig. 6a; Additional file 3: Video S3). While rouleaux is a common finding and usually does not have a clinical impact, it is important to highlight that this can also be frequently observed when there is a proximal venous obstruction, and thus a more proximal DVT must be ruled out.

Error implications A misdiagnosis of DVT only based on rouleaux may lead to higher costs and unnecessary side-effects (bleeding) derived from unnecessary patient anticoagulation. However, depending on the setting, the vessel observed and the patient condition, the rouleaux (or sludge sign) should sometimes induce to extend the observation to the possibility of proximal obstruction. The sludge sign in the inferior vena cava during cardiac arrest with electrical activity and hyperkinetic left cardiac chambers may be a sign of acute right overload [45]. The same sign in the femoral vein, corroborated by asymmetric femoral veins waveforms at color Doppler analysis, may be a sign of isolated iliac thrombus [45].

How to avoid this error In contrast to a real condition of thrombosis, veins with rouleaux formation are compressible. Furthermore, distal compression allows to squeeze the blood and clear the rouleaux while thrombus cannot be released (Fig. 6b; Additional file 3: Video S3). To rule in or out a more proximal venous obstruction in the presence of rouleaux, the operator should look for direct visualization of a thrombus or examine compressibility of the proximal veins. In addition, the use of a spectral Doppler analysis to assess for respiratory flow variations of peripheral veins on both sides may be useful (Fig. 6c, d). More than a pattern of low intensity of the signal, especially, an asymmetric waveform obtained by comparing the two sides, indicates the possibility of a stop between the heart and the site of insonation and induces to extend the US venous study or use more advanced imaging for confirmation.

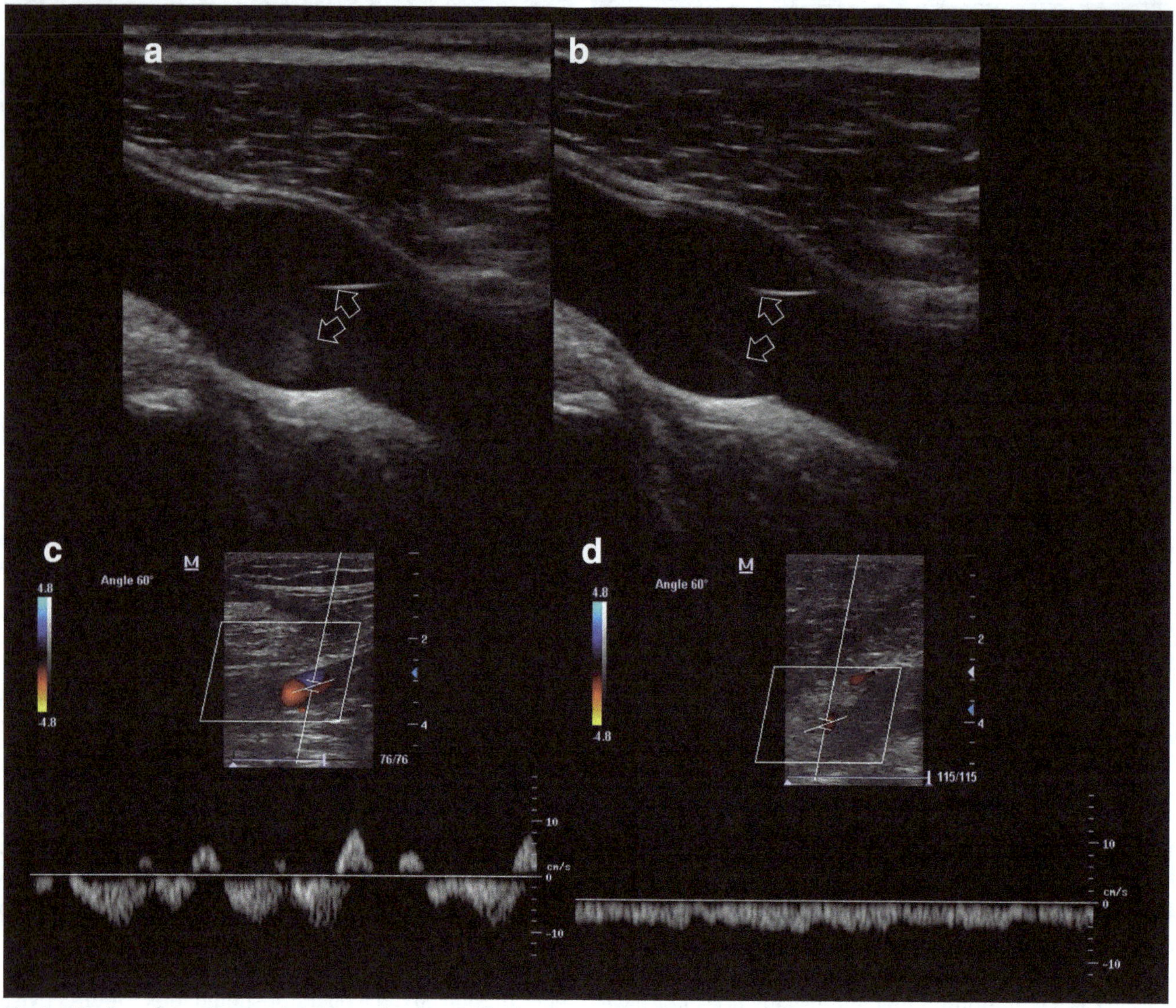

Fig. 6 **a** Rouleaux formation over the venous valves (*arrows*). **b** After distal compression, the blood was squeezed and the rouleaux are finally cleared. *Arrows* venous valves. **c** Normal phasic venous waveform, indicating a non-stopping flow between the heart and the site of insonation. **d** Abnormal non-phasic venous flow, indicating a stop between the heart and the site of insonation

Conclusions

There are some common misleading situations that critical care physicians may encounter in their sonography practice. Following some rules in technique and interpretation, the accuracy of POCUS can be improved and the possibility of dangerous misdiagnoses avoided. It is essential to remember that POCUS does not replace the clinical judgment, physical examination or common sense. POCUS must always be used in a holistic manner to improve the clinical accuracy and patient safety.

Additional files

Additional file 1: Video 1. The inferior vena cava (IVC) in long axis in a patient with massive acute pulmonary embolism (Videos 1 to 3). The view of video 1 shows a significant venous collapse during respiration that is predictive of low venous pressure.

Additional file 2: Video 2. The inferior vena cava (IVC) in long axis in a patient with massive acute pulmonary embolism (Videos 1 to 3). In video 2, the M-mode documents the collapse of IVC during respiration.

Additional file 3: Video 3. The inferior vena cava (IVC) in long axis in a patient with massive acute pulmonary embolism (Videos 1 to 3). The same view (video 3) in long axis performed with the correct technique shows the absence of collapse in the obvious clinical condition of acute right strain. The difference is the correct displaying of the IVC in video 3, which is based on the constant visualization of the inner walls of the vessel.

Additional file 4: Video 4. Normal interphase between the expanding lung and the diaphragm. Note the ultrasonographic tissue pattern of the liver as well as the lung sliding.

Additional file 5: Video 5. Normal interphase between the heart and the expanding lung.

Additional file 6: Video 6. Lung ultrasound in a condition of pneumothorax. The movement of the muscles of the chest wall during the respiratory effort gives the impression of lung sliding. However, the real sliding should be observed against the chest wall and independent from the movement of the intercostal muscles.

Additional file 7: Video 7. Lung ultrasound in a condition of pneumothorax. The pulsing movement of the image is due to an intercostal artery visualized in long axis, giving the impression of a false pulsation of the lung. The real lung pulse should be independent from the movement of the chest wall.

Additional file: Video 8. A case of recurrence of pneumothorax after pleurodesis abrasion. The septa still connecting the lung to the chest wall explain the coexistence of B lines and the absence of sliding in a condition of pneumothorax.

Additional file 9: Video 9. Wash out of rouleaux formation after distal compression, ruling out thrombosis at the site of insonation.

Abbreviations

POCUS: point-of-care ultrasonography; PEF: pericardial effusion; TTE: transthoracic echocardiography; RA: right atrium; RV: right ventricle; LV: left ventricle; LA: left atrium; IVC: inferior vena cava; CT: computerized tomography; DVT: deep vein thrombosis.

Authors' contributions

PB and GV contributed equally to this work. Both authors read and approved the final manuscript.

Author details

[1] Intensive Care Unit, Hospital Dr. Emilio Ferreyra, 4801, 59 St., 7630 Necochea, Argentina. [2] Intensive Care Unit, Clínica Cruz Azul, 2651, 60 St., 7630 Necochea, Argentina. [3] Emergency Medicine, San Luigi Gonzaga University Hospital, 10043 Turin, Italy.

Acknowledgements

PB would like to thank Mrs. Julieta Vigna for the language guidance.

References

1. Frankel HL, Kirkpatrick AW, Elbarbary M, Blaivas M, Desai H, Evans D, Summerfield DT, Slonim A, Breitkreutz R, Price S, Marik PE, Talmor D, Levitov A (2015) Guidelines for the appropriate use of bedside general and cardiac ultrasonography in the evaluation of critically ill patients-part I: general ultrasonography. Crit Care Med 43(11):2479–2502
2. Blanco P (2016) Physical examination along with point-of-care echocardiography: an indisputable right path. Am J Emerg Med 34(3):673
3. Blanco P (2015) A traditional paradigm vs. an ultrasound-supported paradigm in emergency and critical care medicine: a crisis of the mind is needed. J Emerg Med 49(2):e63–e64
4. Álvarez-Fernández JA, Núñez-Reiz A, en representación del Club de Ecografía UCI Madrid de la SOMIAMA (2015) Clinical ultrasound in the ICU: changing a medical paradigm. Med Intensiva 40(4):246–249
5. Ultrasound Certification Task Force on behalf of the Society of Critical Care Medicine. Recommendations for achieving and maintaining competence and credentialing in critical care ultrasound with focused cardiac ultrasound and advanced critical care echocardiography. http://journals.lww.com/ccmjournal/Documents/Critical%20Care%20Ultrasound.pdf. Accessed 02 Jan 2016
6. Via G, Hussain A, Wells M, Reardon R, ElBarbary M, Noble VE, Tsung JW, Neskovic AN, Price S, Oren-Grinberg A, Liteplo A, Cordioli R, Naqvi N, Rola P, Poelaert J, Guliĉ TG, Sloth E, Labovitz A, Kimura B, Breitkreutz R, Masani N, Bowra J, Talmor D, Guarracino F, Goudie A, Xiaoting W, Chawla R, Galderisi M, Blaivas M, Petrovic T, Storti E, Neri L, Melniker L, International Liaison Committee on Focused Cardiac UltraSound (ILC-FoCUS), International Conference on Focused Cardiac UltraSound (IC-FoCUS) (2014) International evidence-based recommendations for focused cardiac ultrasound. J Am Soc Echocardiogr 27(7):683.e1–683.e33
7. Volpicelli G, Elbarbary M, Blaivas M, Lichtenstein DA, Mathis G, Kirkpatrick AW, Melniker L, Gargani L, Noble VE, Via G, Dean A, Tsung JW, Soldati G, Copetti R, Bouhemad B, Reissig A, Agricola E, Rouby JJ, Arbelot C, Liteplo A, Sargsyan A, Silva F, Hoppmann R, Breitkreutz R, Seibel A, Neri L, Storti E, Petrovic T, International Liaison Committee on Lung Ultrasound (ILC-LUS) for International Consensus Conference on Lung Ultrasound (ICC-LUS) (2012) International evidence-based recommendations for point-of-care lung ultrasound. Intensive Care Med 38(4):577–591
8. Expert Round Table on Echocardiography in ICU (2014) International consensus statement on training standards for advanced critical care echocardiography. Intensive Care Med 40(5):654–666
9. Strony R, Linkenheil E (2016) How to delineate pericardial effusion from pleural effusion on bedside ultrasound. J Emerg Med 50(3):495–496
10. Goodman A, Perera P, Mailhot T, Mandavia D (2012) The role of bedside ultrasound in the diagnosis of pericardial effusion and cardiac tamponade. J Emerg Trauma Shock 5(1):72–75
11. Adams JR, Tonelli AR, Rokadia HK, Duggal A (2015) Cardiac tamponade in severe pulmonary hypertension. A therapeutic challenge revisited. Ann Am Thorac Soc 12(3):455–460
12. Cardello FP, Yoon DH, Halligan RE Jr, Richter H (2006) The falciform ligament in the echocardiographic diagnosis of ascites. J Am Soc Echocardiogr 19(8):1074.e3–1074.e4
13. Bertaso AG, Bertol D, Duncan BB, Foppa M (2013) Epicardial fat: definition, measurements and systematic review of main outcomes. Arq Bras Cardiol 101(1):e18–e28
14. Blaivas M, DeBehnke D, Phelan MB (2000) Potential errors in the diagnosis of pericardial effusion on trauma ultrasound for penetrating injuries. Acad Emerg Med 7(11):1261–1266
15. Grifoni S, Olivotto I, Cecchini P, Pieralli F, Camaiti A, Santoro G, Pieri A, Toccafondi S, Magazzini S, Berni G, Agnelli G (1998) Utility of an integrated

clinical, echocardiographic, and venous ultrasonographic approach for triage of patients with suspected pulmonary embolism. Am J Cardiol 82(10):1230–1235
16. The Steering Committee (2012) Single-bolus tenecteplase plus heparin compared with heparin alone for normotensive patients with acute pulmonary embolism who have evidence of right ventricular dysfunction and myocardial injury: rationale and design of the pulmonary embolism thrombolysis (PEITHO) trial. Am Heart J 163(1):33.e1–38.e1
17. Nazerian P, Vanni S, Volpicelli G, Gigli C, Zanobetti M, Bartolucci M, Ciavattone A, Lamorte A, Veltri A, Fabbri A, Grifoni S (2014) Accuracy of point-of-care multiorgan ultrasonography for the diagnosis of pulmonary embolism. Chest 145(5):950–957
18. Volpicelli G, Lamorte A, Tullio M, Cardinale L, Giraudo M, Stefanone V, Boero E, Nazerian P, Pozzi R, Frascisco MF (2013) Point-of-care multiorgan ultrasonography for the evaluation of undifferentiated hypotension in the emergency department. Intensive Care Med 39(7):1290–1298
19. Becattini C, Agnelli G, Vedovati MC, Pruszczyk P, Casazza F, Grifoni S, Salvi A, Bianchi M, Douma R, Konstantinides S, Lankeit M, Duranti M (2011) Multidetector computed tomography for acute pulmonary embolism: diagnosis and risk stratification in a single test. Eur Heart J 32(13):1657–1663
20. Perera P, Mailhot T, Riley D, Mandavia D (2010) The RUSH exam: rapid ultrasound in SHock in the evaluation of the critically Ill. Emerg Med Clin North Am 28(1):29–56
21. Blanco P, Sasai T (2015) Assessment of left ventricle preload by transthoracic echocardiography: an easy task? J Intensive Care 3(1):23
22. Lang RM, Badano LP, Mor-Avi V, Afilalo J, Armstrong A, Ernande L, Flachskampf FA, Foster E, Goldstein SA, Kuznetsova T, Lancellotti P, Muraru D, Picard MH, Rietzschel ER, Rudski L, Spencer KT, Tsang W, Voigt JU (2015) Recommendations for cardiac chamber quantification by echocardiography in adults: an update from the American Society of Echocardiography and the European Association of Cardiovascular Imaging. J Am Soc Echocardiogr 28(1):1e14–39.e14
23. Via G, Tavazzi G, Price S (2015) Ten situations where inferior vena cava ultrasound may fail to accurately predict fluid responsiveness: a physiologically based point of view. Intensive Care Med 42(7):1164–1167
24. Zhang Z, Xu X, Ye S, Xu L (2014) Ultrasonographic measurement of the respiratory variation in the inferior vena cava diameter is predictive of fluid responsiveness in critically ill patients: systematic review and meta-analysis. Ultrasound Med Biol 40(5):845–853
25. Barbier C, Loubières Y, Schmit C, Hayon J, Ricôme JL, Jardin F, Vieillard-Baron A (2004) Respiratory changes in inferior vena cava diameter are helpful in predicting fluid responsiveness in ventilated septic patients. Intensive Care Med 30(9):1740–1746
26. Airapetian N, Maizel J, Alyamani O, Mahjoub Y, Lorne E, Levrard M, Ammenouche N, Seydi A, Tinturier F, Lobjoie E, Dupont H, Slama M (2015) Does inferior vena cava respiratory variability predict fluid responsiveness in spontaneously breathing patients? Crit Care 19:400
27. Lichtenstein D, Mezière G, Biderman P, Gepner A (2000) The lung point: an ultrasound sign specific to pneumothorax. Intensive Care Med 26:1434–1440
28. Volpicelli G, Boero E, Stefanone V, Storti E (2013) Unusual new signs of pneumothorax at lung ultrasound. Crit Ultrasound J 5(1):10
29. Stone MB, Chilstrom M, Chase K, Lichtenstein D (2010) The heart point sign: description of a new ultrasound finding suggesting pneumothorax. Acad Emerg Med 17(11):e149–e150
30. Gillman LM, Alkadi A, Kirkpatrick AW (2009) The "pseudo-lung point" sign: all focal respiratory coupled alternating pleural patterns are not diagnostic of a pneumothorax. J Trauma 67(3):672–673
31. Zhang Z, Chen L (2015) A physiological sign that mimics lung point in critical care ultrasonography. Crit Care 19:155
32. Moreno-Aguilar G, Lichtenstein D (2015) Lung ultrasound in the critically ill (LUCI) and the lung point: a sign specific to pneumothorax which cannot be mimicked. Crit Care 19:311
33. Gelabert C, Nelson M (2015) Bleb point: mimicker of pneumothorax in bullous lung disease. West J Emerg Med 16(3):447–449
34. Campione A, Luzzi L, Gorla A, Terzi A (2010) About ultrasound diagnosis of pulmonary bullae vs. pneumothorax. J Emerg Med 38(3):384–385 **(author reply 385)**
35. Saracino C, Tessaro M (2015) Pneumomediastinum as a sonographic mimic of pneumothorax. J Ultrasound Med 34(8):1521–1522
36. Volpicelli G, Garofalo G, Lamorte A, Frascisco MF (2012) Young man with left thoracic pain. Ann Emerg Med 60(2):e3–e4
37. Malhotra R, Bramante RM, Radomski M, Nelson M (2014) Mirror image artifact mimicking heterotopic pregnancy on transvaginal ultrasound: case series. West J Emerg Med 15(6):712–714
38. Nural MS, Yardan T, Güven H, Baydin A, Bayrak IK, Kati C (2005) Diagnostic value of ultrasonography in the evaluation of blunt abdominal trauma. Diagn Interv Radiol 11(1):41–44
39. Coppolino F, Gatta G, Di Grezia G, Reginelli A, Iacobellis F, Vallone G, Giganti M, Genovese E (2013) Gastrointestinal perforation: ultrasonographic diagnosis. Crit Ultrasound J 5(Suppl 1):S4
40. Mouaqit O, Hibatallah A, Oussaden A, Maazaz K, Taleb KA (2013) Acute intraperitoneal rupture of hydatid cysts: a surgical experience with 14 cases. World J Emerg Surg 8:28
41. Gore RM, Thakrar KH, Newmark GM, Mehta UK, Berlin JW (2010) Gallbladder imaging. Gastroenterol Clin North Am 39(2):265–287
42. Khalili K, Wilson SR (2011) The biliary tree and gallbladder. In: Rumack CM, Wilson SR, Charboneau JW, Levine D (eds) Diagnostic ultrasound, 4th edn. Elsevier Mosby, Philadelphia
43. Volpicelli G, Balik M, Georgopoulos D (2014) Echography is mandatory for the initial management of critically ill patients: no. Intensive Care Med 40(11):1766–1768
44. Charlotte H, Kuntz K, Youngs D (2013) Leg Pain. In: Charlotte H, Kuntz K, Youngs D (eds) Clinical guide to sonography: exercises for critical thinking, 2nd edn. Elsevier Mosby, St Louis
45. Volpicelli G, Mussa A, Frascisco MF (2012) Sonographic diagnosis of pulmonary embolism with cardiac arrest without major dilation of the right ventricle or direct sign of lower limb venous thrombosis. J Clin Ultrasound 40(8):529–533

2

Management of cardiopulmonary assist devices in critically ill patients using point-of-care transthoracic echocardiography

Babar Fiza*, Michael Tang and Michael Maile

Abstract

Point-of-care transthoracic echocardiography is increasingly being utilized by the intensive care physicians in the management of hemodynamically unstable patients. However, its use in the management of critically ill patients requiring cardiopulmonary mechanical device support remains to be well described. In this case series, we present two case reports where point-of-care echocardiography was successfully used by the intensive care team in diagnosing and managing problems related to cardiopulmonary assist device malposition.

Introduction

Traditionally, echocardiography has been performed by cardiologists and cardiac anesthesiologists and, in some hospitals, by sonography technicians with interpretation by cardiologists. Over the past few years, the increasing availability, portability, and better image quality produced by ultrasound machines have resulted in an increased use of transthoracic echocardiogram (TTE) as a point-of-care (POC) ultrasound device. POC TTE is being widely adopted by emergency departments throughout the United States, where its utilization has been demonstrated to achieve great diagnostic capability [1]. In the operative room setting, focused TTE performed by anesthesiologists has been shown to alter management and provide new information in hemodynamically unstable patients [2]. POC echocardiography has even been used as a perioperative screening tool and successfully used in the management of critically ill patients [3, 4]. While the clinical use of POC cardiac ultrasonography continues to expand, this intricate skill requires appropriate education and training, including a comprehensive understanding of its scope and limitations [5].

To date, there are only a few published reports detailing its use in the critical care setting with regard to monitoring of patients with cardiovascular/cardiopulmonary assist devices [6–8]. In the following two case reports, we present the use of POC TTE by the intensive care physicians that resulted in immediate changes in the management of critically ill patients requiring cardiopulmonary mechanical device support.

Case one: Impella® repositioning

A 52-year-old male with history of chronic obstructive pulmonary disease (COPD), severe mitral regurgitation, severe tricuspid regurgitation, and non-ischemic cardiomyopathy (EF 25%) presented to an outside hospital with altered mental status and acute liver failure in the setting of cardiogenic shock. The patient's cardiac index was found to be 1.6 L/min at the time of presentation. Despite maximal medical therapy and subsequent placement of an intra-aortic balloon pump (IABP), there was little improvement in the patient's clinical status. Therefore, an Impella CP® was placed under fluoroscopic guidance in the cardiac catheterization lab. After placement of the Impella device, the patient's cardiac index improved to 2.4 L/min. An improvement in patient's mental status and liver function tests were also noted after placement of the Impella.

*Correspondence: babar@med.umich.edu
Department of Anesthesiology, University of Michigan Hospitals, 1500 East Medical Center Drive, Ann Arbor, MI 48109-5861, USA

The Impella CP® device is an axial flow type of temporary ventricular assist device that, typically, is placed in the femoral artery and positioned across the aortic valve. This allows it to withdraw blood from the left ventricle and eject it into the aorta. The device is placed percutaneously in patients with cardiogenic shock and provides more hemodynamic support than an IABP [9]. Its initial placement is guided by fluoroscopy or echocardiography to ensure that the inflow area is located approximately 3.5 cm below the aortic valve in the left ventricle and the outflow area is located above the aortic valve (Fig. 1). Typically, blood flows of 2.5–3.5 L/min are achieved through the catheter, which assists low native cardiac output states [10].

After undergoing placement of the Impella device, the patient was transferred to our cardiovascular intensive care unit (ICU) for evaluation of a left ventricular assist device placement. On arrival, the patient's hemodynamics were stable and urine was noted to be clear. The placement pressure waveform, a measure of pressure at the outflow of the Impella showed a waveform consistent with an aortic waveform. The motor current, showed good pulsatility, which also indicated correct placement. Next morning, the patient was found to have increasingly dark colored urine, raising concern for hemolysis. Placement waveform signals remained unchanged. A POC TTE performed by the intensive care team showed the Impella® tip to be approximately 5.9 cm below the aortic valve (previously 3.5 cm at the time of placement) in the parasternal long-axis view (Fig. 2). Laboratory workup obtained at this time was consistent with hemolysis and notable for an up-trending lactate dehydrogenase (LDH)

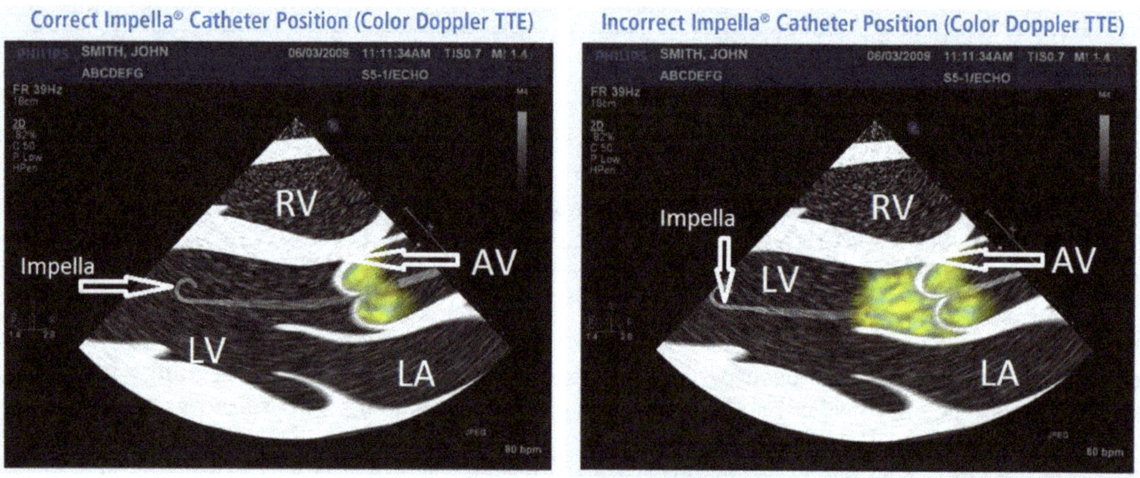

Fig. 1 Illustration showing incorrect and correct positioning of Impella® with color flow. Parasternal long-axis view on transthoracic echo (Illustration). In the incorrectly positioned Impella®, the outflow is seen below the aortic valve. The catheter is also located too deep in the left ventricle compared to a correctly placed catheter. *AV* aortic valve, *LV* left ventricle, *LA* left atrium, *RV* right ventricle. Image reproduced with permission from Abiomed Corporation

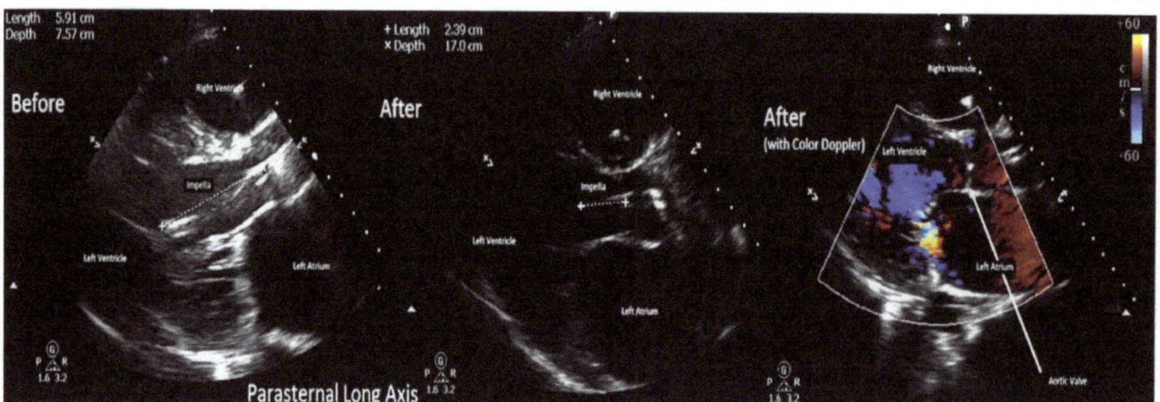

a b c

Fig. 2 Impella positioning visualized on the parasternal long-axis view on the TTE exam. **a** Images acquired at the time of improper positioning. The Impella® (hyperechoic structure) is located 5.9 cm beyond the aortic valve in the left ventricle. **b** Acquired after repositioning. Notice that the length of the Impella® in the left ventricle is now 2.4 cm beyond the aortic valve into the LV. **c** Acquired after repositioning with color Doppler. Flow at the outflow area can be visualized. The outflow area is now located above the aortic valve

and serum-free hemoglobin of 190.3 mg/dL (reference range 1–8 mg/dL for our institution). The cardiac surgery team was notified and subsequently withdrew the Impella by 3 cm. This resulted in resolution of hemolysis as evidenced by clearing of the urine and down-trending LDH and serum-free hemoglobin levels. A repeat POC TTE by the ICU team demonstrated that the catheter was in the correct position, and this was confirmed on color Doppler imaging (Fig. 2; Additional files 1, 2).

Case two: avalon veno-venous extracorporeal membrane oxygenation cannula malpositioning

A 67-year-old male with history of emphysema, chronic obstructive pulmonary disease, and hypertension presented to our ICU after undergoing a thoracoscopic bilateral lung volume reduction surgery. Postoperatively, the patient developed pneumonia and acute respiratory distress syndrome (ARDS) requiring mechanical ventilation. Despite maximal medical therapy and optimization of mechanical ventilator support, the patient's oxygenation worsened. On postoperative day seven, the patient's arterial blood gas analysis was notable for a PaO_2/FIO_2 ratio of 40. The patient was placed on pressure control mode of ventilation with inability to achieve greater than 150 mL of tidal volume on inspiratory pressures of 30 mmHg. The decision was made to place the patient on veno-venous extracorporeal membranous oxygenation (VV-ECMO) via the right internal jugular vein with the use of Avalon Elite Bicaval Dual Lumen catheter (MAQUET Holding B.V. and Co. KG, Rastatt, Germany) under direct fluoroscopic guidance. The patient's oxygenation improved rapidly after VV-ECMO cannulation. ECMO flow was set at 4.0 L/min, sweep at 1 L/min, and ventilation was continued in the same mode as prior to ECMO initiation. Arterial blood gas analysis at this time showed a pH of 7.38, [$PaCO_2$] 39, a PaO_2/FIO_2 ratio of 170, and a mixed venous oxygen saturation of 65%, indicating improved oxygenation.

VV-ECMO can be used as a salvage therapy for patients with severe or refractory hypoxia [11]. Multiple cannula configurations can be used to take blood from and return it to the venous system. The Avalon Elite Bicaval Dual Lumen Cannula® allows this to be accomplished using a single site. The inflow port of this particular catheter draws blood from both the superior and inferior vena cava. This blood flows into the oxygenator and is then returned through a reinfusion port, which is directed toward the tricuspid valve. Fluoroscopy or transesophageal echocardiography is utilized for proper placement of the catheter to ensure that the distal drainage port is located within the IVC, while the proximal drainage port lies in the superior vena cava [11–13].

On ECMO therapy day seven, the patient developed decreased flows, decreased inlet pressures, and chattering of the ECMO tubing. Chattering is vibration of the cannula and tubing that occurs when the drainage cannula abuts the wall of the blood vessel. Chattering most commonly occurs due to inadequate preload due to hypovolemia, or a process causing mechanical obstruction such as tamponade, tension pneumothorax, and abdominal compartment syndrome. Chattering can also occur independent of patient's volume status due to cannula malposition or excessive ECMO pump speeds. [14] Due to history of aggressive fluid diuresis in this patient, initially fluid boluses were administered to correct the chattering, but the patient continued to have problems with low circuit flows. This resulted in the deterioration in oxygenation with patient developing a pulse oximeter saturation of 80% and a mixed venous oxygen saturation of 43%. A POC TTE was performed by the ICU team at this time to identify the cause of decreased flows. On the POC TTE, the patient had normal right and left ventricular function and there was no pericardial effusion. On the subcostal inferior vena cava (IVC) view, it was noted that the catheter's distal tip had migrated into the hepatic vein. The Avalon® catheter was immediately withdrawn by 2–3 cm, and repeat POC TTE showed the cannula tip to be located in the inferior vena cava. Correct placement resulted in rapid improvement in ECMO flows and patient oxygenation with pulse oximeter saturation improving to 90% and mixed venous oxygenation saturation to 69% (Fig. 3; Additional files 3, 4, 5).

Discussion

These two cases illustrate the effective use of POC TTE in rapid diagnosis of clinical problems related to cardiopulmonary mechanical support devices. In the first case, POC echocardiography was used to diagnose Impella malposition. While hemolysis is a documented complication of the Impella device, the underlying mechanism can be related to either the shear stress of the device or improper positioning [15, 16]. The improper positioning of the device can lead to hemolysis as turbulent flow is generated when the outflow of the cannula is too close to the aortic valve or when the outflow of the device is partially below the aortic valve (Fig. 1). Given the different mechanisms that could lead to hemolysis in these patients, it is mandatory to check the cannula position before any therapeutic interventions are undertaken. Unlike the case of malposition, hemolysis related to shear stress would warrant either removal of the device, dependent on the extent of hemolysis, or change in the anticoagulation plan. Bedside TTE thus provides the clinician with the ability to quickly determine if cannula

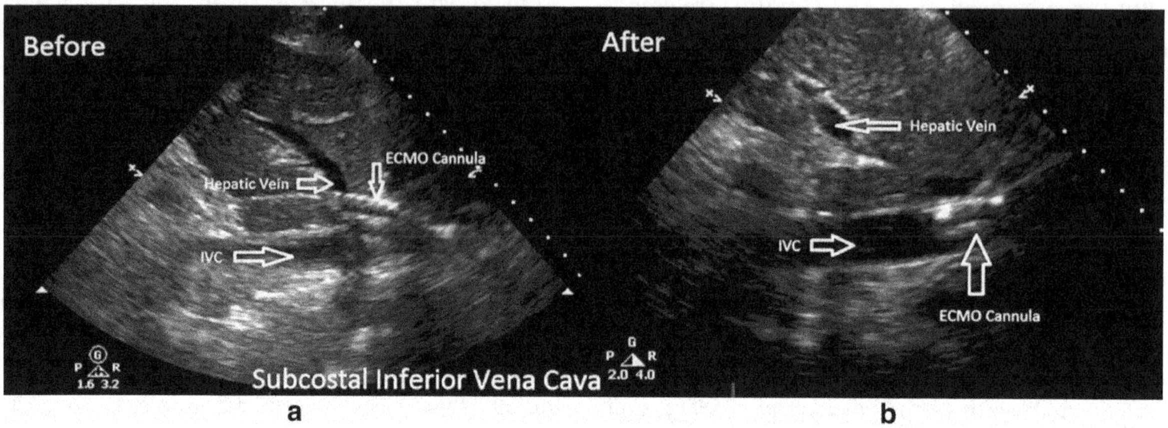

Fig. 3 Still Images taken from the subcostal inferior vena cava view on the TTE exam. **a** Image taken during low flows on the ECMO circuit. The ECMO cannula is visualized as a hyperechoic structure located in the hepatic vein. **b** Resolution of low flows on ECMO circuit after catheter repositioning. The ECMO cannula is now located in the lumen of the inferior vena cava. *IVC* inferior vena cava

malposition is the cause of hemolysis. The bedside availability of TTE for device placement is recommended by the European Expert Group although very few case reports in literature have described the utilization of bedside TTE for Impella device repositioning [17].

Case one also demonstrates the importance of real-time echocardiographic confirmation of device positioning even when device hemodynamic pressure signals do not display evidence of malposition. The Impella device is fitted with a display screen that continuously monitors device position using a waveform calculated from the pressure difference between the inlet and the outlet areas. Based on the changes in this waveform, a proximal or a distal migration of the device can be detected. As the distal pressures are monitored in an open area above the outlet port, migration of the device outlet area into the aortic valve is possible without a change in waveform [15]. We suspect this to be the case in our patient. In this case, even though the device console indicated appropriate device position, the device malposition was evident on the TTE exam.

The second case highlights the important role of bedside echocardiography in daily management of patients requiring VV-ECMO therapy. Traditionally, VV-ECMO support has been achieved via dual cannulation either through femoro-jugular or femoro-femoral venous cannulation. However, VV-ECMO support can now be achieved via single-vessel cannulation at the internal jugular vein with the use of Avalon Elite Bicaval Dual Lumen Cannula®. The advantages of this cannula include less recirculation, improved patient mobility, and decreased risk of infection. However, this catheter like other ECMO catheters when improperly positioned can lead to recirculation, arrhythmias, and a decrease in ECMO flows resulting in hypoxia [7, 8].

As highlighted by our case, echocardiography can assist in determining the cause of inadequate flows and allow clinicians to institute correct therapies. Due to underlying lung pathology, physicians treating these patients generally employ restrictive fluid strategy. This can result in a decrease in ECMO flows due to collapse of the IVC around the cannula. The collapse of the IVC around the catheter combined with signs of hypovolemia can be determined with real-time echocardiography and allow physicians to guide fluid therapy. However, ECMO catheter malpositioning can result in decreased flows as well, in which case the proper therapy would be to reposition the catheter in order to achieve adequate flows. As evidenced by this case, diagnosis of catheter malposition as the cause of decreased flows prevents excessive fluid administration that would otherwise risk worsening of pulmonary function due to volume overload. Additionally, cannula repositioning should always be performed under real-time fluoroscopy or echocardiography guidance as migration of the tip of the cannula into the right ventricle could lead to structural damage and poses risk of arrhythmias [7].

Conclusion

These two case studies show the effective use of POC TTE by the intensive care physicians to diagnose and manage problems arising from complications related to the use of cardiovascular assist devices. Routine imaging such as plain film X-rays can give us limited information and may not necessarily be sufficient to judge proper positioning. Point-of-care echocardiography proved to be invaluable in the presented cases to diagnose improper positioning, resulting in immediate changes in management.

Additional files

Additional file 1. Parasternal long-axis view obtained at time of improper positioning of the Impella®. The Impella® catheter is located 5.9 cm beyond the aortic valve in the left ventricle.

Additional file 2. Parasternal long-axis view obtained after repositioning. The Impella® is now located 2.4 cm beyond the aortic valve into the LV. On color Doppler interrogation flow at the outflow site is now located in the aorta.

Additional file 3. On subcostal inferior vena cava view the ECMO cannula is noted to be located in the hepatic vein.

Additional file 4. Subcostal inferior vena cava view after repositioning of the ECMO cannula. The cannula is now located within the IVC.

Additional file 5. Subcostal inferior vena cava view with color flow Doppler interrogation. Flow is seen in the hepatic vein and the ECMO cannula is located within the IVC.

Abbreviations

TTE: transthoracic echocardiography; POC: point of care; COPD: chronic obstructive pulmonary disease; IABP: intra-aortic balloon pump; EF: ejection fraction; cm: centimeter; ICU: Intensive Care Unit; LDH: lactate dehydrogenase; mg: milligram; dL: deciliter; AV: aortic valve; LV: left ventricle; LA: left atrium; RV: right ventricle; ARDS: acute respiratory distress syndrome; PaO_2: partial pressure of oxygen in arterial blood; FiO_2: fraction of inspired oxygen; mm Hg: millimeters of mercury; $PaCO_2$: partial pressure of carbon dioxide in arterial blood; VV-ECMO: veno-venous extracorporeal membranous oxygenation; ECMO: extracorporeal membrane oxygenation; IVC: inferior vena cava.

Authors' contributions

MT and BF have written the main portion of the manuscript. MM has reviewed and edited the manuscript. BF has been responsible for the discussion of the echo findings in each case and reviewing the imaging portion of the manuscript. All authors read and approved the final manuscript.

Acknowledgements

None.

References

1. Volpicelli G, Lamorte A, Tullio M, Cardinale L, Giraudo M, Stefanone V et al (2013) Point-of-care multiorgan ultrasonography for the evaluation of undifferentiated hypotension in the emergency department. Intensive Care Med 39(7):1290–1298. https://doi.org/10.1007/s00134-013-2919-7
2. Kratz T, Steinfeldt T, Exner M, Orto MCD, Timmesfeld N, Kratz C et al (2017) Impact of focused intraoperative transthoracic echocardiography by anesthesiologists on management in hemodynamically unstable high-risk non-cardiac surgery patients. J Cardiothorac Vasc Anesth 31(2):602–609. https://doi.org/10.1053/j.jvca.2016.11.002
3. Canty DJ, Royse CF, Kilpatrick D, Bowman L, Royse AG (2012) The impact of focused transthoracic echocardiography in the pre-operative clinic. Anaesthesia 67(6):618–625. https://doi.org/10.1111/j.1365-2044.2012.07074.x
4. Manasia AR, Nagaraj HM, Kodali RB, Croft LB, Oropello JM, Kohli-Seth R et al (2005) Feasibility and potential clinical utility of goal-directed transthoracic echocardiography performed by noncardiologist intensivists using a small hand-carried device (SonoHeart) in critically ill patients. J Cardiothorac Vasc Anesth 19(2):155–159. https://doi.org/10.1053/j.jvca.2005.01.023
5. Neskovic AN, Edvardsen T, Galderisi M, Garbi M, Gullace G et al (2014) Focus cardiac ultrasound: the European association of cardiovascular imaging viewpoint. Eur Heart Journal Cardiovascular Imaging 15(9):956–960
6. Uriel N, Morrison KA, Garan AR, Kato TS, Yuzefpolskaya M, Latif F et al (2012) Development of a novel echocardiography ramp test for speed optimization and diagnosis of device thrombosis in continuous-flow left ventricular assist devices. J Am Coll Cardiol 60(18):1764–1775. https://doi.org/10.1016/j.jacc.2012.07.052
7. Ratzlaff RA, Ripoll JG, Cushenbery KA, Lowman PE, Díaz-Gómez JL (2017) Transthoracic echocardiogram-guided avalon catheter repositioning. Anesth Analg 125(1):48–51. https://doi.org/10.1213/ANE.0000000000001909
8. Tanaka D, Pitcher HT, Cavarocchi N, Hirose H (2015) Migrated avalon veno-venous extracorporeal membrane oxygenation cannula: how to adjust without interruption of flow. J Card Surg 30(11):865–868. https://doi.org/10.1111/jocs.12629
9. Ouweneel DM et al (2017) Percutaneous mechanical circulatory support versus intra-aortic balloon pump in cardiogenic shock after acute myocardial infarction. J Am Coll Cardiol 69(3):278–287. https://doi.org/10.1016/j.jacc.2016.10.022
10. Rogers JG, Patel CB, Milano CA (2017) Mechanically assisted circulation. In: Fuster V, Harrington RA, Narula J, Eapen ZJ (eds) Hurst's the heart, 14e. McGraw-Hill Education, New York
11. Napolitano LM (2014) Extracorporeal Lung Support. In: Hall JB, Schmidt GA, Kress JP (eds) Principles of Critical Care, 4e. McGraw-Hill Education, New York
12. Platts David Gerard et al (2012) The role of echocardiography in the management of patients supported by extracorporeal membrane oxygenation. J Am Soc Echocardiogr 25(2):131–141. https://doi.org/10.1016/j.echo.2011.11.009
13. Trimlett RH, Cordingley JJ, Griffiths MJ et al (2011) A modified technique for insertion of dual lumen bicaval cannulae for venovenous extracorporeal membrane oxygenation. Intensive Care Med 37:1036–1037
14. Chung Mabel et al (2014) Monitoring of the adult patient on venoarterial extracorporeal membrane oxygenation. Sci World J 2014:1–10. https://doi.org/10.1155/2014/393258
15. Sibbald M, Džavík V (2012) Severe hemolysis associated with use of the Impella LP 2.5 mechanical assist device. Catheter Cardiovasc Interv 80(5):840–844. https://doi.org/10.1002/ccd.24280
16. Cardozo S, Ahmed T, Belgrave K (2015) Impella induced massive hemolysis: reemphasizing echocardiographic guidance for correct placement. Case Rep Cardiol 2015:1–3. https://doi.org/10.1155/2015/464135
17. Burzotta F, Trani C, Doshi SN, Townend J, van Geuns RJ, Hunziker P, Schiefer B, Karatolios K, Møller JE, Ribichini FL, Schäfer A, Henriques JPS (2015) Impella ventricular support in clinical practice: collaborative viewpoint from a European Expert User Group. Int J Cardiol 201(C):684–691. https://doi.org/10.1016/j.ijcard.2015.07.065

3

A systematic review of the cost-effectiveness of ultrasound in emergency care settings

Brian Lentz[1], Tiffany Fong[2], Randall Rhyne[2] and Nicholas Risko[2*]

Abstract

Background: The use of ultrasound (US) in emergency departments (ED) has become widespread. This includes both traditional US scans performed by radiology departments as well as point-of-care US (POCUS) performed by bedside clinicians. There has been significant interest in better understanding the appropriate use of imaging and where opportunities to enhance cost-effectiveness may exist. The purpose of this systematic review is to identify published evidence surrounding the cost-effectiveness of US in the ED and to grade the quality of that evidence.

Methods: We performed a systematic review of the literature following Preferred Reporting Items for Systematic Review and Meta-Analyses (PRISMA) guidelines. Studies were considered for inclusion if they were: (1) economic evaluations, (2) studied the clinical use of ultrasound, and (3) took place in an emergency care setting. Included studies were critically appraised using the Consolidated Health Economic Evaluation Reporting Standards checklist.

Results: We identified 631 potentially relevant articles. Of these, 35 studies met all inclusion criteria and were eligible for data abstraction. In general, studies were supportive of the use of US. In particular, 11 studies formed a strong consensus that US enhanced cost-effectiveness in the investigation of pediatric appendicitis and 6 studies supported enhancements in the evaluation of abdominal trauma. Across the studies, weaknesses in methodology and reporting were common, such as lack of sensitivity analyses and inconsistent reporting of incremental cost-effectiveness ratios.

Conclusions: The body of existing evidence, though limited, generally demonstrates that the inclusion of US in emergency care settings allows for more cost-effective care. The most definitive evidence for improvements in cost-effectiveness surround the evaluation of pediatric appendicitis, followed by the evaluation of abdominal trauma. POCUS outside of trauma has had mixed results.

Keywords: Ultrasound, Emergency Medicine, Cost-effectiveness, Radiology, Health Economics

Background

Ultrasound (US) is well established as a safe and effective imaging modality for the rapid diagnosis and management of emergency conditions. At the bedside, it also improves success and patient safety during invasive procedures [1–5]. In the wake of technological advances and the increasing availability of imaging technologies, there has been considerable expansion of the use of clinical US—including both radiology-performed consultative studies and point-of-care ultrasound (POCUS) studies [6–11]. A number of initiatives have been promoted to encourage stewardship of imaging resources and the delivery of high-value care. These include the American College of Radiology's "Appropriateness Criteria" which assists referring physicians in the selection of the most efficacious and medically-appropriate imaging [12]; the American Board of Internal Medicine Foundation's "Choosing Wisely" initiative that advocates for use of modalities that are evidence-supported, non-duplicative, harm-free, and truly necessary [13]; and the American Institute of Ultrasound in Medicine's "Ultrasound First" campaign that promotes the practice of ultrasound for its safety, effectiveness, and affordability [14].

*Correspondence: nrisko1@jhmi.edu
[2] Department of Emergency Medicine, Johns Hopkins University School of Medicine, 1800 Orleans St, Baltimore, MD 21287, USA
Full list of author information is available at the end of the article

There is a common assumption that US is cost-effective in emergency care settings as it is diagnostically valuable, rapid, and less expensive than other imaging modalities like computed tomography (CT) and magnetic resonance imaging (MRI) [15]. However, it is unclear whether the published data either support or refute this assertion.

Cost-effectiveness analysis is a tool that combines economic and health outcome data to produce standardized ratios of costs and benefits. The outputs of CEAs allow for comparison of diagnostics that vary by both price and clinical utility, and generate important data to support decisions related to health policy and investment. The validity and reliability of CEAs are highly dependent on the rigor with which they are conducted. In 2013, health economists developed consensus-based guidelines on the conduct and reporting of health economic evaluations, called the Consolidated Health Economic Evaluation Reporting Standards (CHEERS) checklist [16].

We present a systematic review of the published evidence surrounding the cost-effectiveness of US in emergency care settings. Our aim is to characterize the existing knowledge regarding the costs and benefits of emergency US, to examine the quality of cost-effectiveness studies using the CHEERS checklist, and to provide guidance for future research efforts.

Methods

Search strategy

A systematic review of the literature was performed using the Preferred Reporting Items for Systematic Review and Meta-Analyses (PRISMA) guidelines [17]. The review was conducted without date or language restrictions in five major databases (PubMed, Scopus, Embase, Web of Science, and Cochrane). The search terms used are found in Fig. 1.

Selection of studies and data abstraction

All studies were collated and screened for eligibility through Covidence (www.covidence.org), an online platform for systematic review. Studies were considered for inclusion if they were: (1) economic evaluations that assessed costs and outcomes of comparative strategies; (2) studied the clinical use of US; and (3) took place in an emergency care setting. Two reviewers (BL, NR) with experience in reading, writing and reviewing economic evaluations independently assessed titles and abstracts for inclusion in a blinded fashion. Studies progressed to a full-text review if both reviewers agreed on the relevance based on the research question. Studies then underwent full text reviews for eligibility by each reviewer. Disagreements were resolved by consensus. The following information was extracted from each of the studies in the review: country, year of publication, intervention, comparator, time horizon (the time over which the costs and effect are measured), discount rate (the rate at which future costs and benefits are discounted), perspective (which costs are included or excluded), health outcome, sensitivity analyses (an assessment of the level of uncertainty in the modeling), and findings.

Quality assessment

Two reviewers undertook critical appraisal of the included studies using the CHEERS checklist, which comprises 24 items determined by expert consensus to be of importance when reporting economic evaluations of health interventions [16]. The CHEERS checklist was developed to increase transparency and consistency in the reporting of economic evaluations of health interventions, and ultimately lead to better policy, program, and management decisions. A lower score means readers cannot fully understand the modeling assumptions

("Cost-Benefit Analysis"[mh] OR "cost benefit" OR "cost effective" OR "cost effectiveness" OR "cost utility") AND

("Emergency Service, Hospital"[mh] OR "Emergency Medicine"[mh] OR "Emergency medicine"[TW] OR "Emergency services"[TW] OR "Emergency department"[TW] OR "Emergency service"[TW] OR "Emergency departments"[TW] OR "Emergency room"[TW] OR "Emergency rooms"[TW] OR "Emergency ward"[TW] OR "Emergency Unit"[TW] OR "Trauma Centers"[mh] OR "Trauma Center"[TW] OR "Trauma Centers"[TW] OR "emergency health service"[tw] OR "emergency health services"[tw] OR "emergency medical services"[tw] OR "emergency medical service"[tw] OR "accident and emergency"[tw] OR "accident & emergency"[tw] OR "a&e"[tw] OR "A & E"[tw]) AND

("Ultrasonography"[mh] OR "ultrasonography" OR "ultrasound" OR "ultrasounds" OR "echography" OR "sonography" OR "echocardiography"[mh] OR "echocardiography" OR "echocardiogram")

Fig. 1 Search terms

and, therefore, must question the validity and reliability of the presented results. The checklist can also serve to highlight critical gaps in study design, for example when study authors have not described performing a sensitivity analysis to generate confidence intervals it is likely that this step was overlooked.

Results

Overview of included studies

The electronic searches identified 631 potentially relevant articles following the removal of duplicates. After screening titles and abstracts for eligibility, 83 articles remained for full text screening. Of these studies, 35 studies met all inclusion criteria and were eligible for data abstraction. Included studies ranged in publication date from 1996 to 2019, 20 were published in 2014 or later. Studies were excluded in the full-text phase for the following reasons: 39 were not economic evaluations or CEAs, seven were not relevant to the emergency care setting, and two were conference abstracts only. Details are further illustrated in our PRISMA Flow Diagram (Fig. 2).

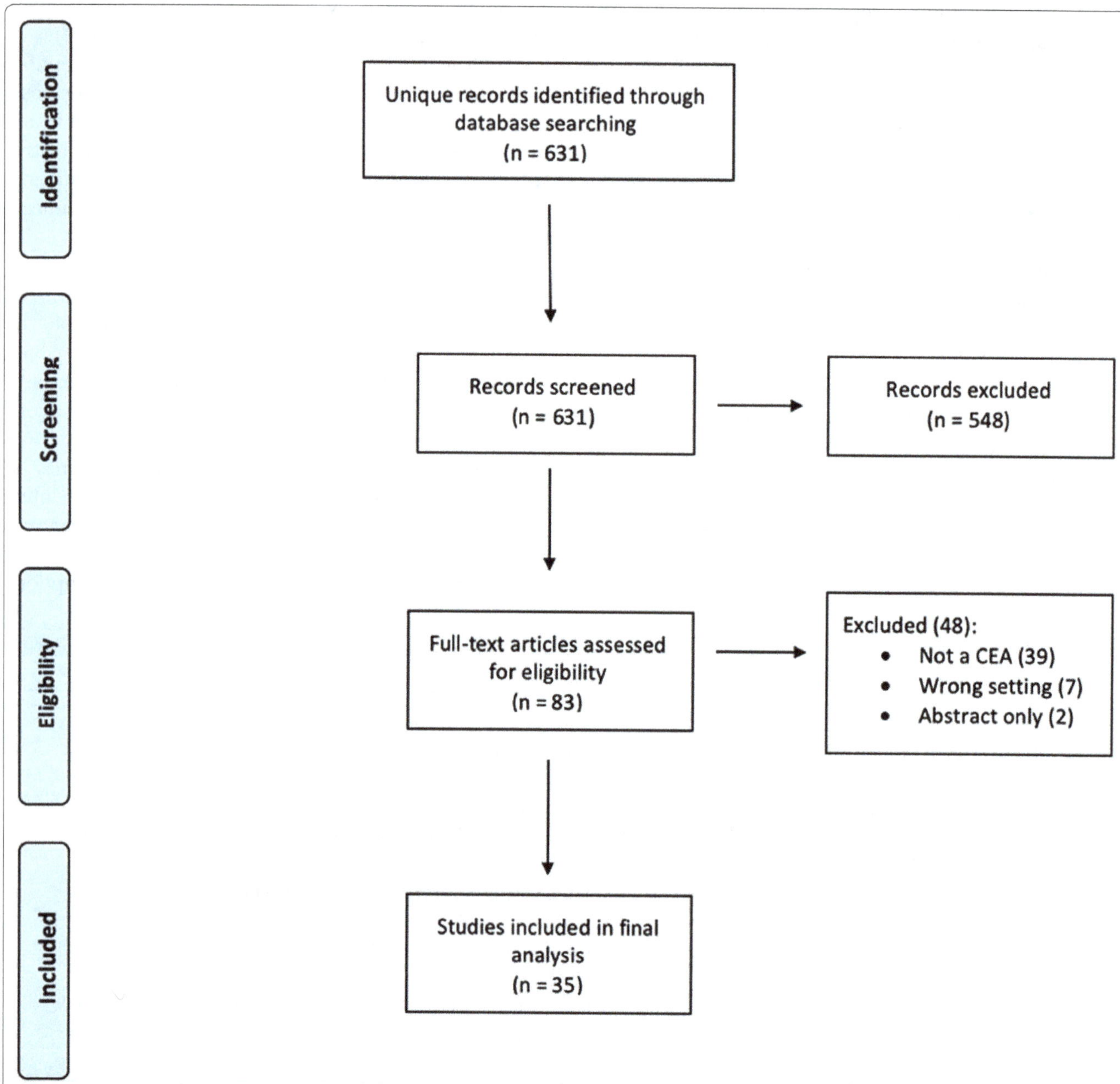

Fig. 2 PRISMA flow diagram

Description of included studies

The 35 included studies covered a broad range of applications within emergency US. The most comprehensive body of evidence surrounds the evaluation of pediatric appendicitis. This is followed by trauma, echocardiography, obstetric/gynecologic (OB/GYN), biliary, venous, and renal applications. A small group of studies also evaluate general US processes and impact in the emergency department (ED). Tables 1, 2, 3, 4, 5 and 6 present the principal findings of each study and our grade of the evidence using the CHEERS score.

Evaluation of pediatric appendicitis

We identified 11 studies that assessed the cost-effectiveness of US in the evaluation of acute appendicitis [18–28]. The impetus to avoid radiation in the pediatric population has sparked substantial research interest in this area. Universally, these studies found that using US as the initial study to evaluate pediatric patients for appendicitis decreased radiation exposure, overall costs, and length of stay. These results held despite significant rates of inconclusive initial scans. The use of clinical decision rules and US quality templates further increased

Table 1 Evaluation of pediatric appendicitis

Study	Year	Findings	CHEERS Score (max 24)
Axelrod [18]	2000	US can be cost-saving as an adjunct to clinical decision making when deciding to observe or discharge benign pediatric abdominal pain; however, it is not cost-saving when appendicitis is strongly suspected	14
Pena [19]	2000	Staged imaging using US first followed by CT when US was negative or equivocal for pediatric appendicitis produced cost-savings compared to standard of care	11
Pershad [20]	2015	Using US and a clinical decision rule prior to CT for evaluation of pediatric appendicitis is more cost-effective than CT alone	17
Van Atta [21]	2015	Staged imaging with US first in pediatric patients with suspected appendicitis reduces overall cost through CT avoidance	10
Wagenaar [22]	2015	Staged imaging with US first in pediatric patients with suspected appendicitis reduces overall cost through CT avoidance and decreased length of stay	8
Gregory [23]	2016	The most cost-effective approach for assessing pediatric appendicitis is use of a clinical decision rule followed by staged imaging with US first	22
Anderson [24]	2017	A protocol using US and MRI for pediatric appendicitis successfully decreased use of CT scan though without any change in health outcomes and increased radiology costs over the study period	13
Imler [25]	2017	A comparison of US or MRI first in the evaluation of young patients for appendicitis showed higher overall costs and longer ED length of stay in the MRI group	10
Kharbanda [26]	2018	A study across nine pediatric EDs showed that in the evaluation of acute abdominal pain, US first sites had 5.2% lower total costs of treatment than CT first sites	17
Kobayashi [27]	2018	Implementation of an US first appendicitis pathway at a general hospital was unsuccessful in decreasing CT utilization due to poor adherence to the pathway	8
Nordin [28]	2018	Using a standardized reporting template to ensure US quality decreased equivocal studies and the need to perform CT scans for appendicitis in a pediatric ED, leading to further cost-savings estimated at nearly $150,000 per year	11

Table 2 Evaluation of trauma

Study	Year	Findings	CHEERS Score (max 24)
Branney [29]	1997	Ultrasound use to evaluate acute abdominal trauma can reduce costs through avoidance of peritoneal lavage and reduced length of stay	10
Partrick [30]	1998	Using US as a triage tool in pediatric blunt abdominal trauma may reduce costs through reduced CT scans	6
Arrillaga [31]	1999	In the evaluation of blunt abdominal trauma US decreases time to disposition and procedural costs	15
Frezza [32]	1999	Residents performing FAST is cost-saving compared to US technicians	8
Melniker [33]	2006	Utilizing FAST in the acute management of trauma patients reduces time to operating room, length of stay and overall costs	7
Hall [34]	2016	Performing the cardiac portion of FAST on blunt trauma patients is only cost-effective if they are hypotensive	23

Table 3 Evaluation of renal, biliary, and venous pathology

Study	Year	Findings	CHEERS Score (max 24)
Durston [35]	2001	Initial POCUS by ED physicians for right-upper quadrant pain followed by radiology department scans if needed, is the most cost-effective approach	12
Goodacre [36]	2006	Assessing for deep vein thrombosis with the Wells score and D-dimer prior to US improves cost-effectiveness by avoiding unnecessary scans	20
Young [37]	2010	There may be a large cost associated with repeating imaging tests for cholecystitis after they have already been performed by proficient ED physicians	9
Ward [38]	2010	In patients with high suspicion for pulmonary embolism but low likelihood of mortality, starting the diagnostic workup with US to assess for deep vein thrombosis and proceeding with only selective CT scanning is cost-effective	22
Melnikow [39]	2016	In patients with suspected kidney stones randomized to initial POCUS, radiology US, or CT there were no significant differences in either outcome or cost	14
Sternberg [40]	2017	An assessment of over 10,000 cases of acute renal colic showed that if US was ordered at the initial visit, overall imaging cost and radiation exposure were lower than if CT scan was ordered initially	9

Table 4 Evaluation of OB/GYN pathology

Study	Year	Findings	CHEERS score (max 24)
Hazlett [41]	1996	Transvaginal US is cost-saving compared to transabdominal as an initial test in the work-up of pelvic pain in the ED with the exception of patients in the second or third trimester of pregnancy with a palpable abdominal mass or with a full bladder	6
Durston [42]	2000	Initial POCUS by ED physicians in rule-out ectopic cases is cost-effective compared to initial radiology department imaging, although this may delay care in those with adnexal mass or tubal rupture	12
Al Wattar [43]	2014	Twenty-four hour US coverage for OB/GYN emergencies can avert admissions and cost-savings depends on volume	4

Table 5 Echocardiography

Study	Year	Findings	CHEERS Score (max 24)
Wyrick [44]	2008	Myocardial contrast echocardiography in the ED on selected chest pain patients may be cost-effective through the prevention of unnecessary admissions	16
Jasani [45]	2018	Patients with low-risk chest pain discharged after stress echocardiography in the ED have lower costs and similar health outcomes compared to similar patients admitted to the hospital	8
Baugh [46]	2019	Large variation exists in ordering practices for tests on older patients with syncope in the ED, with CT head and echocardiogram standing out as expensive tests with relatively low yield	11
Gc [47]	2019	In a modeled scenario based on pilot data, the use of tissue Doppler evaluation of diastolic dysfunction in patients with non-ST elevation acute coronary syndrome produced overall cost-savings by decreasing length of stay	21

cost-effectiveness. One study did not find a significant change because of poor adherence to the US first protocol [27].

Evaluation of trauma

Six studies examined US in the setting of acute trauma [29–34]. They found that US decreases time to the operating room for patients with injury, decreases the use of CT scans in children, decreases length of stay, and decreases invasive procedures such as peritoneal lavage in adults. One study specifically examined the cardiac portion of the focused assessment with sonography in trauma (FAST) exam in blunt trauma patients, finding it was only cost-effective in the setting of hypotension [34].

Evaluation of renal, biliary, and venous pathology

Six studies examined US in the setting of renal, biliary, or venous pathology [35–40]. The use of US to evaluate

Table 6 Miscellaneous studies

Study	Year	Findings	CHEERS Score (max 24)
McGahan [48]	2000	At a single institution, 24-h sonography coverage compared to on-call coverage generated net profit and may have improved patient outcomes	8
Morrow [49]	2015	Ballistics gel can be used to make an effective US training model at a cost-saving with respect to commercially available materials	7
Allen [50]	2017	Downstream imaging after an ED US is increased if the US is performed by a non-radiologist	12
Huang [51]	2017	Introducing a protocol for transcervical US for evaluating pediatric peritonsillar abscess decreased length of stay, surgical procedures and CT scans, however, did not decrease cost	12
Van Schaik [52]	2019	POCUS use in the ED likely produces cost savings by decreasing further diagnostic testing	12

acute flank pain had mixed findings. One study suggested no efficiency gains with US use due to high-numbers of subsequent CT orders, and another found that using US as the initial radiology modality decreases costs and radiation exposure despite a 20% subsequent use of CT to further evaluate patients [39, 40]. Two studies assessed the evaluation of biliary pathology. One study showed that in the evaluation of right-upper quadrant pain, initial POCUS by ED providers followed by radiology department scans if needed was the most cost-effective approach, and a second study described large costs associated with additional imaging after ED POCUS significant for acute cholecystitis [35, 37]. In the evaluation of venous thromboembolism, protocols using clinical screening tools, D-dimer testing, and US to decrease CT usage were the most cost-effective [36, 38].

Evaluation of OB/GYN pathology

Three studies assessed US in the evaluation of emergency OB/GYN complaints [41–43]. One study showed that an initial approach of transvaginal instead of transabdominal US is cost-saving in all patients other than those in the second or third trimester of pregnancy [41]. Another study described benefits and drawbacks of POCUS as the initial test in a rule-out ectopic pregnancy scenario showing higher rates of detection of ectopic pregnancy at the first visit, but with an overall increase in number of US studies performed and the potential of other missed pathology [42]. Finally, a third study found that at high-volume sites 24 h a day US coverage to assess for OB/GYN pathology can avert admissions [43].

Echocardiography

Four studies assessed echocardiography in the emergency care setting [44–47]. Three of the studies focused on decreasing hospitalization using US to provide earlier risk-stratification of patients with acute chest pain or acute cardiac issues [44, 45, 47]. One study assessed the cost-effectiveness of a variety of emergency department modalities to evaluate syncope in older patients, finding that CT head and echocardiography where among the most expensive and least revealing tests that are commonly ordered [46].

Miscellaneous studies

Finally, we identified a collection of studies evaluating the downstream impact of emergency US on resource utilization [48–52]. One study found that patients who had POCUS as opposed to radiology scans were at increased risk of having further confirmatory studies ordered compared to those who had the initial US done by radiology [50]. Another small observational study of POCUS in the ED produced a contrary finding, noting that a bedside US performed by an emergency physician could lead to decreased testing afterwards [52].

Quality assessment of included studies

While we tailored our search criteria to identify formal attempts at CEA, considerable variability remained in the quality of the economic evaluations conducted in the studies we identified. Most studies received about half the possible points on the CHEERS checklist. Inadequacy in the performance or the reporting of study perspectives, preference-based health outcomes (patient-reported preferences for different health states used to calculate metrics such as quality-adjusted life-years), modeling assumptions, transparency of costs, characterization of uncertainty, and incremental cost-effectiveness ratios contributed to the majority of downgrading. For example, only nine of the 35 studies presented any characterization of the uncertainty surrounding their cost-effectiveness results, only seven presented an incremental cost-effectiveness ratio, and only 11 explicitly stated the economic perspective from which they were calculating costs.

Discussion

To our knowledge, this is the first systematic review to broadly evaluate the cost-effectiveness of US in the emergency care setting across all applications, including both radiology-performed and POCUS exams. The body of literature identified through this systematic review is fairly consistent in supporting the increased cost-effectiveness of integrating US in emergency care settings across a variety of applications. Healthcare systems have begun to focus on value-based approaches throughout the hospital including the ED [53], and the demonstration of cost-effectiveness of US has the potential to lead to an expansion of its role in ED patient care.

Of the studies identified in this systematic review, those pertaining to the cost-effectiveness of US in the ED evaluation for pediatric appendicitis were the most plentiful and consistent in demonstration of cost-effectiveness gains, particularly when used in conjunction with clinical decision rules [18–28]. Three of the studies identified in this review were amongst the most rigorous we identified using CHEERS methodology [20, 23, 26]. When combined with the decreased radiation exposure of this approach, these studies add to the case for the widespread adoption of an US first approach in the ED evaluation of pediatric appendicitis.

Use of POCUS evaluation of trauma is ubiquitous and recommended by the American College of Surgeons [54]. The six studies we identified demonstrated consistent cost-effectiveness gains when POCUS is used in the evaluation of trauma [29–34]. These studies, however, generally had poor cost-effectiveness methodology and reporting, with the exception of the investigation by Hall et al. which concluded that in blunt trauma patients the cardiac component of the FAST exam is only cost-effective when a patient is hypotensive [34].

Cost-effectiveness of consultative ED US was demonstrated across a variety of applications, including echocardiography, appendicitis, venous thromboembolism, renal, and obstetric. This is consistent with a prior narrative review that demonstrated increased cost-efficiency of US across the spectrum of clinical medicine [55].

The studies identified in this review generally support the cost-effectiveness of POCUS, although some reach the alternative conclusion. The aforementioned studies evaluating POCUS in trauma consistently demonstrated cost savings. Additionally, multiple studies demonstrated potential cost savings in POCUS for biliary and OB/GYN applications [35, 37, 42]. However, one study failed to identify cost savings in POCUS for patients with suspected kidney stones and another demonstrated additional downstream imaging after initial POCUS [39, 50]. Contrarily, a separate study identified in this review demonstrated that POCUS leads to decreased downstream testing and can lower direct and indirect costs associated with diagnostic workups [52]. Given the large number of supporting studies publication bias should be considered, but an assessment of this falls outside of the scope of our manuscript.

None of the studies included in this systematic review specifically address the widely-inferred cost-effectiveness of POCUS due to increased efficiency (US scans are both performed and interpreted at the bedside in real time by a clinician who can immediately integrate the results into patient management) and patient throughput, or the decreased adverse iatrogenic events due to US guidance of procedures [56–59]. This highlights a gap that could be addressed by future research.

This systematic review sought to identify all relevant articles by searching five databases without language or date restrictions; however, it remains possible that pertinent articles were missed. Multiple independent reviewers were utilized at each step of the study selection and data abstraction process to minimize the likelihood of excluding relevant studies. Additionally, the mixed quality of methodology and reporting surrounding the economic evaluations conducted in these studies is notable. Most authors did not frame their analysis as a formal cost-effectiveness study, which may have led to the lack of robust methodology. Both past and recent reviews of cost-effectiveness studies in radiology have highlighted the need for standardized approaches [60, 61]. This limited utilization of established health economics modeling and reporting standards calls into question the reliability of results and makes comparability across studies difficult.

Conclusions

In summary, the body of existing evidence, though limited, is generally supportive of the cost-effectiveness of US in the emergency care setting. The strongest evidence of cost-effectiveness of ultrasound in the ED exists in the evaluation of pediatric appendicitis and of abdominal trauma. Further study, using established best-practice standards in the methodology of cost-effectiveness analysis, is needed to definitively establish the cost-effectiveness of consultative and POCUS across a variety of applications in emergency care settings.

Abbreviations

CEA: Cost-effectiveness analysis; ED: Emergency Department; FAST: Focused Assessment with Sonography in Trauma; POCUS: Point-of-Care Ultrasound; US: Ultrasound; CT: Computed Tomography; PRISMA: Preferred Reporting Items for Systematic Review and Meta-Analyses; CHEERS: Consolidated Health Economic Evaluation Reporting Standards; OB/GYN: Obstetric/Gynecologic; MRI: Magnetic Resonance Imaging.

Acknowledgements

Not applicable.

Authors' contributions

NR conceived the project. NR & BL undertook critical appraisal of the included studies using the CHEERS checklist. All authors performed analysis of the scored studies and contributed to writing the manuscript. All authors read and approved the final manuscript.

Author details

[1] Department of Emergency Medicine, Highland Hospital-Alameda Health System, 1411 E. 31st Street, QIC 22123, Oakland, CA 94602, USA. [2] Department of Emergency Medicine, Johns Hopkins University School of Medicine, 1800 Orleans St, Baltimore, MD 21287, USA.

References

1. Bioeffects Committee of the American Institute of Ultrasound in Medicine (2008) American Institute of Ultrasound in Medicine consensus report on potential bioeffects of diagnostic ultrasound: executive summary. J Ultrasound Med 27:503–515
2. Bierig SM, Jones A (2009) Accuracy and cost comparison of ultrasound versus alternative imaging modalities, including CT, MR, PET, and angiography. J Diagn Med Sonogr 25:138–144
3. Moore CL, Copel JA (2011) Point-of-care ultrasonography. N Engl J Med 364:749–757
4. Shekelle PG, Wachter RM, Pronovost PJ et al (2013) Making health care safer II: an updated critical analysis of the evidence for patient safety practices. Evid Rep Technol Assess 211:1–945
5. Lamperti M, Bodenham AR, Pittiruti M et al (2012) International evidence-based recommendations on ultrasound-guided vascular access. Intensive Care Med 38(7):1105–1117
6. Smith-bindman R, Miglioretti DL, Johnson E et al (2012) Use of diagnostic imaging studies and associated radiation exposure for patients enrolled in large integrated health care systems, 1996–2010. JAMA 307(22):2400–2409
7. Smith-bindman R, Kwan ML, Marlow EC et al (2019) Trends in use of medical imaging in US health care systems and in Ontario, Canada, 2000–2016. JAMA 322(9):843–856
8. Moore CL, Molina AA, Lin H (2006) Ultrasonography in community emergency departments in the United States: access to ultrasonography performed by consultants and status of emergency physician-performed ultrasonography. Ann Emerg Med 47(2):147–153
9. Sanders J, Noble VE, Raja AS et al (2015) Access to and use of point-of-care ultrasound in the emergency department. West J Emerg Med 16(5):747–752
10. Leschyna M, Hatam E, Britton S et al (2019) Current state of point-of-care ultrasound usage in Canadian emergency departments. Cureus. https://doi.org/10.7759/cureus.4246
11. Chamberlain MC, Reid SR, Madhok M (2011) Utilization of emergency ultrasound in pediatric emergency departments. Pediatr Emerg Care 27(7):628–632
12. American College of Radiology (2020) ACR Appropriateness Criteria. https://acsearch.acr.org/list. Accessed Feb 15 2020.
13. American Board of Internal Medicine Foundation (2020) Choosing Wisely Initiative. https://www.choosingwisely.org. Accessed Feb 15 2020.
14. American Institute of Ultrasound in Medicine (2020) Ultrasound First. http://www.ultrasoundfirst.org. Accessed Feb 15 2020.
15. Sistrom CL, McKay NL (2005) Costs, charges, and revenues for hospital diagnostic imaging procedures: differences by modality and hospital characteristics. J Am Coll Radiol 2(6):511–519
16. Husereau D, Drummond M, Petrou S et al (2013) Consolidated health economic evaluation reporting standards (CHEERS) statement. Int J Technol Assess Health Care 29(2):117–122
17. Liberati A, Altman DG, Tetzlaff J et al (2009) The PRISMA statement for reporting systematic reviews and meta-analyses of studies that evaluate health care interventions: explanation and elaboration. Ann Intern Med 151(4):W65-94
18. Axelrod DA, Sonnad SS, Hirschl RB (2000) An economic evaluation of sonographic examination of children with suspected appendicitis. J Pediatr Surg 35(8):1236–1241
19. Peña BM, Taylor GA, Fishman SJ, Mandl KD (2000) Costs and effectiveness of ultrasonography and limited computed tomography for diagnosing appendicitis in children. Pediatrics 106(4):672–676
20. Pershad J, Waters TM, Langham MR, Li T, Huang EY (2015) Cost-effectiveness of diagnostic approaches to suspected appendicitis in children. J Am Coll Surg. 220(4):738–746
21. Van atta AJ, Baskin HJ, Maves CK, et al (2015) Implementing an ultrasound-based protocol for diagnosing appendicitis while maintaining diagnostic accuracy. Pediatr Radiol 45(5):678–685
22. Wagenaar AE, Tashiro J, Wang B et al (2015) Protocol for suspected pediatric appendicitis limits computed tomography utilization. J Surg Res 199(1):153–158
23. Gregory S, Kuntz K, Sainfort F, Kharbanda A (2016) Cost-effectiveness of integrating a clinical decision rule and staged imaging protocol for diagnosis of appendicitis. Value Health 19(1):28–35
24. Anderson KT, Bartz-kurycki M, Austin MT et al (2017) Approaching zero: implications of a computed tomography reduction program for pediatric appendicitis evaluation. J Pediatr Surg 52(12):1909–1915
25. Imler D, Keller C, Sivasankar S et al (2017) Magnetic resonance imaging versus ultrasound as the initial imaging modality for pediatric and young adult patients with suspected appendicitis. Acad Emerg Med 24(5):569–577
26. Kharbanda AB, Christensen EW, Dudley NC et al (2018) Economic analysis of diagnostic imaging in pediatric patients with suspected appendicitis. Acad Emerg Med 25(7):785–794
27. Kobayashi E, Johnson B, Goetz K, Scanlan J, Weinsheimer R (2018) Does the implementation of a pediatric appendicitis pathway promoting ultrasound work outside of a children's hospital? Am J Surg 215(5):917–920
28. Nordin AB, Sales S, Nielsen JW, Adler B, Bates DG, Kenney B (2018) Standardized ultrasound templates for diagnosing appendicitis reduce annual imaging costs. J Surg Res 221:77–83
29. Branney SW, Moore EE, Cantrill SV, Burch JM, Terry SJ (1997) Ultrasound based key clinical pathway reduces the use of hospital resources for the evaluation of blunt abdominal trauma. J Trauma 42(6):1086–1090
30. Partrick DA, Bensard DD, Moore EE, Terry SJ, Karrer FM (1998) Ultrasound is an effective triage tool to evaluate blunt abdominal trauma in the pediatric population. J Trauma 45(1):57–63
31. Arrillaga A, Graham R, York JW, Miller RS (1999) Increased efficiency and cost-effectiveness in the evaluation of the blunt abdominal trauma patient with the use of ultrasound. Am Surg 65(1):31–35
32. Frezza EE, Ferone T, Martin M (1999) Surgical residents and ultrasound technician accuracy and cost-effectiveness of ultrasound in trauma. Am Surg 65(3):289–291
33. Melniker LA, Leibner E, Mckenney MG, Lopez P, Briggs WM, Mancuso CA (2006) Randomized controlled clinical trial of point-of-care, limited ultrasonography for trauma in the emergency department: the first sonography outcomes assessment program trial. Ann Emerg Med 48(3):227–235
34. Hall MK, Omer T, Moore CL, Taylor RA (2016) Cost-effectiveness of the cardiac component of the focused assessment of sonography in trauma examination in blunt trauma. Acad Emerg Med 23(4):415–423
35. Durston W, Carl ML, Guerra W et al (2001) Comparison of quality and cost-effectiveness in the evaluation of symptomatic cholelithiasis with different approaches to ultrasound availability in the ED. Am J Emerg Med 19(4):260–269
36. Goodacre S, Stevenson M, Wailoo A, Sampson F, Sutton AJ, Thomas S (2006) How should we diagnose suspected deep-vein thrombosis? QJM 99(6):377–388
37. Young N, Kinsella S, Raio CC et al (2010) Economic impact of additional radiographic studies after registered diagnostic medical sonographer (RDMS)-certified emergency physician-performed identification of cholecystitis by ultrasound. J Emerg Med 38(5):645–651
38. Ward MJ, Sodickson A, Diercks DB, Raja AS (2011) Cost-effectiveness of lower extremity compression ultrasound in emergency department patients with a high risk of hemodynamically stable pulmonary embolism. Acad Emerg Med 18(1):22–31
39. Melnikow J, Xing G, Cox G et al (2016) Cost analysis of the STONE randomized trial: can health care costs be reduced one test at a time? Med Care 54(4):337–342
40. Sternberg KM, Littenberg B (2017) Trends in imaging use for the evaluation and followup of kidney stone disease: a single center experience. J Urol 198(2):383–388
41. Hazlett KS, Wagner A, Guidi C, Victoria D, Weir S, Wise S (1996) Cost effectiveness of pelvic sonogram in the emergency room: endovaginal vs. transabdominal examination. Emergency Radiol 3(5):231–235

42. Durston WE, Carl ML, Guerra W, Eaton A, Ackerson LM (2000) Ultrasound availability in the evaluation of ectopic pregnancy in the ED: comparison of quality and cost-effectiveness with different approaches. Am J Emerg Med 18(4):408–417
43. Al Wattar BH, Frank M, Fage E, Gupta P (2014) Use of ultrasound in emergency gynaecology. J Obstet Gynaecol 34(2):172–173
44. Wyrick JJ, Kalvaitis S, Mcconnell KJ, Rinkevich D, Kaul S, Wei K (2008) Cost-efficiency of myocardial contrast echocardiography in patients presenting to the emergency department with chest pain of suspected cardiac origin and a nondiagnostic electrocardiogram. Am J Cardiol 102(6):649–652
45. Jasani G, Papas M, Patel AJ et al (2018) Immediate stress echocardiography for low-risk chest pain patients in the emergency department: a prospective observational cohort study. J Emerg Med 54(2):156–164
46. Baugh CW, Sun BC, Syncope Risk Stratification Study Group (2019) Variation in diagnostic testing for older patients with syncope in the emergency department. Am J Emerg Med 37(5):810–816
47. Gc VS, Alshurafa M, Sturgess DJ et al (2019) Cost-minimisation analysis alongside a pilot study of early tissue doppler evaluation of diastolic dysfunction in emergency department non-ST elevation acute coronary syndromes (TEDDy-NSTEACS). BMJ Open. https://doi.org/10.1136/bmjopen-2018-023920
48. Mcgahan JP, Cronan MS, Richards JR, Jones CD (2000) Comparison of US utilization and technical costs before and after establishment of 24-hour in-house coverage for US examinations. Radiology 216(3):788–791
49. Morrow DS, Broder J (2015) Cost-effective, reusable, leak-resistant ultrasound-guided vascular access trainer. J Emerg Med 49(3):313–317
50. Allen B, Carrol LV, Hughes DR, Hemingway J, Duszak R, Rosenkrantz AB (2017) Downstream imaging utilization after emergency department ultrasound interpreted by radiologists versus nonradiologists: a medicare claims-based Study. J Am Coll Radiol 14(4):475–481
51. Huang Z, Vintzileos W, Gordish-dressman H, Bandarkar A, Reilly BK (2017) Pediatric peritonsillar abscess: outcomes and cost savings from using transcervical ultrasound. Laryngoscope 127(8):1924–1929
52. Van Schaik GWW, Van Schaik KD, Murphy MC (2019) Point-of-care ultrasonography (POCUS) in a community emergency department: an analysis of decision making and cost savings associated with POCUS. J Ultrasound Med 38(8):2133–2140
53. Farmer SA, Brown NA (2017) Value-based approaches for emergency care in a new era. Ann Emerg Med 69(6):684–686
54. American College of Surgeons (2018) Advanced trauma life support: student course manual, 10th edn. Illinois, Chicago
55. Bierig SM, Jones A (2009) Accuracy and cost comparison of ultrasound versus alternative imaging modalities, including CT, MR, PET, and angiography. J Diagn Med Sonography 25(3):38–144
56. Blaivas M, Harwood RA, Lambert MJ (1999) Decreasing length of stay with emergency ultrasound examination of the gallbladder. Acad Emerg Med 6:1020–1023
57. Burgher SW, Tandy TK, Dawdy MR (1998) Transvaginal ultrasonography by emergency physicians decreases patient time in the emergency department. Acad Emerg Med 5:802–807
58. Leung J, Duffy M, Finckh A (2006) Real-time ultrasonographically guided internal jugular vein catheterization in the emergency department increases success rates and reduces complications: a randomized, prospective study. Ann Emerg Med 48:540–547
59. Randolph AG, Cook DJ, Gonzales CA, Pribble CG (1996) Ultrasound guidance for placement of central venous catheters: a meta-analysis of the literature. Crit Care Med 24:2053–2058
60. Zhou A, Yousem DM, Alvin MD (2018) Cost-effectiveness analysis in radiology: a systematic review. J Am Coll Radiol 15(11):1536–1546. https://doi.org/10.1016/j.jacr.2018.06.018 (**Epub 2018 Jul 26**)
61. Otero HJ, Rybicki FJ, Greenberg D, Neumann PJ (2008) Twenty years of cost-effectiveness analysis in medical imaging: are we improving? Radiology 249(3):917–925. https://doi.org/10.1148/radiol.2493080237

4

Venous Doppler ultrasound in critically Ill COVID-19 patients: game changer in anticoagulation therapy

Marta Alfageme[1*], Jorge González Plaza[1], Santiago Méndez[1], Juan A. Gómez Patiño[1], María L. Collado[1], José M. Abadal[2], Rocío González Costero[1], Teresa Fontanilla[3] and Agustín García Suárez[1]

Abstract

Background: COVID-19 infection has been associated with a high rate of thrombotic events, such as deep vein thrombosis (DVT) and acute pulmonary embolism (APE).

Methods: The purpose of our retrospective study was to evaluate the prevalence of asymptomatic DVT in lower limbs in critically ill COVID-19 patients ($n=23$) with severe respiratory failure and high levels of D-dimer by bedside Doppler ultrasound (DU).

Results: DVT was diagnosed in 14 cases (60.87%), 5 in proximal venous territory and 9 in infrapopliteal veins. Computed Tomography Pulmonary Angiography (CTPA) was performed in six patients and all of them showed acute pulmonary embolism (APE) at segmental or subsegmental branches of pulmonary arteries. These patients (APE or DVT confirmed) were treated with therapeutic doses of anticoagulant therapy.

Conclusion: In critically COVID-19 ill ICU patients with severe respiratory failure and elevated D-dimer, the incidence of asymptomatic DVT is high. We propose that DU allows detection of DVT in asymptomatic patients, adding a factor that may balance the decision to fully anticoagulate these patients.

Introduction

COVID-19 infection has been associated with a high rate of thrombotic events, such as deep vein thrombosis (DVT) and acute pulmonary embolism (APE) in patients admitted to intensive care unit (ICU) [1].

Several studies report a high risk of DVT in COVID-19 critically ill patients with pneumonia despite adequate thromboprophylaxis [2] and have suggested the use of anticoagulant therapy in therapeutic range [3].

The purpose of our study was to evaluate the prevalence of asymptomatic DVT in lower limbs in critically ill COVID-19 patients with severe respiratory failure and high levels of D-dimer by bedside Doppler ultrasound (DU).

Materials and methods

This is an observational descriptive retrospective study performed at a third level hospital in Madrid between the 1st and 10th of April 2020. DU was performed on all consecutive confirmed COVID-19 patients admitted to the Intensive Care Unit (ICU) with the diagnosis of severe pneumonia (with radiological pattern compatible with COVID-19 and extensive involvement in chest X-ray), who developed acute severe respiratory failure, requiring invasive mechanical ventilation and with elevated D-dimer levels > 0.5 µg/ml (normal range < 0.5 µg/ml).

Computed tomography pulmonary angiography (CTPA) could not be performed due to the risk of unstable patient transfer to the radiology, so DU was

*Correspondence: marta.alfageme@gmail.com
[1] Department of Interventional Radiology, Hospital Universitario Puerta de Hierro, Majadahonda, España
Full list of author information is available at the end of the article

carried out at patient bedside to screen venous thromboembolic disease.

Nevertheless, later respiratory and clinical improvement of 6 patients permitted CTPA.

Patients were excluded if they were under full-dose anticoagulant therapy or if they developed symptomatic DVT.

Several patients showed alterations in coagulation parameters, so International Society of Thrombosis and Haemostasis (ISTH) score, a scoring system for disseminated intravascular coagulation (DIC), was calculated.

All patients at ICU received thromboprophylaxis with subcutaneous low molecular weight heparin (LMWH) (enoxaparin 40 mg/24 h), adjusted for renal insufficiency (creatinine clearance < 30 ml/min) and overweight patients (> 100 Kg).

DU examinations were practiced by two radiologists with more than 10-year of experience (Samsung HS50 ® equipment US and with a multifrequency linear probe). DU protocol includes grayscale, color and spectral Doppler evaluation. The examination included the deep venous system of the thigh, calf and both saphenous. DVT was diagnosed in cases of increased vein diameter, presence of echogenic material, non-compressibility of the veins and absence of color and spectral Doppler signal (Figs. 1, 2, 3).

Formal approval from the Medical Ethics Review Committee was not required as the Medical Research Involving Human Subjects Act (WMO) did not apply for this observational study.

Regarding descriptive statistical analysis, categorical data were expressed as relative and absolute frequencies, while numerical data were reported as the mean and standard deviation (SD) if there was a normal distribution or median and interquartile range (IQR) if they have a non-normal distribution. Qualitative variables were presented by the frequency distribution and percentages.

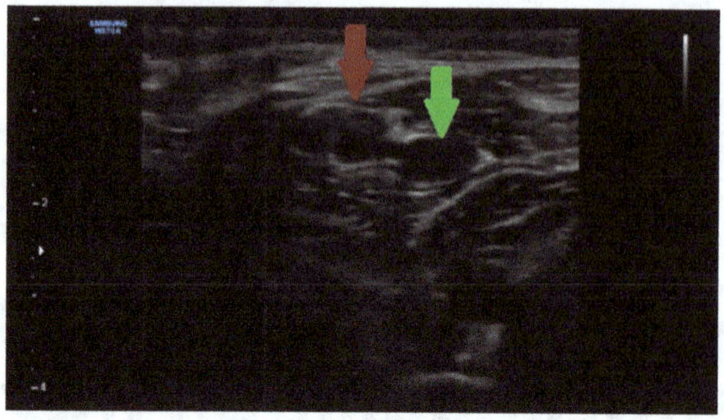

Fig. 2 Absence of collapse after compression with the ultrasound transducer. With the transducer in the same position as Fig. 1, pressure is exerted. In the absence of thrombosis, the veins should collapse. In this case, they not collapse (arrows). This maneuver helps to confirm thrombosis of the right side vein (green arrow)

Results

Initially, we had included 27 patients, but we excluded 4 patients from this study: 2 of them because they were already treated with therapeutic anticoagulant therapy and other 2 patients as they developed symptomatic DVT. Thus, the study comprised 23 patients, 16 males (69.57%) and 7 females (30.43%). Mean patient age was 59.17 ± 12.9 (DS).

DVT was diagnosed in 14 cases (60.87%) (Table 1). Five in proximal venous territory and nine in infrapopliteal veins. No proximal and distal thrombosis was found simultaneously in the same patient.

CTPA was performed in six patients and all of them showed acute pulmonary embolism (APE) at segmental or subsegmental branches of pulmonary arteries. None of them showed thrombus in the main or lobar

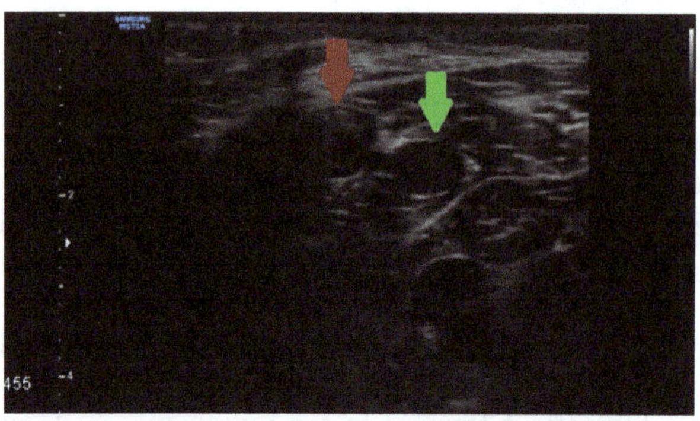

Fig. 1 Gastrocnemius veins thrombosis. Echogenic content is identified within the veins. The content is better visualized in the vein on the left (red arrow) than in the right (green arrow)

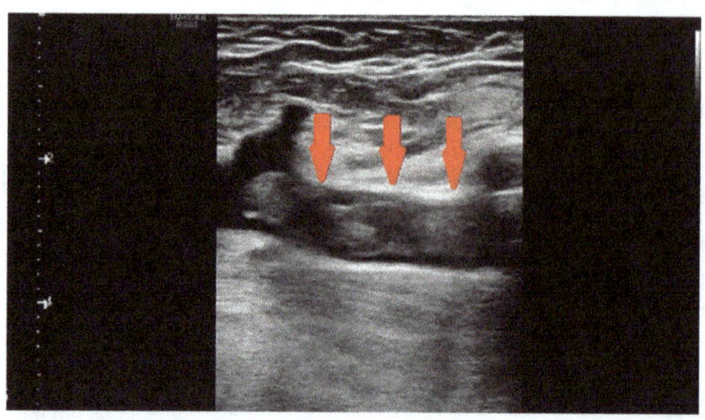

Fig. 3 Longitudinal image of the posterior tibial vein. It is enlarged and with echogenic content in relation to acute venous thrombosis (arrows)

Table 1 Characteristics of COVID-19 patients included in the study

AGE (years)	SEX[a]	DVT[b]	D-DIMER (μg/ml)	ISTH score	CTPA[c]
55	1	1	13.99	2	1
34	1	1	18.47	3	n/a
51	1	0	10.11	2	n/a
64	1	0	2.94	1	n/a
57	1	1	93.24	3	1
48	1	1	12.14	3	n/a
77	1	1	49.88	3	1
59	0	1	59.60	3	1
73	1	1	12.08	1	n/a
43	0	1	8.74	1	1
63	0	1	15.07	2	n/a
53	1	0	3.25	1	n/a
41	1	0	13.82	3	n/a
72	0	1	3.51	1	n/a
76	1	1	57.48	2	n/a
75	1	0	9.30	3	n/a
64	1	1	12.31	2	1
49	0	0	4.60	4	n/a
72	1	1	18.79	3	n/a
52	0	0	4.79	2	n/a
71	0	0	4.30	1	n/a
71	1	1	17.26	3	n/a
41	1	0	13.82	1	n/a

All patients presented extensive and bilateral lung involvement on Chest-X-Ray

DVT deep venous thrombosis, *ISTH* International Society of Thrombosis and Hemostasis Criteria for Disseminated intravascular Coagulation (DIC), *ICU* Intensive Care Unit

[a] Sex: 1 = male, 0 = female, [b]DVT: 1 = positive, 0 = negative [c]Computed Tomography Pulmonary Angiography: 1 = positive, 0 = negative, n/a = not available

pulmonary arteries. DU confirmed DVT in these 6 cases. In five of them the thrombosis was distal.

The median of D-Dimer was 12.31 μgr/ml (IQR 6.75–17.86 μg/ml). Patients with DVT had higher D-Dimer 16.16 μg/ml (IQR 12.18–42.03) μg/ml than patients without DVT 4.79 μg/ml (IQR 4.3–10.11) μg/ml.

All the patients presented ISTH score < 5, suggesting non-overt or low grade DIC (Table 1).

Patients with APE (n = 6) or confirmed DVT were treated with therapeutic doses of anticoagulant therapy (1 mg of enoxaparin/kg every 12 h), adjusted to weight and renal function.

Major hemorrhagic complications occurred in 3/23 patients (13%), two of them developed inferior epigastric artery bleeding and one patient presented middle hemorrhoidal artery bleeding, requiring in all cases endovascular embolization. One of the patients with epigastric bleeding had infrapopliteal thrombosis. The other two patients had proximal DVT.

Discussion

COVID-19 has been associated with a higher risk of thrombotic events like DVT and APE [4–6]. Some studies propose that thromboembolic events could be secondary to a systemic procoagulant response (excessive inflammation, hypoxia, platelet activation and endothelial dysfunction) to COVID-19 infection [7, 8]. The evidence to date supports the concept that the thrombotic manifestations of severe COVID-19 are due to the ability of SARS-CoV-2 to invade endotelial cells via ACE-2 (angiotensin-converting enzyme 2), which is expressed on the endothelial cell surface. However, in patients with COVID-19, the subsequent endothelial inflammation, complement activation, thrombin generation, platelet, and leukocyte recruitment, and the initiation of innate and adaptive immune responses culminate in immunothrombosis, ultimately causing (micro)thrombotic complications, such as deep vein thrombosis, pulmonary embolism, and stroke [9]. The frequency of these complications increases in critically ill patients admitted to the ICU [1, 2]. The results of autopsy studies indicate the presence of pulmonary.

endothelial damage and microthrombosis. In a case series of 4 autopsies of COVID-19-infected patients from New Orleans with sudden respiratory decompensation, it was shown that there were no thromboembolisms in the major pulmonary arteries, but small thrombi were present in sections of the peripheral lung parenchyma [10]. It is not clear from the clinical studies whether the thrombotic pulmonary complications are APE or primary pulmonary thrombosis. The presence of distal and microthrombosis in many patients suggests local pathology, which does not exclude the possibility of embolic events [11]. In view of this, some groups recommend full dose anticoagulant therapy for patients with unfavorable evolution and worst prognosis, especially in those with sepsis, elevated levels of D-dimer and disseminated intravascular coagulopathy [3, 12]. Another study found lower mortality rate in critically ill patients under anticoagulant therapy [13].

In our study, we found an increased incidence of asymptomatic DVT (60.87%), mostly in the infrapopliteal venous system in selected COVID-19 patients (elevated D-Dimer and severe respiratory failure). The presence of APE was also documented in the six patients who CTPA was performed. One of the limitations of our study is the lack of CTPA of all the patients.

A recently study also found an increased frequency of distal DVT up to 85% of the COVID-19 ICU patients [5]. Multiple studies reported a high incidence of DVT in critically ill COVID-19 patients, one of them found an incidence of 47%, but all critically patients were included, not only the severe patients [1]. In another study, the incidence was 20% but the authors did not specify whether asymptomatic patients were also studied [2].

Despite our study has limitations as small sample size, the results suggest a higher incidence of asymptomatic DVT in critically ill COVID-19 patients than reported by others studies in non-COVID-19 critically ill patients where the incidence was around 10% [14, 15].

There is not a consensus on the use of anticoagulant therapy on asymptomatic infrapopliteal DVT no COVID-19 patients because of the lower probability of thrombus migration into the lungs and some groups prefer an expectant management [16] while others propose to use anticoagulant therapy (17). The indication of treatment depends on the clinical context of each patient. In our critically ill COVID-19 patients, documenting the DVT helped tip the balance to full anticoagulation.

Therefore, we propose the use of bedside ultrasound to detect DVT including infrapopliteal, especially in ICU patients who cannot be mobilized to perform CTPA.

Conclusion

In critically COVID-19 ill ICU patients with severe respiratory failure and elevated D-dimer, the incidence of asymptomatic DVT is high.

DU allows detection of DVT in asymptomatic patients, adding a factor that may influence the decision to fully anticoagulate these patients.

Abbreviations

DVT: Deep vein thrombosis; ICU: Intensive care unit; APE: Acute pulmonary embolism; DU: Doppler ultrasound; CTPA: Computed tomography pulmonary angiography; ISTH: International Society of Thrombosis and Haemostasis; DIC: Disseminated intravascular coagulation; LMWH: Low molecular weight heparin; SD: Standard deviation; IQR: Interquartile range; N/A: Not available.

Acknowledgements

Not applicable.

Authors' contributions

All the authors of the article are responsible for concept and writing. All authors read and approved the final manuscript.

Author details

[1] Department of Interventional Radiology, Hospital Universitario Puerta de Hierro, Majadahonda, España. [2] Department of Interventional Radiology, Hospital Universitario Severo Ochoa, Leganés, España. [3] Department of Radiology, Hospital Universitario Puerta de Hierro, Majadahonda, España.

References

1. Middeldorp S, Coppens M, van Haaps TF et al (2020) Incidence of venous thromboembolism in hospitalized patients with COVID-19. J Thromb Haemost. https://doi.org/10.1111/jth.14888
2. Klok FA, Kruip MJHA, van der Meer NJM et al (2020) Incidence of thrombotic complications in critically ill ICU patients with COVID-19. Thromb Res. https://doi.org/10.1016/j.thromres.2020.04.013
3. Casini A, Alberio L, Angelillo-Scherrer A, Fontana P, Gerber B et al (2020) Thromboprophylaxis and laboratory monitoring for in-hospital patients with Covid-19 - a Swiss consensus statement by the Working Party Hemostasis. Swiss Med Wkly 150:w20247. https://doi.org/10.4414/smw.2020.20247
4. Chen J, Wang X, Zhang S, Liu B, Wu X, Wang Y et al (2020) Findings of acute pulmonary embolism in COVID-19 Patients. Lancet Infect Dis. https://doi.org/10.2139/ssrn.3548771
5. Ren B, Yan F, Deng Z et al (2020) Extremely high incidence of lower extremity deep venous thrombosis in 48 patients with severe COVID-19 in Wuhan. Circulation. https://doi.org/10.1161/CIRCULATIONAHA.120.047407
6. Zhang L, Feng X, Zhang D et al (2020) Deep Vein Thrombosis in Hospitalized Patients With Coronavirus Disease 2019 (COVID-19) in Wuhan. Prevalence, Risk Factors, and Outcome. Circulation, China. https://doi.org/10.1161/CIRCULATIONAHA.120.046702
7. Bikdeli B, Madhavan MV, Jimenez D et al (2020) COVID-19 and thrombotic or thromboembolic disease: implications for prevention, antithrombotic therapy, and follow-up. J Am Coll Cardiol S0735–1097(20):35008–35017. https://doi.org/10.1016/j.jacc.2020.04.031
8. Luo W, Yu H, Gou J et al (2020) Clinical pathology of critical patient with novel coronavirus pneumonia (COVID-19). Preprints 2020:2020020407
9. McFadyen JD, Stevens H et al (2020) (2020) The Emerging Threat of (Micro)Thrombosis in COVID-19 and Its Therapeutic Implications. Circ Res. 127(4):571–587. https://doi.org/10.1161/CIRCRESAHA.120.317447
10. Fox S, Akmatbekov A, Harbert J, Li G et al (2020) (2020) Pulmonary and cardiac pathology in African American patients with COVID-19: an autopsy series from New Orleans. Lancet Respir Med 8(7):681–686. https://doi.org/10.1016/S2213-2600(20)30243-5
11. Miesbach W, Makris M (2020) COVID-19: coagulopathy, risk of thrombosis, and the rationale for anticoagulation. Clin Appl Thromb Hemost 26:1076029620938149. https://doi.org/10.1177/1076029620938149
12. Tang N, Li D, Wang X, Sun Z (2020) Abnormal coagulation parameters are associated with poor prognosis in patients with novel coronavirus pneumonia. J Thromb Haemost 18(4):844–847. https://doi.org/10.1111/jth.14768
13. Tang N, Bai H, Chen X, Gong J, Li D, Sun Z (2020) Anticoagulant treatment is associated with decreased mortality in severe coronavirus disease 2019 patients with coagulopathy. J Thromb Haemost 18(5):1094–1099. https://doi.org/10.1111/jth.14817
14. Arabi YM, Burns KEA, Alsolamy SJ et al (2020) Surveillance or no surveillance ultrasonography for deep vein thrombosis and outcomes of critically ill patients: a pre-planned sub-study of the PREVENT trial. Intensive Care Med 46:737–746. https://doi.org/10.1007/s00134-019-05899-1
15. Harris LM, Curl GR, Booth FV, Hassett JM Jr, Leney G, Ricotta JJ (1997) Screening for asymptomatic deep vein thrombosis in surgical intensive care patients. J Vasc Surg 26(5):764–769. https://doi.org/10.1016/S0741-5214(97)70088-0
16. Fleck D, Albadawi H, Wallace A, Knuttinen G, Naidu S, Oklu R (2017) Below-knee deep vein thrombosis (DVT): diagnostic and treatment patterns. Cardiovasc Diagn Ther 7(Suppl 3):S134–S139. https://doi.org/10.21037/cdt.2017.11.03
17. Franco L, Giustozzi M, Agnelli G, Becattini C (2017) Anticoagulation in patients with isolated distal deep vein thrombosis: a meta-analysis. J Thromb Haemost 15(6):1142–1154. https://doi.org/10.1111/jth.13677

5

Comparison of ultrasonographic versus infrared pupillary assessment

Christian D. Yic[1*], Gabriel Prada[3], Sergio I. Paz[2], Leandro Moraes[1], Julio C. Pontet[2], Marcos E. Lasso[1] and Alberto Biestro[1]

Abstract

Objectives: To evaluate the correlation between ultrasonographic and infrared pupillary assessments in critically ill patients, including neurocritically ill patients.

Design: Prospective, observational study.

Setting: Tertiary teaching hospital intensive care unit (ICU) in Montevideo, Uruguay.

Patients: Twenty-six adults patients with age 18 or older admitted to the intensive care unit with and without neurologic pathology. A total of 212 pupillary measures were made between ultrasonographic pupillary assessment (UPA) and infrared pupillary assessment (IPA).

Interventions: This was a study that utilized non-invasive (minimal risk) ultrasonographic and infrared pupillary assessment in patients admitted to the ICU. Time between UPA and IPA in a single patient was consistently less than 3 min.

Measurements and main results: There was a strong positive association between UPA and IPA (right eye [OD]: $r=$ de 0.926, p-value < 0.001; left eye [OS], $r=0.965$, p-value < 0.001), also observed in the group of neurocritically ill patients (OD: $r=0.935$, p-value < 0.001; OS: $r=$ de 0.965, p-value < 0.001). Taking IPA as reference measure, the percent error for all subjects was 2.77% and 2.15% for OD and OS, respectively, and for neurocritically ill patients it was 3.21% and 2.44% for OD and OS, respectively.

Conclusions: Ultrasonographic pupillary assessment is strongly correlated with infrared pupillary assessment in critically ill patients, including neurocritically ill patients. Ultrasonographic pupillary assessment is a quick, feasible, non-invasive method that allows accurate pupillary assessment, particularly neurologic function, in patients in whom a more precise measurement of the pupil is required or eye opening is not possible (e.g., periorbital edema due to traumatic brain injury).

Keywords: Ocular ultrasonography, Ocular ultrasound, Pupillometry, Pupillary assessment, Traumatic brain injury, Brain herniation

Introduction

Pupillary assessment (i.e., bilateral evaluation of pupils size, shape, symmetry, and reactivity) is a cornerstone of the neurologic physical examination in the critically ill, particularly the neurocritically ill. Systematic pupillary assessments are routinely performed in the critically ill because they can render early signs of neurologic deterioration, which, in some cases, may be the only clinically obtainable sign. The Brain Trauma Foundation's guidelines for the management of severe traumatic brain injury acknowledge the evaluation of pupils' size and reactivity to light as source for early prognostic signs of neurologic pathology [1].

*Correspondence: docyic@hotmail.com
[1] Department of Critical Care Medicine, Hospital de Clínicas, Montevideo, Uruguay
Full list of author information is available at the end of the article

There are reports of pupillary assessment as far back as 1929, when Otto Lowestein first developed a technique based on the analysis of simple, direct, visual evaluations [2]. Nonetheless, despite remarkable technologic advances and substantial improvements on the understanding of the central nervous system, the pupillary examination has not much changed during the last century. Regarding the conventional, visual pupillary assessment, there is considerable intra- and inter-observer variability due to inconsistency on several factors, such as illumination of patient's room, examiner's visual acuity and experience, and intensity and technique of light stimuli. Therefore, alternative techniques have been proposed [3, 4].

The most accepted alternative technique is the infrared pupillary assessment (IPA), first described in 1958 by Lowestein himself, and then, as from 1993, extensively studied by Merlin Larson; by these means, both of Lowestein and Larson ended up elucidating the association between pupillary abnormalities and brainstem injuries or pharmacologic effects [5, 6]. In 2003, Taylor et al., using an infrared pupillometer, established an association between intracranial pressure and pupillary abnormalities in patients with acute brain injury [7]. In 2011, Chen et al. using the infrared pupillometer, described a significant inverse relationship between decreasing pupil reactivity and increasing intracranial pressure; the first evidence of pupil abnormalities occurred, on average, 15.9 h prior to the time of the peak of intracranial pressure [8]. Today, the IPA is being increasingly adopted as a routine part of the neurologic examination, supported by a growing body of literature demonstrating its reliability, accuracy, and ease of use. Automated pupillometry allows rapid, non-invasive, reliable, and quantifiable assessment of pupillary function which may allow rapid diagnosis of intracranial pathology that affects clinical decision-making [9, 10].

On the other hand, the first report of ocular ultrasound was made in 1956 [11]. Technologic advances in ultrasound devices have since allowed implementing ocular ultrasound in the evaluation of several ophthalmologic pathologies such as ocular trauma and intraocular foreign body identification [12–14]. However, the ultrasonographic evaluation of the pupillary diameter and pupillary light reflex has not been well studied, let alone implemented. In cases when direct visualization of the pupil is not possible due to soft tissue injury that precludes eye opening, alternative techniques such as IPA and LED-based perimetric pupillometry have been proposed; unfortunately, most of these techniques do not overcome the physical barrier placed by the soft tissue, rely on advanced devices that are not generally available in emergency situations, and require of specialized technical support [15–17]. In this context, UPA is particularly useful because it offers a simple yet accurate alternative that can be performed with small, portable devices at the point of care.

To the authors' knowledge, few reports have been published regarding UPA application and clinical relevance, mostly in emergency medicine and critical care medicine. Nevertheless, none of them have evaluated and compared UPA's accuracy to standard techniques such as IPA [18–21].

Objective

To evaluate the correlation between ultrasonographic and infrared pupillary assessments in critically ill patients, including neurocritically ill patients.

Methods

Study design and study population

This was a prospective, observational study following the Helsinki Declaration and approved by the institutional review board. Patients older than 18 years who were admitted to the ICU of the Hospital de Clínicas, Montevideo, Uruguay, from October 1, 2018 to March 1, 2019 were included. Exclusion criteria were patients with ophthalmologic or periorbital pathology, including abnormal pupillary anatomy or neurologic assessment at baseline, or with facial or periorbital soft tissue edema that precluded eye opening, and therefore adequate IPA.

Upon admission to the ICU, consent was obtained from patients' family members. Disease severity was determined following the Glasgow Coma Scale, and electronic medical records were reviewed to obtain demographics (age, gender, race), vital signs (heart rate, respiratory rate, blood pressure, temperature), and hemodynamic parameters (if any).

Non-invasive (minimal risk) ultrasonographic and infrared pupillary assessments were performed during same visit to the patient. Lights in patients' room were turned off and windows and curtains were closed, thereby ensuring homogeny in rooms' illumination regardless of time of the day.

Because UPA required manual measurement of pupillary diameter, we performed UPA first and then IPA, thereby reducing potential source of observer bias. The time frame between UPA and IPA was less than 3 min, during which there was no administration of new medications or physical maneuvers or activities on the patient. The examinations, both UPA and IPA, were performed at any time during ICU stay, by three authors (C.Y, S.P and M.L) who were experienced in UPA and IPA. On some patients, two or more pupillary examinations (UPA and IPA) were performed, each on different days while still in the ICU. The ultrasound and infrared devices and the information they yielded were used as standard of care; however, the devices themselves were not investigated.

Ultrasonographic pupillary assessment (UPA)

The ultrasonographic pupillary assessment included evaluation of bilateral pupillary diameter and pupillary light reflex. With the ultrasound machine on "small parts" preset and the patient in a supine, semi-recumbent position, a linear 7.5–15 MHz transducer was gently placed over the lower edge of the closed eye for a trans-palpebral tangential view, with the probe marker pointed toward the right side of the patient (Fig. 1).

Following FDA regulations for mechanical index and thermal index for ophthalmic ultrasound, we used values less than 0.23 for the mechanical index and less than 1.0 for the thermal index. Although we use the preset small parts, we lowered the mechanical index below 0.23 by changing the acoustic power.

Subsequent tilting movement of the probe was applied until the pupil is visualized. Then, on each eye at a time, over the closed eye and across the eyelid, a light stimulus was shown first ipsilateral to assess for direct pupillary light reflex. Only motion-mode (M-mode) ultrasonographic modality was used for the measurements (Fig. 2). The overall time for UPA per patient, including right and left eye, was never more than 3 min. Although the ultrasound machine is designed to produce minimal risk to the user and the patient, adverse events, such as eye discomfort, irritation, redness or pain, due to superficial pressure exerted by the transducer or due to eyelid and/or eye contact with the sonographic gel, if any, were documented.

Infrared pupillary assessment (IPA)

The infrared pupillary assessment included evaluation of bilateral pupillary diameter and pupillary light reflex. The infrared pupillometer is a monocular, stand-alone, handheld, battery-operated instrument, which captures and analyzes the images in less than 3 s. When placed over the eye, the infrared pupillometer shows a light stimulus over the open eye in order to assess for the pupillary light reflex (Fig. 3). The overall time for IPA per patient, including right and left eye, was never more than 1 min. The infrared pupillometer machine is designed to produce minimal risk to the user and the patient. The only designated mechanical contact point with the patient is the headrest. All levels of radiation fall below threshold values recommended by the International Commission on Non-Ionizing Radiation Protection.

For both UPA and IPA, normal values of pupillary diameter were 2 to 4 mm. A pupillary diameter less than 2 mm was documented as miosis, whereas a pupillary diameter greater than 4 mm was documented as mydriasis. The pupillary light reflex was determined by the percentage of reduction in size of pupil diameter immediately after light stimuli. Such a light stimuli was given by the flashlight of a mobile phone model iPhone 6, iPhone 7, iPhone 8 or iPhone X, at an approximate distance of 8 to 12 cm from the eye, and at an angle of 90 degrees (i.e., perpendicular) to the coronal plane of the

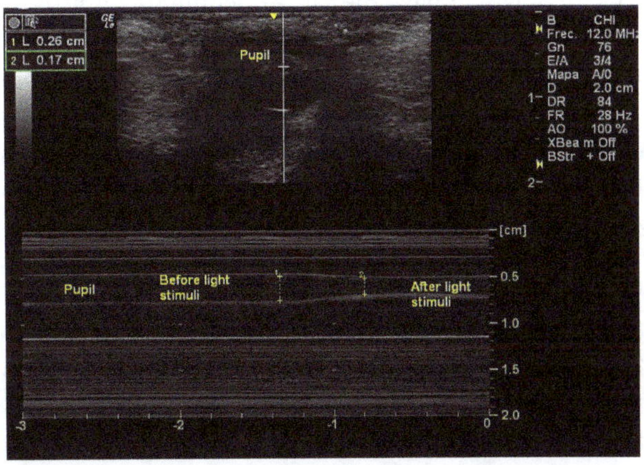

Fig. 2 Ocular ultrasound on 2D (top) and M-mode (bottom) showing pupil before light stimuli and after light stimuli. Pupillary on M-mode tracing is highlighted by two white, horizontal, straight, parallel lines

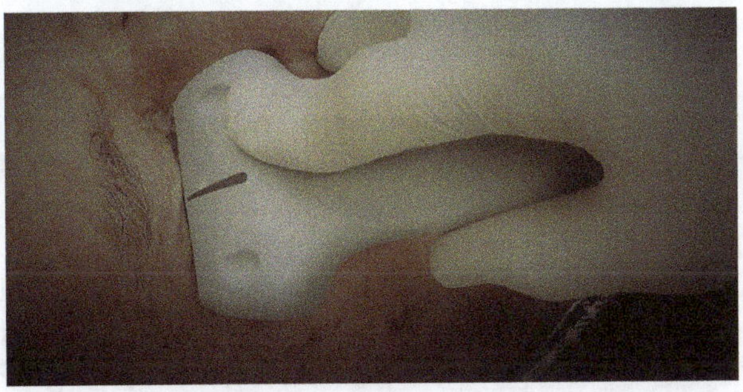

Fig. 1 Ultrasonographic pupillary assessment. The 7.5–15 MHz linear transducer gently placed over the lower edge of the closed eye for a trans-palpebral tangential view

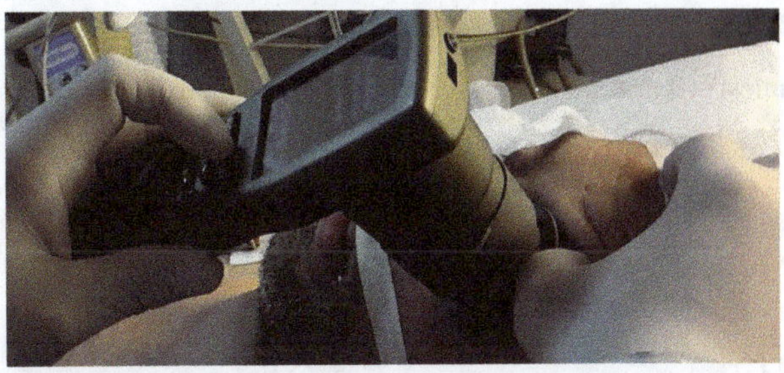

Fig. 3 Infrared pupillary assessment. The pupillometer is placed over the open eye, which shows a light stimulus to assess for the pupillary light reflex

pupil, all of which have the same documented luminosity, regardless of remaining battery, according to Apple Inc. and were available to the research staff.

The reduction in pupillary diameter was calculated as follows: (maximum resting aperture − minimum aperture)/maximum resting aperture; where maximum resting aperture was the maximal pupillary diameter recorded before light stimuli was shown, minimum aperture was the minimal pupillary diameter recorded after light stimuli was shown. A normal pupillary light reflex was considered as percentage of reduction in size of pupil diameter after light stimuli of 10% or more according to a large study by Taylor et al. [7].

Statistical analysis

For the comparison between UPA and IPA, Bland–Altman and dispersion plots, simple linear regression models, and the Chi-square test were used. The Shapiro–Wilk test and Q–Q plots were used to corroborate normal distribution of the data. All calculations were done using the R programming language and statistical software (version 3.5.1).

Results

Total of patients included were 26, most were men (60.0%), with a mean age of 45,05 (range 18–84) years, and mean glasgow coma score at the moment of the pupillary assessment of 8,69 (range 3–15). A total of 212 pupillary measures were obtained, of which 106 were on each eye (i.e., right and left eyes), and 108 were in neurocritically ill patients. Table 1 shows patients classified according to main pathology for ICU admission.

Frequencies and percentages of patients according to main pathology for intensive care unit admission.

Ultrasonographic pupillary assessment was feasible in all patients. There was a strong positive correlation between measures of reduction in pupillary diameter (pupillary light reflex) obtained by IPA and UPA ($r_{OD}=0.926$, 95% CI 0.893–0.949, p-value < 0.001; $r_{OS}=0.965$, 95% CI 0.949–0.976, p-value < 0.001) (Fig. 4a, b).

Table 1 Absolute frequency represents the number of times the value is present for each variable

Clinical categorization	Absolute frequency (*n*)	Relative frequency (%)
Medical	106	50.0
Medical and surgical	66	31.2
Neurocritical	16	7.5
Surgical	24	11.3
Total	212	100.0

The relative frequency indicates the proportion of the population that correspond to that variable value

In the subgroup of patients with critical neurological pathology, a total of 108 measures were obtained with UPA and IPA (54 for OD, 54 for OS) in 8 patients. There was found a strong positive association between UPA and IPA (rOD = 0.935, p value < 0.001; rOS = 0.965, p value < 0.001) (Fig. 4c, d).

Adjusted analysis through simple linear regression models showed good concordance between IPA and UPA (regression line for OD, $y=1,\ 013x+0,\ 0192$; regression line for OS, $y=0.8915x+0.0806$). Upon evaluation of normal distribution of the data, 11 measures for OD (differences between-technique measures greater than 0, 3 mm) and 7 for OS (differences between-technique measures less than −0, 3 mm) were discarded. Taking IPA as reference measure, the percent error for all subjects was 2.77% and 2.15% for OD and OS, respectively (Fig. 5a, b). Regarding concordance between IPA and UPA for measures of reduction in pupillary diameter that were less than 10% (i.e., abnormal), techniques differed in 1 observation for OD and 3 observations for OS, over a total of 106 observations for each eye.

In the subgroup of patients with critical neurological pathology, adjusted analysis through simple linear regression models showed good concordance between IPA and UPA (regression line for OD, $y=0,\ 986x+0.0134$; regression line for OS, $y=0,\ 9089x+0,\ 0483$). Taking IPA as reference measure, the percent error for all subjects was 3.21% and 2.44% for OD and OS, respectively (Fig. 5c, d). Regarding concordance between IPA and UPA for measures of reduction in pupillary diameter that were less than 10% (i.e., abnormal), techniques differed in 1 observation for OD and none for OS, over a total of 54 observations for each eye.

In cases of patients with anisocoria (11 observations), defined as a difference of at least 1 mm between resting pupillary diameter, there was also a strong positive association between UPA and IPA ($r=0.91$, 95% CI 0.68–0.98, p-value < 0.001 OD; $r=0.954$, 95% CI 0.828–0.988, p-value < 0.001 OS).

Discussion

This study found a strong correlation between ultrasonographic and infrared pupillary assessments in critically ill patients, including those with neurologic pathology. UPA could, therefore, be utilized for the evaluation of pupillary diameter and pupillary light reflex in critically ill patients in whom eye opening is not possible. To the authors' knowledge, this is the first study comparing UPA with IPA.

Unfortunately, the fact that there were very few cases of patients with anisocoria precludes the authors from

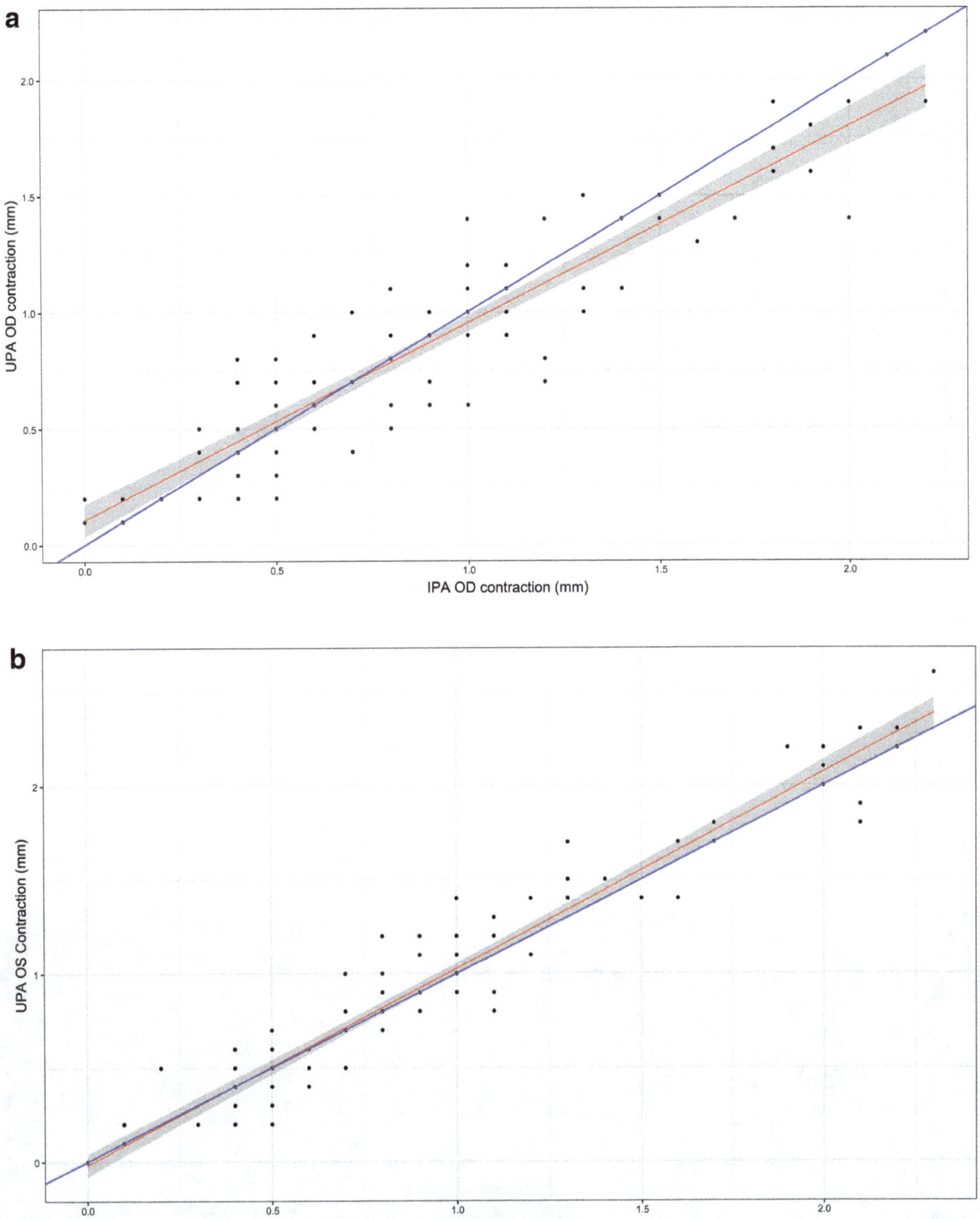

Fig. 4 Scatterplot. Panels **a** and **b** demonstrate correlation between UPA and IPA for OD and OS, respectively. Panels **c** and **d** demonstrate correlation between UPA and IPA for OD and OS, respectively, in neurocritically ill patients. The blue line would be the perfect match between both techniques. The red line is the fit of a regression on the set of points

drawing further conclusions about the role of UPA in this specific patient population. Further studies with a larger patient population are needed.

Regarding the small differences between UPA and IPA, the authors hypothesize that they could be related to the less-intense light stimuli in the case of UPA, because the

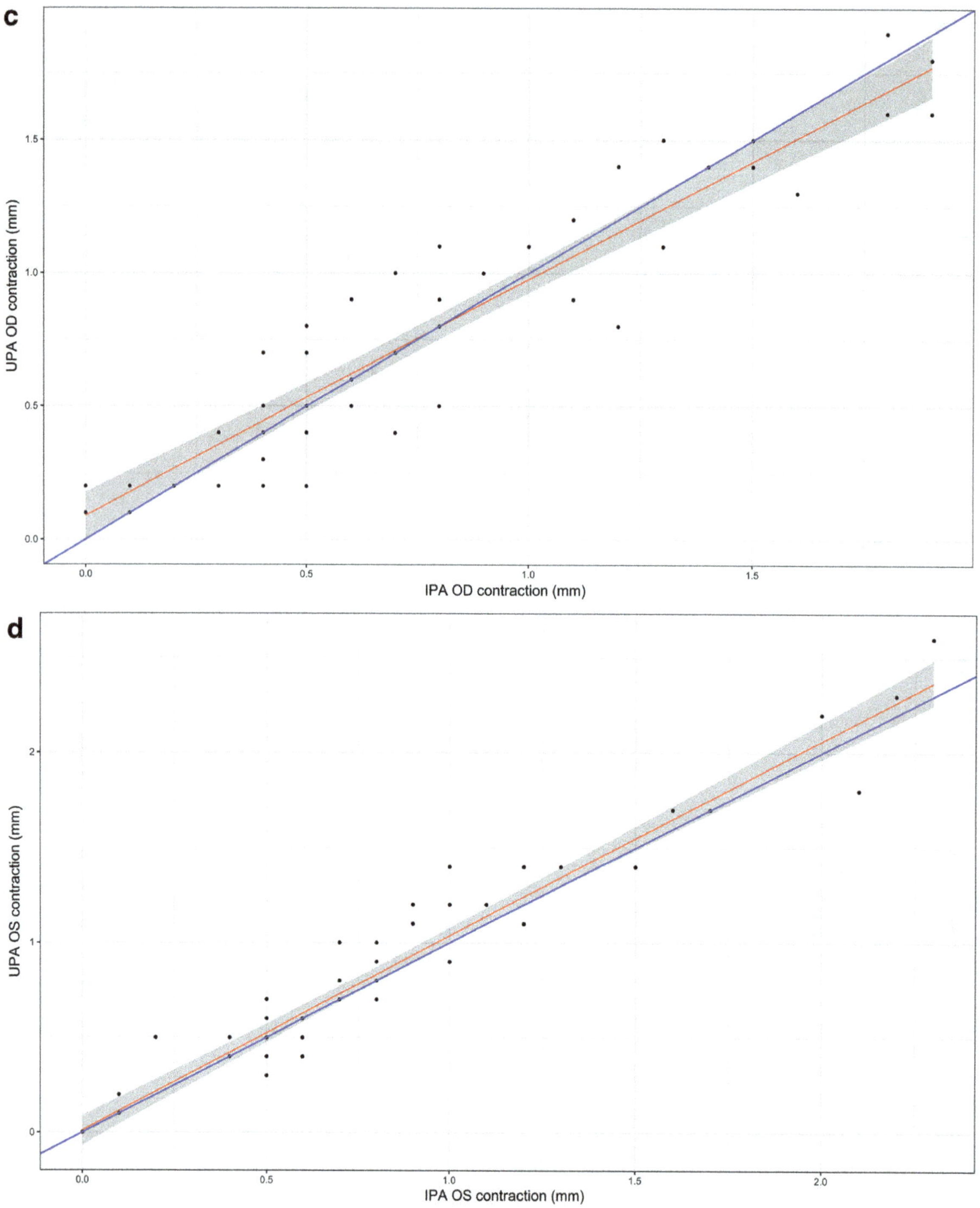

Fig. 4 continued

light stimuli is shown over the closed eye, as opposed to the light stimuli shown directly over the open eye for IPA.

This study shows that UPA is a quick, non-invasive, point-of-care, practical method that provides reliable information, when compared to IPA, regarding pupillary size and pupillary light reflex, which permits assessment of brain herniation. In patients at high risk of brain herniation, UPA becomes particularly useful because it removes the intra- and inter-observer variability inherent to direct visualization of the pupil (i.e., conventional

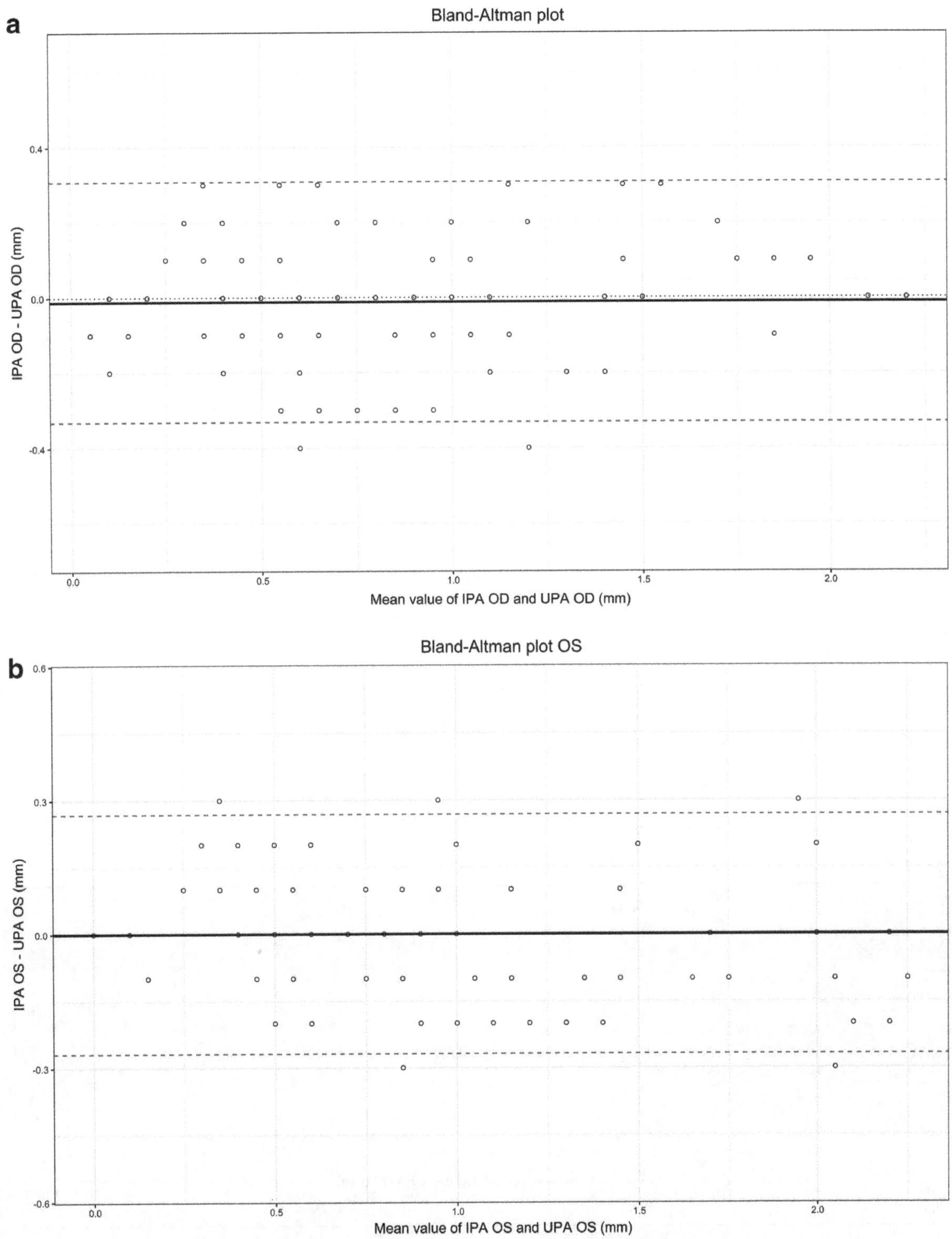

Fig. 5 Bland–Altman graphs show the agreement between the IPA and UPA. Panels **a** and **b** demonstrate the agreement between UPA and IPA for OD and OS, respectively. Panels **c** and **d** demonstrate the agreement between UPA and IPA for OD and OS, respectively, in neurocritically ill patients. The solid lines represent the average of the differences; dashed lines indicate limits of agreement (mean ± 1.96 times the standard deviation)

pupillary physical exam). The most important application of UPA would be to provide accurate pupillary assessment in patients in whom eye opening is not possible (e.g., periorbital soft tissue edema) as well as in patients with significant eyelid edema as usually occurs in those with extensive burn injuries. It is not uncommon that

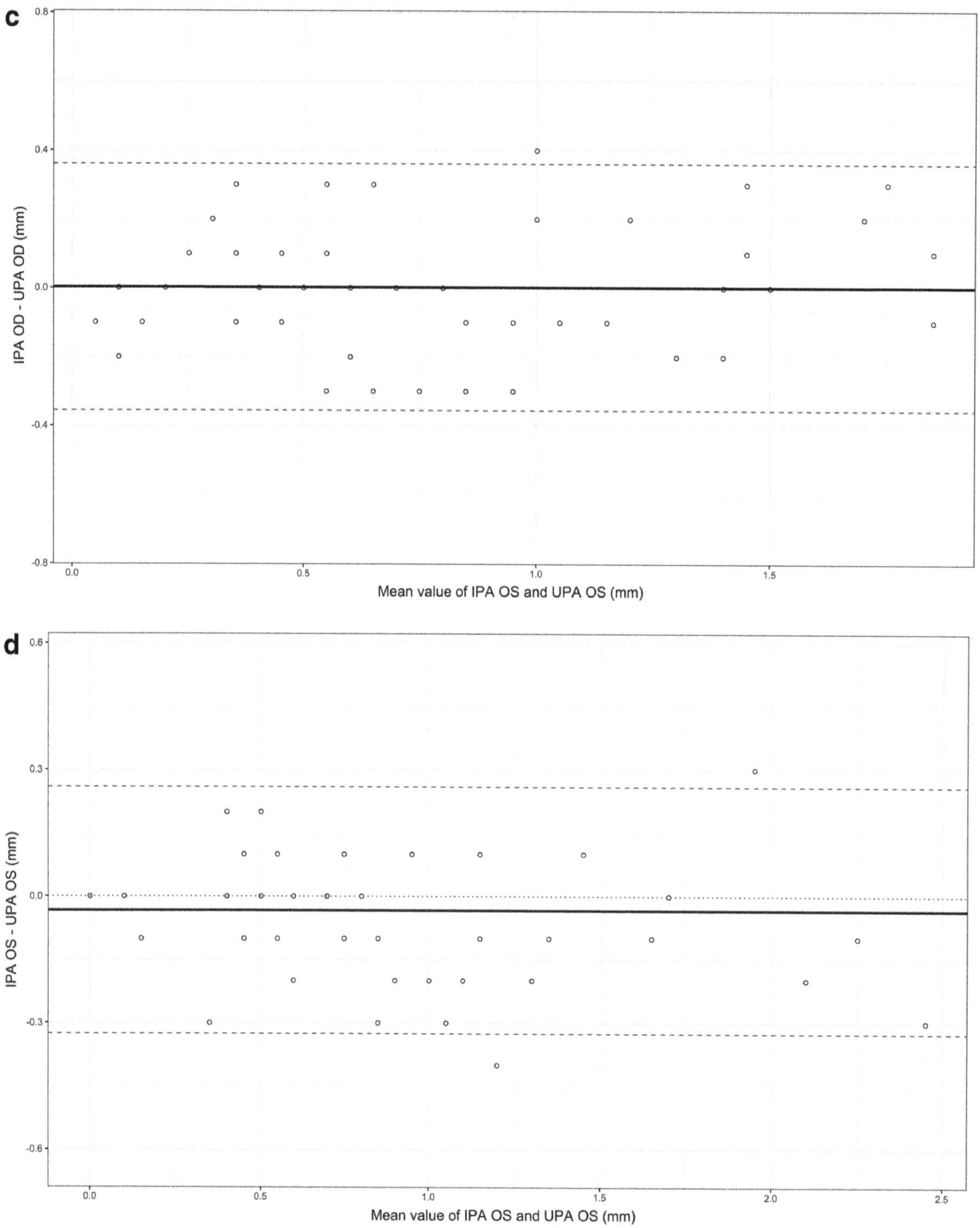

Fig. 5 continued

patients at risk of or under suspicion of critical neurologic pathology such as brain herniation have concurrent peri-orbital edema (e.g., traumatic brain injury). UPA could be performed while waiting for computer tomography in the emergency department, ICU, operating room, as well as in emergency pre-hospital settings or underserved areas wherein computed tomography or resonance magnetic imaging is not available.

Limitations

The small patient population of this study is its major limitation. The greater limitation for UPA is the experience of the operator, for the reliability and accuracy of UPA are directly related to operator skills. Finally, we used different iPhone models that have different technologies generating the flash light used as light stimulus; however, it is unclear whether minor variations in intensity and type of light can significantly affect the assessment of the pupillary light reflex.

Conclusion

Ultrasonographic pupillary assessment is strongly correlated with infrared pupillary assessment in critically ill patients, including neurocritically ill patients. Ultrasonographic pupillary assessment is a quick, feasible, non-invasive method that allows accurate evaluation of pupillary size and pupillary light reflex in patients in whom a more precise measurement of the pupil is required or eye opening is not possible (e.g., periorbital edema due to traumatic brain injury).

Acknowledgements
Matias Muñoz for his immense contribution in the statistical analysis.

Authors' contributions
The examinations, both UPA and IPA were performed by three authors (CY, SP and ML) who were experienced in UPA and IPA. CY, GP, LM, JP and AB performed the analysis of the results. CY and GP were the main contributors in writing the manuscript. All authors read and approved the final manuscript.

Author details
[1] Department of Critical Care Medicine, Hospital de Clínicas, Montevideo, Uruguay. [2] Department of Critical Care Medicine, Hospital Pasteur, Montevideo, Uruguay. [3] Department of Critical Care Medicine, Mayo Clinic, Jacksonville, USA.

References

1. Carney N, Totten AM, O'Reilly C et al (2017) Guidelines for the management of severe traumatic brain injury, fourth edition. Neurosurgery. 80(1):6–15. https://doi.org/10.1227/neu.0000000000001432
2. Thompson HS (2005) Otto lowenstein, pioneer pupillographer. J Neuroophthalmol 25(1):44–49. https://doi.org/10.1097/00041327-200503000-00012
3. Couret D, Boumaza D, Grisotto C et al (2016) Reliability of standard pupillometry practice in neurocritical care: an observational, double-blinded study. Crit Care. 20:99. https://doi.org/10.1186/s13054-016-1239-z)
4. Martínez-Ricarte F, Castro A, Poca MA, Aparicio J (2013) Pupilometría por infrarrojos. Descripción y fundamentos de la técnica y su aplicación en la monitorización no invasiva del paciente neurocrítico. Neurologia (Barcelona, Spain) 28 (1): 41–51
5. Larson MD, Sessler DI, Washington DE, Merrifield BR, Hynson JA, McGuire J (1993) Pupillary response to noxious stimulation during isoflurane and propofol anesthesia. Anesth Analg 76(5):1072–1078. https://doi.org/10.1213/00000539-199305000-00028
6. Lowenstein O, Loewenfeld IE (1958) Electronic pupillography; a new instrument and some clinical applications. AMA Arch Ophthalmol. 59(3):352–363
7. Taylor WR, Chen JW, Meltzer H et al (2003) Quantitative pupillometry, a new technology: normative data and preliminary observations in patients with acute head injury. Technical note. J Neurosurg. 98(1):205–213. https://doi.org/10.3171/jns.2003.98.1.0205
8. Chen JW, Gombart ZJ, Rogers S, Gardiner SK, Cecil S, Bullock RM (2011) Pupillary reactivity as an early indicator of increased intracranial pressure: the introduction of the Neurological Pupil index. Surg Neurol Int. 2:82. https://doi.org/10.4103/2152-7806.82248
9. Phillips SS, Mueller CM, Nogueira RG, Khalifa YM (2019) A systematic review assessing the current state of automated pupillometry in the neuroICU. Neurocrit Care 31(1):142–161. https://doi.org/10.1007/s12028-018-0645-2
10. Lussier BL, Olson DM, Aiyagari V (2019) Automated pupillometry in neurocritical care: research and practice. Curr Neurol Neurosci Rep 19:71. https://doi.org/10.1007/s11910-019-0994-z
11. Fledelius HC (1997) Ultrasound in ophthalmology. Ultrasound Med Biol. 23:365–375
12. Fisher YL (1975) The current status of ophthalmic B-scan ultrasonography. J Clin Ultrasound 3:219–223
13. Fisher YL (1989) Advances in contact ophthalmic ultrasonography: ocular trauma and intraocular foreign body patients. Dev Ophthalmol 18:69–74. https://doi.org/10.1159/000417090
14. Hassani SN, Bard RL (1978) Real time ophthalmic ultrasonography. Radiology 127:213–219
15. Ellis CJ (1981) The pupillary light reflex in normal subjects. Br J Ophthalmol 65(11):754–759. https://doi.org/10.1136/bjo.65.11.754
16. Fankhauser F 2nd, Flammer J (1989) Puptrak 1.0–a new semiautomated system for pupillometry with the Octopus perimeter: a preliminary report. Doc Ophthalmol. 73(3):235–248. https://doi.org/10.1007/bf00155093
17. Hasegawa S (1989) Ishikawa S [age changes in pupillary light reflex. A demonstration by means of a pupillometer]. Nippon Ganka Gakkai zasshi 93:955–961
18. Galinski M, Manikeo M, Tazarourte K, Lapostolle F (2013) Ultrasound pupillary assessment in the critical patient. Intensive Care Med 39(11):2034–2035. https://doi.org/10.1007/s00134-013-3051-4
19. Harries A, Shah S, Teismann N, Price D, Nagdev A (2010) Ultrasound assessment of extraocular movements and pupillary light reflex in ocular trauma. Am J Emerg Med 28(8):956–959. https://doi.org/10.1016/j.ajem.2009.06.026
20. Chiao L, Sharipov S, Sargsyan AE et al (2005) Ocular examination for trauma; clinical ultrasound aboard the International Space Station. J Trauma 58(5):885–889. https://doi.org/10.1097/01.ta.0000162456.37962.01
21. Chen JW, Vakil-Gilani K, Williamson KL, Cecil S (2014) Infrared pupillometry, the Neurological Pupil index and unilateral pupillary dilation after traumatic brain injury: implications for treatment paradigms. Springerplus. 3:548. https://doi.org/10.1186/2193-1801-3-548

6

Real-time ultrasound-guided thoracentesis in the intensive care unit: prevalence of mechanical complications

David Rene Rodriguez Lima[1*], Andrés Felipe Yepes[2], Claudia Inés Birchenall Jiménez[2], Mario Andrés Mercado Díaz[2] and Darío Isaías Pinilla Rojas[2]

Abstract

Background: The use of thoracic ultrasound during thoracentesis reduces complications. The aim of this study was to determine the prevalence of complications for real-time ultrasound-guided thoracentesis performed by intensivists. As a secondary objective, the change in oxygenation before and after the procedure was evaluated.

Patients and methods: An observational prospective study was conducted. A total of 81 cases of real-time ultrasound-guided thoracentesis performed by intensivists in the intensive care unit (ICU) of Méderi Major University Hospital, Bogotá, Colombia, between August 2018 and August 2019 were analyzed. Thoracentesis performed by interventional radiologists and using techniques different from the focus of this study were excluded from the analysis.

Results: There was one pneumothorax, for a prevalence rate of mechanical complications in this population of 1.2%. The mean partial oxygen pressure to inspired oxygen fraction ratio (PaO_2/FiO_2) prior to the procedure was 198.1 (95% CI 184.75–211.45), with a PaO_2/FiO_2 after the procedure of 224.6 (95% CI 213.08–226.12) ($p < 0.05$).

Conclusions: Real-time ultrasound-guided thoracentesis performed by intensivists is a safe procedure and leads to a significant improvement in oxygenation rates. Future studies are required to determine the impact of these results on other outcomes, such as mortality, ICU stay, and days of mechanical ventilation.

Keywords: Ultrasound, Thoracentesis, Complications, Intensive care

Background

Pleural effusion is a frequent finding in the intensive care unit (ICU), and it can cause hypoxemia and alterations in lung mechanics [1].

The prevalence of pleural effusion in the ICU can vary between 40 and 60% [2]. The commonly reported causes of pleural effusion in this population are infectious exudates (43%), non-infectious exudates (33%) and transudates (24%) [3]. In postoperative patients undergoing cardiovascular surgery, up to 7% present with pleural effusion, the most common cause being hemothorax in up to 50% of cases, with dyspnea as the predominant symptom [4].

Pleural effusions with documented volumes greater than 500 ml affect gas exchange, hemodynamic stability and respiratory work, and it has been demonstrated that drainage of pleural effusions in ICU patients under mechanical ventilation is related to improved oxygenation indices, increased end-expiratory volume and decreased transpulmonary pressure [5]. A recent meta-analysis that included 31 studies with 2265 patients showed that drainage of pleural fluid produces improvement in PaO_2/FiO_2 as an oxygenation index and tends to increase end-expiratory volume [6].

Thoracentesis is a percutaneous procedure for collecting pleural fluid, and it has diagnostic utility and therapeutic applications. It is recommended for pleural

*Correspondence: drrodriguezl@hotmail.com
[1] Emergency Medicine and Critical and Intensive Care Medicine, Hospital Universitario Mayor Méderi–Universidad del Rosario, Bogotá, Colombia
Full list of author information is available at the end of the article

effusions of unknown cause, because it allows defining the cause of the effusion and has therapeutic utility in large-volume pleural effusions associated with respiratory distress [7]. Thoracentesis should not be performed for bilateral effusions in a clinical picture strongly suggestive of transudate (e.g., cardiac failure), unless the presentation is atypical or does not respond to clinical management [8, 9].

Complications related to the performance of blind thoracentesis include a high incidence of pneumothorax (11%) [10]; for this reason, the use of ultrasound guidance is strongly recommended for performing interventions in the pleural space and using small-diameter catheters [11, 12]. In turn, the diagnostic sensitivity of ultrasound for pleural effusion is higher compared to that of chest X-ray and allows identifying the pleural fluid characteristics that differentiate complicated and uncomplicated effusions and homogeneous and heterogeneous effusions [13]. In addition, the routine implementation of pulmonary ultrasound in the ICU decreases the number of chest X-rays, with a reduction in medical costs and radiation exposure, without affecting the clinical results [14].

Various techniques have been developed to estimate the volume of pleural fluid by ultrasound, with a good correlation between the drained liquid and that calculated prior to the procedure, finding that distances between the diaphragm and the visceral pleura greater than 30 mm are related to pleural effusions greater than 500 ml [15]. Balik et al. described a formula to calculate the pleural effusion volume by ultrasound by measuring the maximal interpleural distance (Sep) in millimeters (mm) in end-expiration at the lung base in a posterior axillary line and multiplying this value by 20, quantifying the pleural fluid volume (Vpl) in milliliters (ml) [16]. The method described by Balik et al. was validated in patients under invasive mechanical ventilation in a supine position with mild trunk elevation at 15°; however, the mean prediction error of this equation is high (158 ± 160 ml) [16, 17]. The position of the patient influences the volume calculated by this method because when elevating the headboard, the free pleural fluid experiences the effects of gravity and can increase the interpleural distance [18]. In Balik et al.'s original work, no difference in correlation of interpleural distance with the right- and left-side drained volumes was found [16]; however, other studies have found a better correlation on the right side [19, 20]. This is secondary to the fact that on the left side, the heart increases the level of a pleural effusion, like a stone in a container with water, leading to overestimation of the interpleural distance [18].

The aim of this observational study was to determine the prevalence of complications of real-time ultrasound-guided thoracentesis performed by intensivists. As a secondary objective, the change in oxygenation before and after the procedure was evaluated.

Patients and methods

Méderi Major University Hospital (*Hospital Universitario Mayor Méderi*) is a Colombian high-complexity hospital with 780 hospital beds and 97 adult ICU beds where routine use of ultrasound for the performance of guided procedures by intensivists has been implemented for 5 years.

During a period of 13 months (between August 2018 and August 2019), data were collected prospectively from 81 consecutive real-time ultrasound-guided thoracentesis performed by intensivists in the ICU of Méderi Major University Hospital, Bogota, Colombia. Patients undergoing thoracentesis using methods other than real-time ultrasound-guided techniques and those in whom thoracentesis was performed by interventional radiologists were excluded from the analysis. Authorization for this study was granted by the Institutional Human Research Ethics Committee of Del Rosario University (DVO005 1068-CV1177).

All thoracentesis were performed by intensivists with more than 5 years of experience, who during their graduate education had at least 1 month of certified ultrasound training. The decision to perform thoracentesis was made only for clinical reasons and was not based on the protocol.

Pleural effusion is diagnosed by portable chest X-ray findings (anteroposterior view and supine position), pleural ultrasound or chest tomography according to the clinical applicability for each patient. If the treating physician considered the patient to be a candidate for drainage, an assessment was performed by an intensivist with experience in thoracic ultrasound. This professional performed the thoracic ultrasound, evaluating the chest wall in eight areas as recommended by the International Evidence-Based Recommendations for point-of-care lung ultrasound [21] to confirm the presence of pleural effusion and to determine whether it was susceptible to drainage.

Estimation of the pleural effusion volume (Vpl) in ml was performed similarly to the method described by Balik et al.: Vpl (ml) = Sep (mm) * 20; however, the majority of patients included in this study were not under mechanical ventilation and showed little tolerance to the supine position at 15°, and therefore, the investigators decided to perform the measurement with the trunk elevated to 30° regardless of whether the patient was under invasive mechanical ventilation or spontaneous breathing.

The technique used is similar to that described by Vertrugno et al. [22] and was carried out as follows:

For the procedure, a SonoSite M-Turbo ultrasound machine with a 5-MHz small-footprint convex transducer and a 13-MHz linear transducer were used. The real-time ultrasound-guided thoracentesis technique used for the patients included in this study is described below (Figs. 1, 2 and 3):

1. The thoracentesis kit, which contains antiseptic solution, sterile gloves, sterile gauze, local anesthetic, intramuscular needle, subcutaneous needle, 5-, 10-, and 50-ml syringes, 3-way stopcock, 16 gauge thoracentesis needle, 6-French pigtail thoracic drainage catheter, 0.38″ × 80 J-tip metal guide, 6Fr dilator, scalpel, silk to fasten the catheter and collection bag, is prepared.

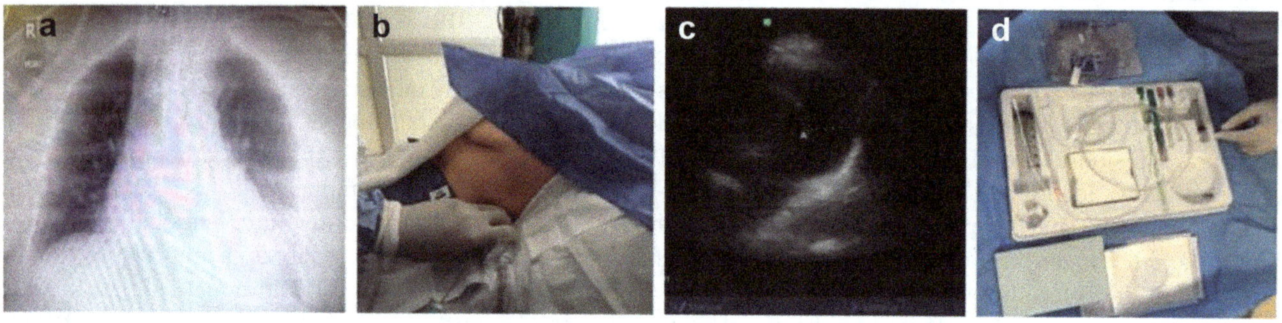

Fig. 1 **a** Chest X-ray of the patient with left pleural effusion during the postoperative period of myocardial revascularization. **b** Patient in the supine position with the head at 30°; ultrasound assessment in the lower thorax on the posterior axillary line. **c** Quantification of the pleural effusion with a 5-MHz convex transducer; measurement of the distance between the visceral pleura and the posterior wall of the thorax in the transverse axis. In this case, the distance is 26 mm, with an approximate calculated volume of 520 ml by the Balik method. **d** Thoracentesis kit

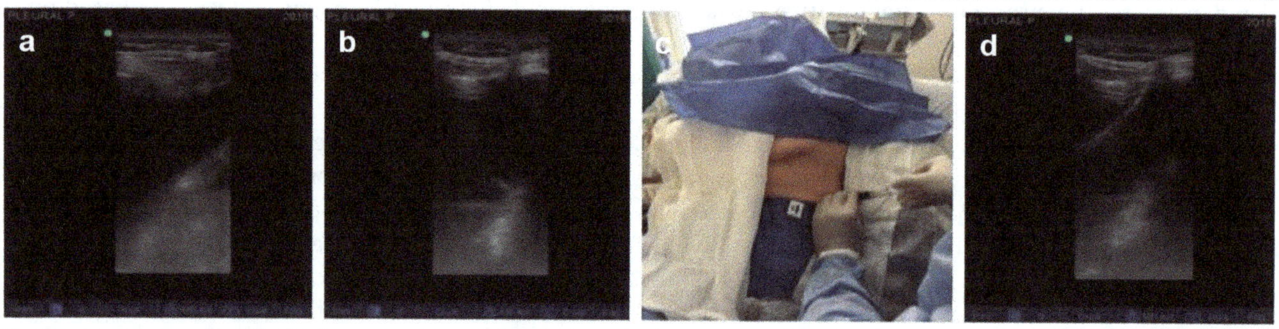

Fig. 2 **a** Assessment, with a 13-MHz linear transducer, of the effusion in the lower aspect of the thorax on the posterior axillary line, visualizing the upper and lower ribs, intercostal space, pleural fluid, and diaphragm. **b** After verifying no interposition of vessels with color Doppler, needle puncture is performed; needle passage into the pleural cavity is visualized in real time. **c** Pleural fluid return is verified, in this case blood. **d** Passage of the guide toward the pleural cavity on the diaphragm

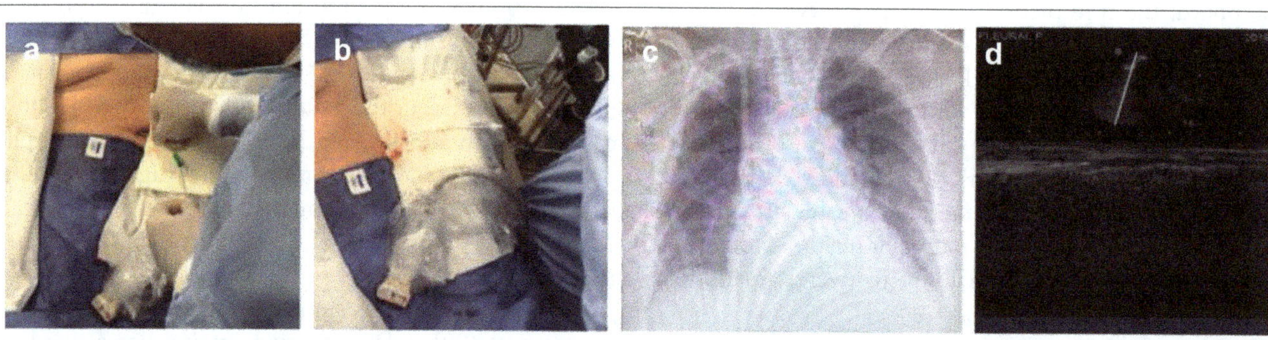

Fig. 3 **a** Passage of the dilator (between 1 and 2 cm), depending on thoracic wall thickness. **b** Passage of the pigtail catheter to begin drainage. **c** Chest X-ray after drainage showing a fluid-free pleural cavity. **d** Ultrasound verification, with a sector transducer, of a fluid-free pleural cavity, also dismissing the presence of pneumothorax ("sand-on-the-beach" sign)

2. The patient is placed in the supine position with the headboard at 30°.
3. The pleural effusion is visualized with a 5-MHz convex transducer in longitudinal position at the lung base in a posterior axillary line.
4. Once the pleural effusion is visualized, the transducer is rotated to obtain a transverse view.
5. The distance between the visceral pleura and the posterior chest wall is measured.
6. If the distance is greater than 15 mm, the patient is a candidate for the procedure.
7. After asepsis and antisepsis, with the linear transducer in the longitudinal direction, the transducer is positioned on the posterior axillary line in order to obtain an image of the diaphragm between two ribs.
8. Using color Doppler, it is verified that there is no blood vessel interposition.
9. Thoracentesis needle puncture (16 gauge) is performed over the center of the transducer in real time by visualizing needle insertion the entire time.
10. Once the pleural cavity is entered and fluid is collected, the metal guide is inserted, and its position is verified sonographically.
11. Then, the dilator is passed by inserting it 1 to 2 cm, depending on the thickness of the chest wall.
12. The dilator is removed, and the pigtail catheter is inserted over the guide.
13. Once the pigtail catheter is inserted, the drainage system is connected to a 3-way stopcock with one connection directed toward the drainage bag and the other toward a 50-ml syringe. Active drainage is started with the 50-ml syringe, without creating negative pressure that exceeds $-$ 20 cmH_2O to avoid complications [10]. Importantly, during thoracentesis, the pleural and intrathoracic pressure decrease and the left ventricular afterload increases with a decrease in left ventricular systolic performance, and patients with moderate-to-severe left ventricular dysfunction can develop pulmonary edema [23]. After the procedure, ultrasound is used to determine if residual fluid remains and to rule out the presence of pneumothorax. A chest X-ray performed within 24 h of the procedure is reviewed.

Demographic and clinical variables (macroscopic description of the pleural fluid, amount of drained fluid, interpleural distance, and possible cause), complications and procedure indications were analyzed. The presence of complications was ruled out by performing a lung ultrasound at the end of the procedure and reviewing a chest X-ray performed within 24 h after the thoracentesis. In cases of hemothorax in postoperative cardiac surgery patients, given that there could be confusion as to whether it was residual or associated with thoracentesis, after draining blood from the pleural space, no recurrence of hemothorax after the procedure was verified by ultrasound and on the chest X-ray taken on the following day. The indications for the procedure were classified as diagnostic if the objective of the procedure was only sampling to clarify the etiology of the effusion and as therapeutic if thoracentesis was performed because the patient was considered to have respiratory distress or hypoxemia secondary to the effusion.

A univariate analysis of categorical and continuous variables was performed; normality was tested with the Kolmogorov–Smirnov test. The paired samples t test or the Wilcoxon signed rank test was performed. A value of $p<0.05$ was considered significant. The analysis was performed in STATA 14.

Results

A total of 81 ultrasound-guided thoracentesis were performed with the described technique. In the study period, 61.7% of the patients were men, and 38.3% were women; the mean age of the observed group was 67 years (SD $\pm$ 14 years). In 96% of cases, the indication for thoracentesis was therapeutic, and only 3.7% of patients underwent the procedure as part of their diagnostic algorithm. The diagnoses presented by these patients were, for the most part, postoperative cardiovascular surgery (56.8%), followed by heart failure (16%), pneumonia (12.3%) and others (14.8%), among which paraneoplastic pleural effusion was noteworthy (Table 1).

The following macroscopic characteristics of the drained fluid were observed: evidence of a hemothorax (55.6%), citrine (29.6%), chylous (6.2%), purulent (7.4%) and paraneoplastic (1.2%). Of the 46 cardiovascular surgery patients who underwent thoracentesis, 38 (82%) had a hemothorax (Table 2).

Table 1 Diagnoses presented in ICU patients that led to thoracentesis

	Absolute frequency (n=81)	Relative frequency (n=81)	Accumulated percentage (n=81)
Principal diagnosis			
Cardiovascular surgery	46	56.8	56.8
Heart failure	13	16.0	72.8
Pneumonia	10	12.3	85.2
Other	12	14.8	100.0

Table 2 Appearance of the pleural fluid drained from the ICU patients

	Absolute frequency ($n=81$)	Relative frequency ($n=81$)	Accumulated percentage ($n=81$)
Appearance of the drainage			
Hemothorax	45	55.6	55.6
Citrine	24	29.6	85.2
Chylous	5	6.2	91.4
Purulent	6	7.4	98.8
Paraneoplastic	1	1.2	100.0

All performed thoracentesis were successful, with one pneumothorax and no hemothorax observed, for a prevalence rate of mechanical complications in this population of 1.2%. The pneumothorax presented in a 77-year-old man not receiving mechanical ventilation, who required diagnostic thoracentesis, had a maximal interpleural distance of 15 mm and, for management, required the passage of a chest tube with drainage of 200 cc of purulent fluid.

The mean PaO_2/FiO_2 presented positive variations in relation to the measurement at admission ($p < 0.05$). Prior to the procedure, the PaO_2/FiO_2 was 198.1 (SD ± 12.3) (95% CI 184.75–211.45), and after the procedure, it was 224.6 (SD ± 52.9) (95% CI 213.08–226.12) (Table 3, Fig. 4). The stratified analysis showed that this improvement in PaO_2/FiO_2 was maintained in the subgroups regardless of the diagnosis ($p < 0.05$).

Regarding the characteristics of the procedure, drainage was located on the right side in 54.3% and on the left side in 45.7%. Drainage was therapeutic in 96.3% of cases, the median amount drained was 900 ml (95% CI 900–1100 ml), and the pleural effusion volume estimated by the Balik et al. equation was 710 ml (95% CI 600–1000 ml) (Table 4). Spearman's rho correlation analysis showed a moderate positive relationship between the amount drained and the estimated volume pre-thoracentesis (rho = 0.573) ($p < 0.05$); when differentiating the sides, the correlation between the drained amount and the estimated volume was significant only for the right side (rho = 0.7308, $p < 0.05$), i.e., not for the left side (rho = 0.3776, $p > 0.05$).

Of the total number of patients undergoing thoracentesis, 28.4% were on mechanical ventilation, and the median time to extubation was 6 days (95% CI 5–12 days). For the 23 patients on mechanical ventilation, the PaO_2/FiO_2 prior to the procedure was 184.3 (±48.37) (95% CI 163.39–205.22), with a PaO_2/FiO_2 after the procedure of 205.82 (±57.38) (95% CI 181.01–230.64), maintaining the positive variation but without statistical significance ($p = 0.08$). Of these 23 patients, 11 (47.8%) returned to spontaneous breathing within 7 days after thoracentesis, and in 10 (43.4%), mechanical ventilation was prolonged beyond 1 week. Two patients (8.7%) died in this period. For the 11 patients who achieved early extubation after drainage, the mean PaO_2/FiO_2 before and after the procedure was 222.81 (SD ± 40.67) (95% CI 195.49–250.13) and 240.44 (SD ± 50.77) (95% CI 206.33–274.55), respectively. For the 10 patients in whom early extubation was not achieved after drainage, the mean PaO_2/FiO_2 values before and after the procedure were 196.40 (SD ± 60.46) (95% CI 153.15–239.65) and 228.12 (SD ± 70.66) (95% CI 177.58–278.60), respectively.

Discussion

This study shows that real-time ultrasound-guided thoracentesis performed by intensivists at the bedside is a safe procedure, with a prevalence rate of complications of 1.2%, lower than that reported in the literature when blind pleural aspiration is performed, where the presence of pneumothorax ranges from 10 to 18% [12, 24, 25].

The safety of ultrasound-guided thoracentesis has been evaluated in other studies, and it is the recommended technique for this procedure by different international guidelines [12]. Barnes et al. [24] and Gervais et al. [26], in retrospective studies on ultrasound-guided thoracentesis performed by interventional radiologists, reported pneumothorax rates of 4.9% and 2.3%, respectively. Petersen et al. [27] reported a series of 338 ultrasound-guided thoracentesis in the ICU, with four pneumothoraces (1.2%). Lichtenstein et al. [28] and Mayo et al. [29] reported pneumothorax rates in patients receiving mechanical ventilation of 0 and 1.3%, respectively.

Table 3 Pre- and post-thoracentesis oxygenation parameters in the ICU patients

	Mean ($n=81$)	Standard deviation ($n=81$)	Minimum ($n=81$)	Maximum ($n=81$)
PaO_2/FiO_2 prior to the procedure	198.1	61.3	74.0	385.0
PaO_2/FiO_2 after the procedure	224.6	52.9	110.0	385.0
Change in PaO_2/FiO_2	29.1	46.4	– 84.0	157.0

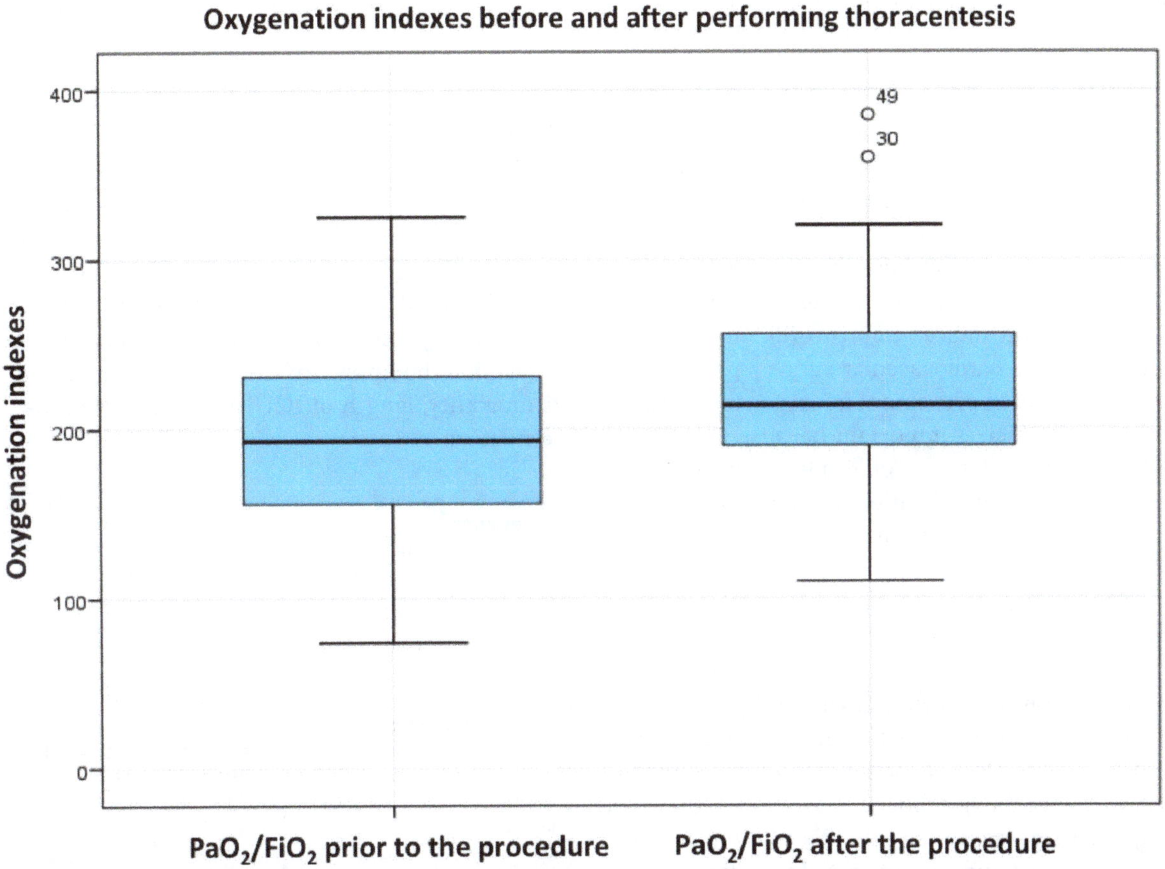

Fig. 4 Oxygenation indexes before and after performing thoracentesis. The average PaO_2/FiO_2 before the procedure was 198.1, and the average PaO_2/FiO_2 after the procedure was 224.6, $p<0.05$

Table 4 Amount of drainage in milliliters (ml), interpleural distance prior to procedure in millimeters (mm), volume estimated using Balik's method

	Median ($n=81$)	Median 95% CI ($n=81$)	Interquartile range ($n=81$)
Drained amount (ml)	900	900–1100	550–1100
Distance (mm)	35.5	30–50	28–58.5
Estimated volume (ml)	710.0	600–1000	560–1170
Drained amount, right (ml)	900	650–1000	550–1150
Distance, right (mm)	32.5	26.86–50.83	25–62
Estimated volume, right (ml)	650	537.21–1016.72	500–1240
Drained amount, left (ml)	800	700–947.13	550–1100
Distance, left (mm)	47.5	30–54.95	30–57
Estimated volume, left (ml)	950	600–1099.05	600–1140

In these two studies, the procedure was performed in patients under mechanical ventilation. In comparison with those studies, the prevalence of complications reported in the present study is similar or lower.

Another important finding is the impact on oxygenation indexes after pleural drainage, evidencing post-procedure improvement in the PaO_2/FiO_2 ($p<0.05$), in agreement with that reported by Vertrugno et al. [10] and Goligher et al. [30]. In this study, the group of patients on mechanical ventilation was small (28.4%), and of those in whom extubation was achieved in the first 7 days after thoracentesis, the PaO_2/FiO_2 post-procedure was higher, but not statistically significant, than in those with prolonged mechanical ventilation. These data suggest that patients in whom drainage led to a greater increase in PaO_2/FiO_2 were successfully weaned from mechanical ventilation earlier, as reported by Vertrugno et al. [20]. Further studies are needed to evaluate the importance of oxygenation indices in clinical benefits and outcomes after thoracentesis.

The median volume of drained fluid was 900 ml, and it is known that when volumes greater than 500 ml are drained, oxygenation indices improve [8]. Interestingly, in the postoperative cardiovascular surgery patient subgroup, the benefit of improvement in oxygenation indices was maintained, which is important because it has been reported that the incidence of clinically significant pleural effusion in this group of patients is approximately 7% and in whom almost 50% of the fluid drained is hemorrhagic [4].

Spearman's rho correlation analysis showed a moderate positive linear relationship (rho = 0.573) between the drained amount and the estimated volume; however, this correlation was lower than that described by Balik et al. [16], which can be explained by the fact that in this study, the estimate was applied to patients with spontaneous breathing and with the headboard at 30°. However, when analyzing each side separately, the correlation between the drained amount and the estimated volume was significant only on the right side (rho = 0.7308) and not on the left side (rho = 0.3776), which can be explained by the presence of the heart, as it increases the pleural effusion level, leading to an overestimation of the calculated volume [17, 18].

The intensivists who performed thoracentesis during this study have more than 5 years of experience in the use of ultrasound at the bedside, and during their residency program, they were trained to perform ultrasound-guided procedures, which helps to explain the low rate of complications reported in this study. To begin performing thoracentesis in real scenarios, we first recommend the development of this skill in phantom models of lung anatomy [31].

This study has the strength of being the first series in which the majority of thoracentesis procedures were performed under ultrasound guidance in real time by intensivists, confirming the safety of this technique and the improvement in oxygenation indices.

This study is observational and has limitations. A lung ultrasound was not performed on all ICU patients during the study period; therefore, the proportion of pleural effusions that required drainage could not be reported. This study also does not allow assessing the safety of thoracentesis performed by other ultrasound-guided techniques, such as radiological marking and subsequent drainage by a different physician or marking and immediate puncture.

Conclusions

Real-time ultrasound-guided thoracentesis performed by intensivists is a safe procedure with a low complication rate compared to that for blind techniques, has a complication rate similar to that for other ultrasound-guided techniques and leads to significant improvement in oxygenation rates. Future studies are needed to determine the impact of these results on outcomes such as mortality, length of ICU stay and days of mechanical ventilation.

Abbreviations

ICU: Intensive care unit; SD: Standard deviation; ml: Milliliters; mm: Millimeters; PaO_2/FiO_2: Partial pressure arterial oxygen/fraction of inspired oxygen; Sep: Maximal interpleural distance; Vpl: Pleural fluid volume.

Acknowledgements

Does not apply.

Authors' contributions

DRRL, AFY, MAMD, DIPR collected data and contributed to writing the manuscript. CIBJ performed the statistical analysis of the information and contributed to writing the manuscript. All authors read and approved the final manuscript.

Author details

[1] Emergency Medicine and Critical and Intensive Care Medicine, Hospital Universitario Mayor Méderi–Universidad del Rosario, Bogotá, Colombia. [2] Critical and Intensive Care Medicine, Hospital Universitario Mayor Méderi–Universidad del Rosario, Bogotá, Colombia.

References

1. Nishida O, Arellano R, Cheng DC, DeMajo W, Kavanagh BP (1999) Gas exchange and hemodynamics in experimental pleural effusion. Crit Care Med 27(3):583–587. https://doi.org/10.1097/00003246-199903000-00040
2. Mattison LE, Coppage L, Alderman DF, Herlong JO, Salm SA (1997) Pleural effusions in the medical ICU: prevalence, causes and clinical implications. Chest 111(4):1018–1023. https://doi.org/10.1378/chest.111.4.1018
3. Fartoukh M, Azoulay E, Galliot R, Le Gall JR, Baud F, Chevret S, Schlemmer B (2002) Clinically documented pleural effusions in medical ICU patients: how useful is routine thoracentesis? Chest 121(1):178–184. https://doi.org/10.1378/chest.121.1.178
4. Labidi M, Baillot R, Dionne B, Lacasse Y, Maltais F, Boulet LP (2009) Pleural effusions following cardiac surgery: prevalence, risk factors, and clinical features. Chest 136(6):1604–1611. https://doi.org/10.1378/chest.09-0689
5. Razazi K, Boissier F, Neuville M, Jochmans S, Tchir M, May F, de Prost N, Brun-Buisson C, Carteaux G, Mekontso Dessap A (2018) Pleural effusion during weaning from mechanical ventilation: a prospective observational multicenter study. Ann Intensive Care. https://doi.org/10.1186/s13613-018-0446-y
6. Vetrugno L, Bignami E, Orso D, Vargas M, Guadagnin GM, Saglietti F, Servillo G, Volpicelli G, Navalesi P, Bove T (2019) Utility of pleural effusion drainage in the ICU: An updated systematic review and META-analysis. J Crit Care 52:22–32. https://doi.org/10.1016/j.jcrc.2019.03.007
7. Brogi E, Gargani L, Bignami E, Barbariol F, Marra A, Forfori F, Vetrugno L (2017) Thoracic ultrasound for pleural effusion in the intensive care unit: a narrative review from diagnosis to treatment. Crit Care. https://doi.org/10.1186/s13054-017-1897-5

8. Thomsen TW, DeLaPena J, Setnik GS (2006) Videos in clinical medicine. Thoracentesis. The New Engl J Med 355(15):e16. https://doi.org/10.1056/nejmvcm053812
9. Hooper C, Lee YCG, Maskell N (2010) Investigation of a unilateral pleural effusion in adults: British Thoracic Society pleural disease guideline 2010. Thorax. https://doi.org/10.1136/thx.2010.136978
10. Seneff MG, Corwin RW, Gold LH, Irwin RS (1986) Complications associated with thoracocentesis. Chest 90(1):97–100. https://doi.org/10.1378/chest.90.1.97
11. Ingelfinger JR, Feller-Kopman D, Light R (2018) Pleural disease. N Engl J Med 378(8):740–751. https://doi.org/10.1056/nejmra1403503
12. Havelock T, Teoh R, Laws D, Gleeson F (2010) Pleural procedures and thoracic ultrasound: British Thoracic Society pleural disease guideline 2010. Thorax. https://doi.org/10.1136/thx.2010.137026
13. Xirouchaki N, Magkanas E, Vaporidi K, Kondili E, Plataki M, Patrianakos A, Akoumianaki E, Georgopoulos D (2011) Lung ultrasound in critically ill patients: Comparison with bedside chest radiography. Intensive Care Med 37(9):1488–1493. https://doi.org/10.1007/s00134-011-2317-y
14. Brogi Etrusca, Bignami E, Sidoti A, Shawar M, Gargani L, Vetrugno L, Volpicelli G, Forfori F (2017) Could the use of bedside lung ultrasound reduce the number of chest x-rays in the intensive care unit? Cardiovasc Ultrasound 15(1):23. https://doi.org/10.1186/s12947-017-0113-8
15. Usta E, Mustafi M, Ziemer G (2010) Ultrasound estimation of volume of postoperative pleural effusion in cardiac surgery patients. Interact Cardiovasc Thorac Surg 10(2):204–207. https://doi.org/10.1510/icvts.2009.222273
16. Balik M, Plasil P, Waldauf P, Pazout J, Fric M, Otahal M, Pachl J (2006) Ultrasound estimation of volume of pleural fluid in mechanically ventilated patients. Intensive Care Med 32(2):318–321. https://doi.org/10.1007/s00134-005-0024-2
17. Vetrugno L, Brogi E, Barbariol F, Forfori F, Bignami E (2018) A message in the bottle. Anesthesiol J Am Soc Anesthesiol 128(3):677. https://doi.org/10.1097/aln.0000000000002039
18. Vetrugno L, Bove T (2018) Lung ultrasound estimation of pleural effusion fluid and the importance of patient position. Ann Intensive Care 8(1):8–10. https://doi.org/10.1186/s13613-018-0471-x
19. Vignon P, Chastagner C, Berkane V, Chardac E, François B, Normand S, Bonnivard M, Clavel M, Pichon N, Preux PM, Maubon A, Gastinne H (2005) Quantitative assessment of pleural effusion in critically ill patients by means of ultrasonography. Crit Care Med 33(8):1757–1763. https://doi.org/10.1097/01.ccm.0000171532.02639.08
20. Vetrugno L, Guadagnin GM, Barbariol F, D'Incà S, Delrio S, Orso D, Girometti R, Volpicelli G, Bove T (2019) Assessment of pleural effusion and small pleural drain insertion by resident doctors in an intensive care unit: an observational study. Clin Med Insights Circ Respir Pulm Med. https://doi.org/10.1177/1179548419871527
21. Volpicelli G, Elbarbary M, Blaivas M, Lichtenstein DA, Mathis G, Kirkpatrick AW, Melniker L, Gargani L, Noble VE, Via G, Dean A, Tsung JW, Soldati G, Copetti R, Bouhemad B, Reissig A, Agricola E, Rouby JJ, Arbelot C, Liteplo A, Sargsyan A, Silva F, Hoppmann R, Breitkreutz R, Seibel A, Neri L, Storti E, Petrovic T, International Liaison Committee on Lung Ultrasound (ILC-LUS) for International Consensus Conference on Lung Ultrasound (ICC-LUS) (2012) International evidence-based recommendations for point-of-care lung ultrasound. Intensive Care Med 38(4):577–591. https://doi.org/10.1007/s00134-012-2513-4
22. Vetrugno L, Guadagnin GM, Orso D, Boero E, Bignami E, Bove T (2018) An easier and safe affair, pleural drainage with ultrasound in critical patient: a technical note. Crit Ultrasound J 10(1):1–10. https://doi.org/10.1186/s13089-018-0098-z
23. Mokotedi CM, Balik M (2017) Is the mechanism of re-expansion pulmonary oedema in a heart-lung interaction? BMJ Case Rep 2017:1–5. https://doi.org/10.1136/bcr-2017-219340
24. Barnes TW, Morgenthaler TI, Olson EJ, Hesley GK, Decker PA, Ryu JH (2005) Sonographically guided thoracentesis and rate of pneumothorax. J Clin Ultrasound 33(9):442–446. https://doi.org/10.1002/jcu.20163
25. Raptopoulos V, Davis LM, Lee G, Umali C, Lew R, Irwin RS (1991) Factors affecting the development of pneumothorax associated with thoracentesis. Am J Roentgenol 156(5):917–920. https://doi.org/10.2214/ajr.156.5.2017951
26. Gervais DA, Petersein A, Lee MJ, Hahn PF, Saini S, Mueller PR (1997) US-guided thoracentesis: requirement for postprocedure chest radiography in patients who receive mechanical ventilation versus patients who breathe spontaneously. Radiology 204(2):503–506. https://doi.org/10.1148/radiology.204.2.9240544
27. Petersen S, Freitag M, Albert W, Tempel S, Ludwig K (1999) Ultrasound-guided thoracentesis in surgical intensive care patients. Intensive Care Med 25(9):1029. https://doi.org/10.1007/s001340051004
28. Lichtenstein D, Hulot JS, Rabiller A, Tostivint I, Mezière G (1999) Feasibility and safety of ultrasound-aided thoracentesis in mechanically ventilated patients. Intensive Care Med 25(9):955–958. https://doi.org/10.1007/s001340050988
29. Mayo PH, Goltz HR, Tafreshi M, Doelken P (2004) Safety of ultrasound-guided thoracentesis in patients receiving mechanical ventilation. Chest 125(3):1059–1062. https://doi.org/10.1378/chest.125.3.1059
30. Goligher EC, Leis JA, Fowler RA, Pinto R, Adhikari NKJ, Ferguson ND (2011) Utility and safety of draining pleural effusions in mechanically ventilated patients: a systematic review and meta-analysis. Crit Care. https://doi.org/10.1186/cc10009
31. Vetrugno L, Volpicelli G, Barbariol F, Toretti I, Pompei L, Forfori F, Della Rocca G (2016) Phantom model and scoring system to assess ability in ultrasound-guided chest drain positioning. Crit Ultrasound J 8(1):1–7. https://doi.org/10.1186/s13089-016-0038-8

7

Ultrasound-guided peripheral venous cannulation in critically ill patients: a practical guideline

Pablo Blanco*

Abstract

Background: Up to one-third of critically ill patients have difficult intravenous access (DIVA). This occurs often in obese patients, those with generalized edemas or in patients with previous venous cannulations. In DIVA patients, the conventional technique often fails. In contrast, ultrasound-guided cannulation has demonstrated a high success rate, improving patient satisfaction and even a reduction in the need of central venous lines. However, a high rate of premature catheter failure has been shown in cannulations performed by ultrasound guidance and thus a comprehensive knowledge of several aspects related to this procedure is mandatory to improve cannulation success, avoid complications and lengthen the survival of the catheter.

Main text: Several practical issues related to peripheral venous cannulation are described: peripheral venous anatomy, vein size and catheter selection, distance from skin to vein, insertion angle and selection of the catheter length, cannulation technique itself (out-of-plane or in-plane) and checking catheter position.

Conclusion: Key concepts regarding ultrasound-guided peripheral vein cannulation should be well known for practitioners, aiding in improving cannulation success and catheter dwell time, and avoiding complications.

Keywords: Ultrasound, Point-of-care, Peripheral venous catheterization

Background

Peripheral venous cannulation is essential to provide care for the patients in the emergency department or critical care unit. While most intravenous catheters are placed using the conventional technique (i.e., seeing and/or palpating the vein), up to one-third of the patients have difficult intravenous access (DIVA) [1]. This group often involves patients with generalized edemas, obese, those with multiple previous cannulations or intravenous drug users [2–5]. For patients who have DIVA, ultrasound (US)-guided cannulation has shown an overall success rate higher than 90%, compared to 25–30% using the conventional technique [2–4, 6], and also aids in reducing the need for central venous lines [4, 5]. Patient satisfaction also improves using US guidance [2]. In spite of that, the rate of premature catheter failure (PCF), which may account for as high as 50% within 24 h of catheter placement, is higher with US-guided cannulations (45–56%) compared to the conventional technique (19–25%) [1, 6, 7]. Infiltration is the leading cause of catheter failure; catheter dislodgement and thrombophlebitis are also common [1, 6]. Key concepts regarding veins, catheters and the technique itself should be considered by practitioners to improve success, reduce complications and improve dwell times in US-guided peripheral intravenous cannulation, and these are provided in this article, and are summarized in Table 1 as well. Basic general knowledge for US-guided vascular cannulation is shown in Fig. 1.

Key concept 1: Select superficial veins

Anatomically, peripheral veins may be superficial or epifascial (i.e., above the fascia), and deep or subfascial (i.e., below the fascia). Superficial veins are found close

*Correspondence: ohtusabes@gmail.com
Intensive Care Unit, Clínica Cruz Azul, 2651, 60 St, 7630 Necochea, Argentina

Table 1 Key concepts for ultrasound-guided peripheral venous cannulation

Key concept	Description	Considerations
Must know	Basic general knowledge for ultrasound-guided vascular cannulation	Selection of the transducer and preset; image orientation; basic image optimization; distinguishing veins versus arteries; managing techniques of cannulation (out-of-plane and in-plane technique)
1	Select superficial veins (i.e., epifascial)	Superficial veins: short pathway to reach the vein; high probability that a great proportion of the catheter will dwell in the vein Deep veins: inherent risks of needle-stick injury of the artery or the nerve; frequent catheter dislodgment
2	Patent veins	Anechoic lumen; fully compressible Do not misinterpret stagnant blood in the vein lumen with thrombus (distal compression is useful)
3	Vein size: anteroposterior diameter ≥ 4 mm	AP diameter (mm) = maximum Fr catheter size (e.g., 4 mm = up to 4-Fr catheter)
4	Vein depth: up to 16 mm (short axis)	Real distance to reach the vein (45° insertion angle)*: 1.4 × vertical distance *Ideally measure real distance in long axis and select the best angle of insertion ≥ 2.75 cm of the catheter must dwell in the vein Consider using ultra-long peripheral (6.3 cm) and midline (8–20 cm) catheters to minimize catheter failure
5	Select the technique: in-plane or out-of-plane technique	Both are useful, although it seems to be a greater success rate with the out-of-plane technique Learning and using both techniques is encouraged
6	Checking catheter position	Direct: double hyperechoic line into the lumen vein Indirect: saline flush test (two-dimensional and/or color Doppler)

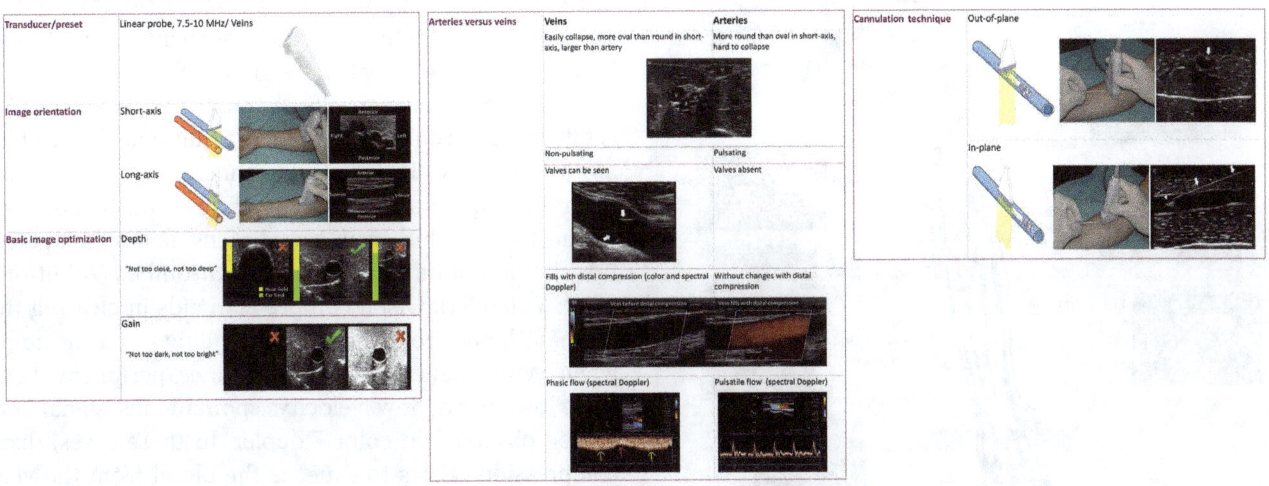

Fig. 1 Basic general knowledge for ultrasound-guided vascular cannulation: selection of the transducer and preset, image orientation, basic image optimization, distinguishing veins versus arteries and the two techniques of cannulation used in practice: the out-of-plane and the in-plane technique

to the skin and travel without an accompanying artery or nerve. In contrast, deep veins (which may be paired, as seen in brachial veins) are found at the neurovascular bundle, and thus are accompanied by an artery and a nerve (Fig. 2 and Additional file 1: Video S1). From these anatomical points, some key concepts advocate for the use of superficial veins instead of deep veins. Using superficial veins provides a short pathway to cannulation, leads to dwell a higher proportion of the catheter inside the vein (an issue intimately related to PCF, see below) and as a safe issue, avoids needle-stick injury of the artery or nerve. Cannulation of deep veins is also associated with a greater risk of catheter dislodgment when compared to cannulation of superficial

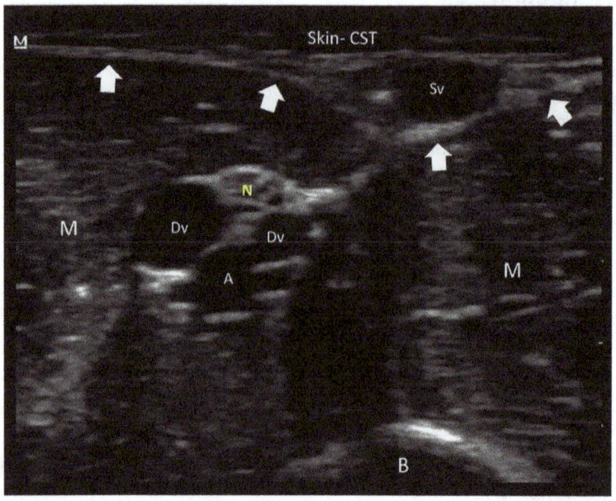

Fig. 2 Ultrasound anatomy applied to cannulation of the peripheral veins of the upper limbs. Superficial veins (Sv) are found above fascia (delineated by arrows) in the cellular subcutaneous tissue (CST), and deep veins below fascia, or subfascial. As noted, deep veins are paired (brachial veins in this case), and are accompanied by an artery (A, brachial artery in this example) and a nerve (N, median nerve in this case) in the neurovascular bundle. The muscle (M) and the bone (B) are also found in the subfascial compartment. Superficial veins should be selected for cannulation

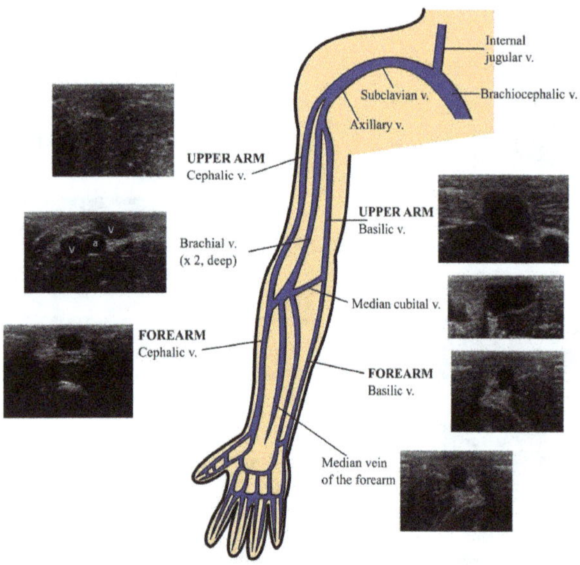

Fig. 3 Anatomy of the peripheral veins of the upper limbs. *v* vein

veins [3, 8]. The superficial veins of the upper limbs which can be cannulated are the basilic (found medial, in the upper arm and in the forearm), and the cephalic (found lateral, in the upper arm and in the forearm).The median vein of the forearm and the median cubital vein are other veins which often have an adequate size for US-guided cannulation (Fig. 3).

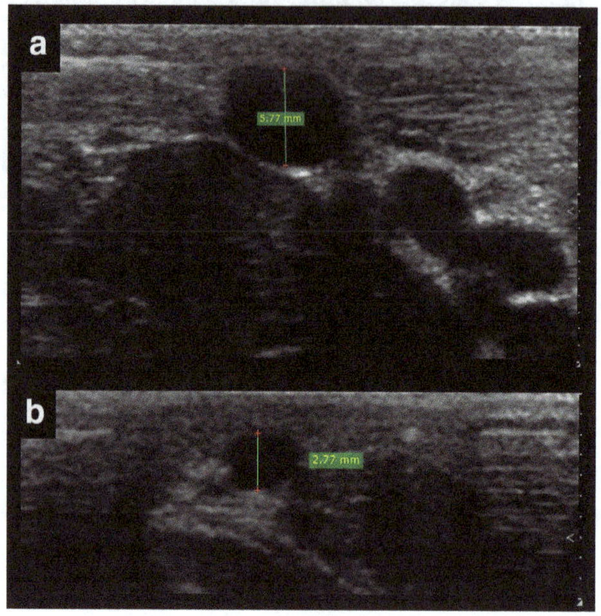

Fig. 4 Two different anteroposterior diameters of the vein for US-guided cannulation. The vein in **a** has an excellent diameter for cannulation (>4 mm), in contrast with the smaller vein in **b**

Key concept 2: Select patent veins

A fully patent vein is sine qua non for cannulation. This is demonstrated by applying slight compression forces over the skin with the transducer and observing veins that collapse easily (Additional file 2: Video S2). In contrast, a thrombosed vein is partially or totally non-compressible, is filled with thrombotic material (Additional file 3: Video S3) and thus is discarded for cannulation. After applying a tourniquet, a stagnant blood flow may be observed within the vein lumen in two-dimensional imaging, and this should not be confused with a thrombus (Additional file 4: Video S4). Distal compression aids in clearing this stagnant blood from the vein and ruling out a thrombus when vein patency is in doubt. Since peripheral veins have low blood flow velocity, spontaneous signal may not be observed in color Doppler. In these cases, distal compression allows to squeeze the blood from the vein, elevate blood flow velocity, thus aiding in the demonstration of flow in patent veins.

Key concept 3: Determine vein size–catheter size

An optimal vein size is required to improve cannulation, and the size recommended in the literature is at least 4 mm in anteroposterior (AP) diameter [9] (Fig. 4). This suggested vein diameter, although important, should not be used in practice in a strict manner, since smaller veins can still be cannulated successfully, as seen in some studies [4, 6]. The vein size fulfills not only an established role in cannulation success (i.e., large veins are easily

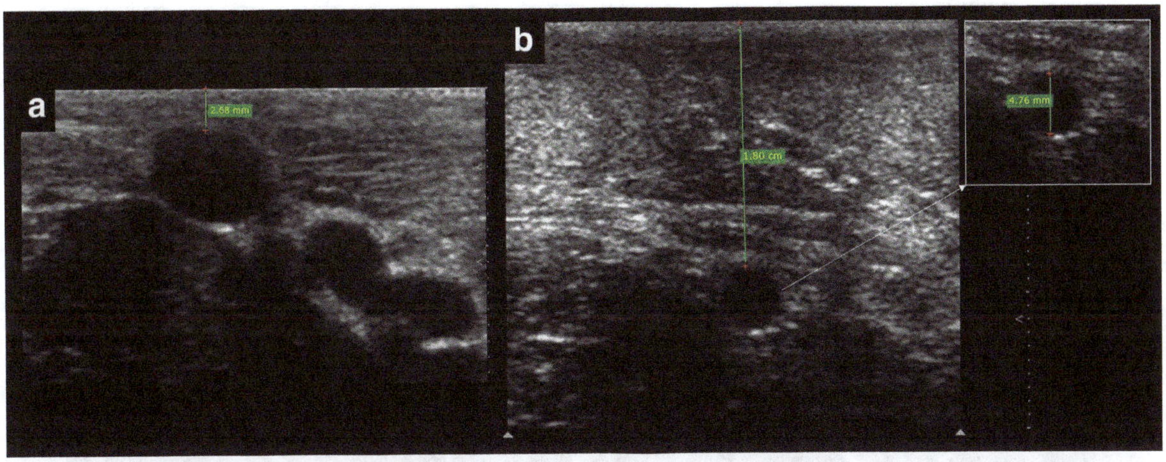

Fig. 5 Distance from skin to vein for US-guided cannulation. In **a**, it is < 12 mm (ideal), while in **b** is > 16 mm. Since the vein in **b** has a diameter > 4 mm, it could still be cannulated using longer catheters than usual, for example, a midline catheter

observed, as well as the needle within the vessel), but also aids in guiding catheter selection. As a rule of thumb, AP diameter indicates the upper limit of the external diameter of the catheter which can be used, considering that up to one-third of the vein lumen should be occupied by the catheter [10]. Thus, for example, a 4-Fr catheter (with an external diameter of 1.3 mm) is the maximum size for a 4-mm vein.

Key concept 4: Determine vein depth–insertion angle–catheter length

As mentioned before, apart from avoiding the injury of the artery or nerve, practitioners should select superficial veins to guarantee a short pathway to cannulate the vein. The maximum suggested distance from skin to vein is < 16 mm [9, 11], while < 12 mm can be considered ideal [1] (Fig. 5). This distance supposes a 90° needle insertion related to the vessel, and thus, the real or "corrected" distance of the needle traveling to reach the vein can be approached performing Pythagorean assumptions, which are entirely true for a needle insertion angle of 45°. This distance is equal to 1.4 multiplied by the vertical distance (Fig. 6). For example, a vertical distance of 12 mm equals 16.8 mm using a 45° insertion. However, in practice, this length varies with the use of shallower (increased distance) or more sloped (decreased distance) needle insertions. Without the need to make calculations, practitioners can directly get this distance in the long axis, offering a big picture regarding the real distance to reach the vein when using different angles of insertion (Fig. 7). Of note, knowing this distance is of paramount importance to minimize PCF, given that a large proportion of the catheter must dwell in the vein [1, 6], and thus, a large distance to vein will result in a large proportion of the catheter outside the vein using standard-length catheters (SLC). A recent investigation using SLC showed that when < 30% (or one-third) of the catheter resides in the vein, all catheters failed. On the other hand, when > 65% (or two-thirds) of the catheter resides in the vein, none of the catheters failed. When 30–64% of the catheter was in the vein, 32.4% of intravenous catheters were lost [6]. More recently, comparing standard 4.78-cm-long catheters versus 6.35-cm-long catheters, Bahl et al. showed a significantly increased catheter survival when > 2.75 cm of the catheter resided in the vessel [12] (Fig. 8). This is coherent with the previous study, since 2.75 cm is closest to the 65% of an SLC. Thus, as a rule of thumb, achieving at least 2.75 cm of the catheter dwelling in the vein should be the cut-off used to mitigate catheter failure. This means, for example, that for an SLC of 4.78 cm, the "real" distance to reach the vein must be lower than 2 cm. To achieve this, several strategies can be used, for example, selecting vessels at the lowest possible depth, using sloped insertion angles, and inserting catheters which are longer than usual, such as ultra-long peripheral catheters (ULPC, 18-20G, 6.35 cm in length) and midline catheters (8–20 cm in length) [1, 8, 12, 13]. Using catheters which are longer than the standard size aids in minimizing PFC, allowing operators to use shallower insertion angles to improve needle visualization and also to select veins which are even deeper than 16 mm. Advantages of ULPC over midline are its low costs and the fact that they do not require advanced skills such as managing the Seldinger technique, so they can be inserted by nurses or technicians.

Key concept 5: Select the cannulation technique: out-of-plane or in-plane technique

Practitioners should remember that each technique has advantages and disadvantages and thus learning and

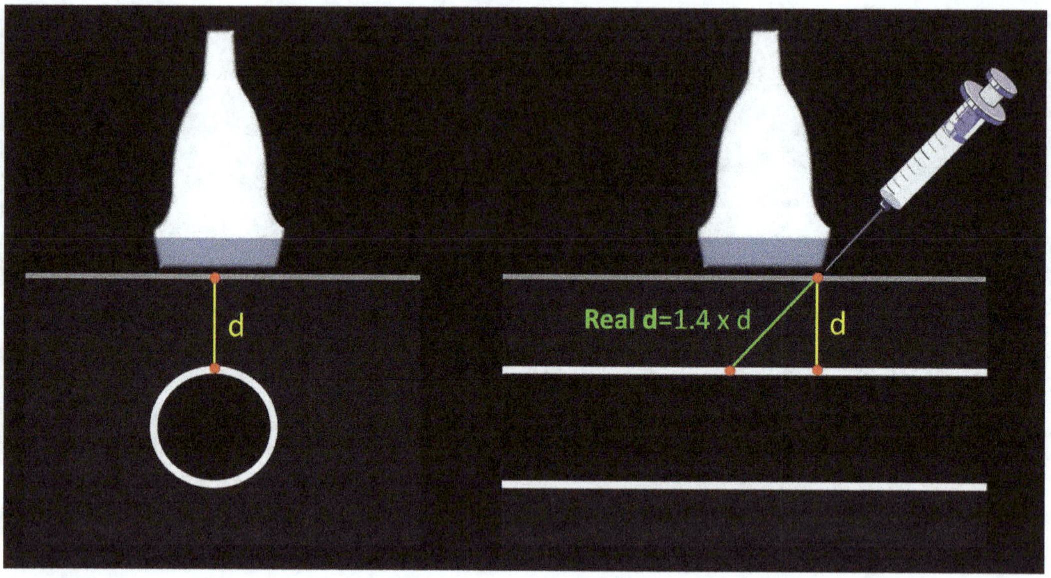

Fig. 6 Explaining the distance from skin to vessel in ultrasound-guided cannulation. While this distance (*d*) is estimated in the short axis, the real distance to reach the vein depends on the insertion angle. Assuming a 45° insertion angle, this real distance is equal to *d* multiplied by 1.4. Of note, the real distance decreases with sloped insertions, and increases using shallower insertions

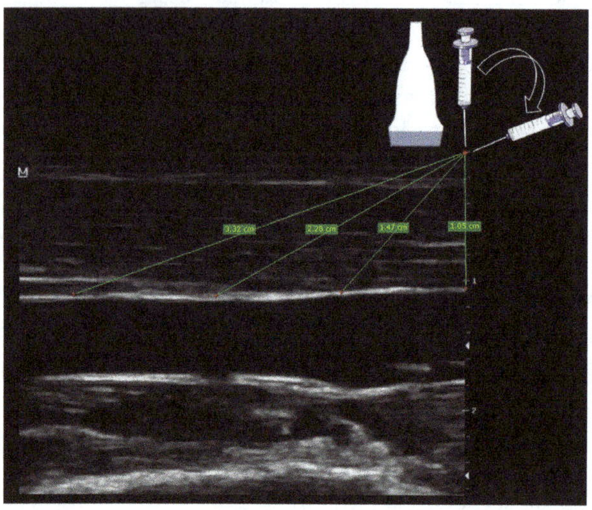

Fig. 7 Real distance from skin to vein measured directly in the long axis. As shown, shallowest insertions determine a longest pathway to reach the vein, resulting in a large proportion of the catheter dwelling outside the vein and ultimately leading to catheter failure. In contrast, sloped insertions lead to shortening the distance to reach the vein, and aid in increasing the proportion of the catheter dwelling in the vein lumen

using both techniques are encouraged (Additional file 5: Video S5 and Additional file 6: Video S6), since they can select one or the other based on the situation [14, 15]. In a recent systematic review and meta-analysis, greater success has been shown with the out-of-plane technique compared to the in-plane technique [16]. However, for the out-of-plane technique, the visualization of the needle tip is an important limitation, having shown a higher rate of posterior wall perforations, compared to in-plane technique, which shows a clear delineation of the needle shaft and needle tip as it is advanced from superficial tissues into the vein [17, 18]. Using the "walk-down" maneuver (i.e., "follow the tip technique") improves visualization of the needle tip when using out-of-plane insertions [14] and should be considered for using in practice. Side-lobe artifact is common when performing the in-plane technique, which simulates that the needle is inserted into the vein lumen, when is in fact close to it [14]. The learning curve for the in-plane technique seems to be longer compared to the out-of-plane technique [15].

Key concept 6: Demonstrate the catheter is in the vein lumen and perform a saline flush test

After cannulating the vein, it is useful to check if the catheter is in the vein lumen, since is not infrequent that the infused solution passes easily to the subcutaneous tissue without any warning signs, thus delaying the institution of intravenous therapies. The catheter is observed as two parallel hyperechoic lines in the short, the long or both axes (Fig. 9a, b). In midline catheter insertions, the guidewire, seen as a hyperechoic linear structure, should be demonstrated before inserting the catheter (Fig. 9c). Finally, a saline flush test may be performed through the catheter, observing bubbles in the lumen vein in correctly

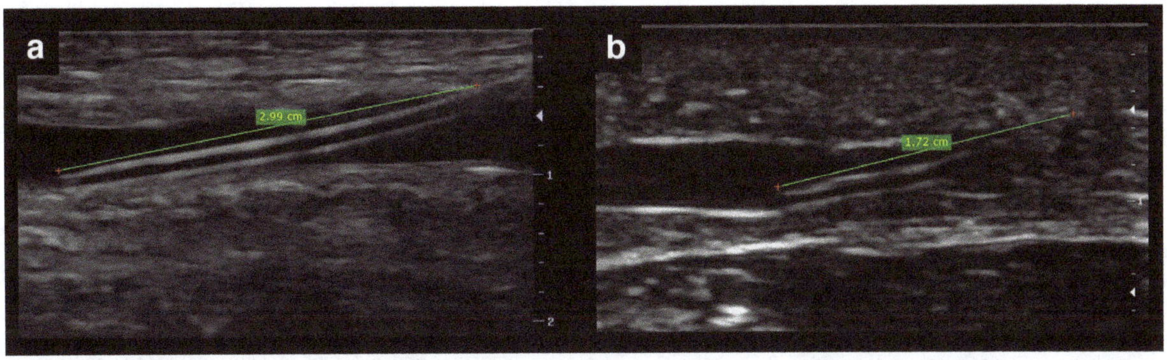

Fig. 8 Amount of catheter residing in the vein. In **a.** the catheter dwelling in the vein is > 2.75 cm, in contrast with **b.** To achieve at least 2.75 cm of the catheter dwelling in the vein, several strategies can be used, for example, selecting veins at the lowest depth possible, using sloped insertion angles, and inserting catheters which are longer than usual, such as ultra-long peripheral catheters or midline catheters

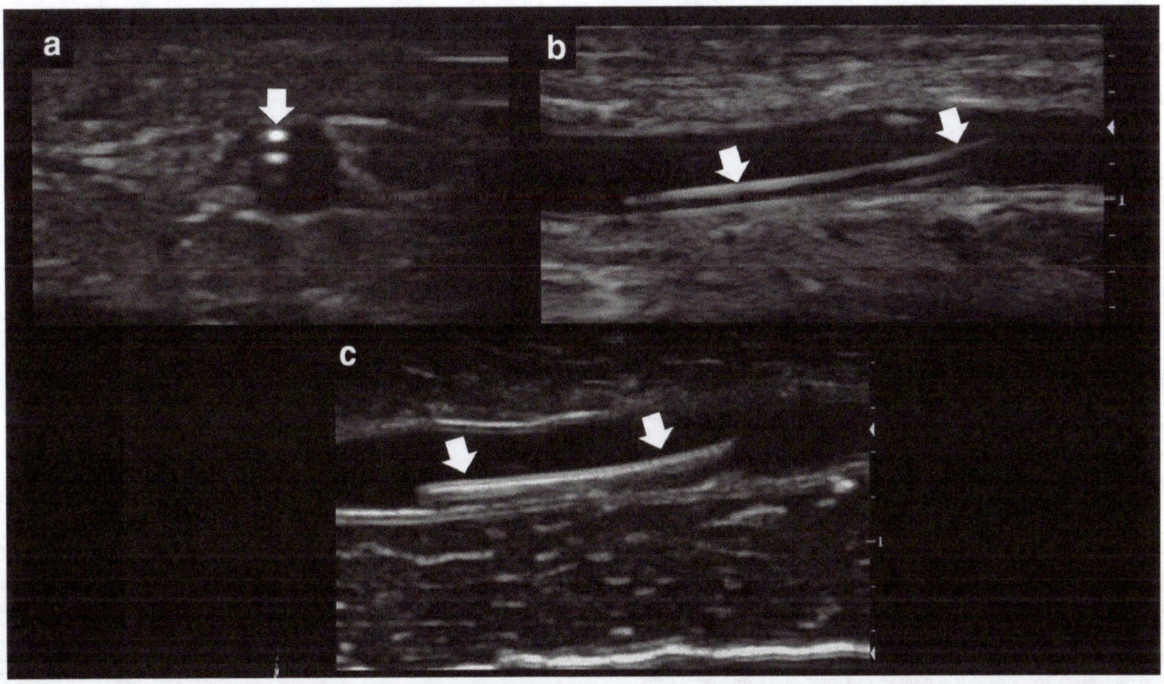

Fig. 9 **a**, **b** Demonstration of the catheter (arrows) entering the vein lumen in short (**a**) and long axis (**b**); **c** demonstration of the guidewire entering the lumen vein (arrows) in the long axis, when using a midline catheter

positioned catheters (Additional file 7: Video S7); color Doppler can be used for this purpose as well [19].

Conclusions

Practitioners should consider several issues when inserting intravenous peripheral catheters under ultrasound guidance, aiming to improve success rate, avoid complications and lengthen the survival of the catheter. Based on available data and everyday practice, all indicate that catheters longer than standard size are needed for US-guided peripheral venous cannulation, with the purpose of minimizing premature catheter failure. This is a call for attention to catheter manufacturers, since a more affordable solution at hand is expected from them shortly.

Supplementary information

Additional file 1: Video S1. Real-time cross-section two-dimensional ultrasound imaging of the upper limb showing the anatomy of the peripheral veins and its relation to the fascia. Sv: superficial vein; Dv: deep vein; A: artery; N: nerve. As shown, superficial veins are epifascial, while deep veins are subfascial, and are accompanied by an artery and a nerve (in this case the deep veins are the paired brachial veins, the brachial artery and the median nerve).

Additional file 2: Video S2. Real-time two-dimensional ultrasound imaging showing patency of the peripheral veins, which are fully compressible.

Additional file 3: Video S3. Real-time two-dimensional and duplex ultrasound imaging showing a thrombosed superficial vein, which is noncompressible and filled by thrombotic material.

Additional file 4: Video S4. Real-time two-dimensional ultrasound imaging in long axis showing stagnant blood within the vein lumen after applying a tourniquet.

Additional file 5: Video S5. Real-time imaging showing the out-of-plane technique for ultrasound-guided vascular cannulation. The most relevant pros and cons of this technique are highlighted.

Additional file 6: Video S6. Real-time imaging showing the in-plane technique for ultrasound-guided vascular cannulation. The most relevant pros and cons of this technique are highlighted.

Additional file 7: Video S7. Saline flush test. Real-time two-dimensional ultrasound imaging in long axis showing bubbles appearing in the vein lumen immediately after flushing saline through the catheter, indicating a correctly positioned catheter.

Abbreviations

DIVA: difficult intravenous access; PCF: premature catheter failure; US: ultrasound; SLC: standard-length catheters; ULPC: ultra-long peripheral catheters.

Acknowledgements

None.

Authors' contributions

The author PB wrote the manuscript, and edited the multimedia material. The author read and approved the final manuscript.

References

1. Bahl A, Hang B, Brackney A, Joseph S, Karabon P, Mohammad A, Nnanabu I, Shotkin P (2019) Standard long IV catheters versus extended dwell catheters: a randomized comparison of ultrasound-guided catheter survival. Am J Emerg Med 37(4):715–721
2. Costantino TG, Parikh AK, Satz WA, Fojtik JP (2005) Ultrasonography-guided peripheral intravenous access versus traditional approaches in patients with difficult intravenous access. Ann Emerg Med 46(5):456–461
3. Keyes LE, Frazee BW, Snoey ER, Simon BC, Christy D (1999) Ultrasound-guided brachial and basilic vein cannulation in emergency department patients with difficult intravenous access. Ann Emerg Med 34(6):711–714
4. Gregg SC, Murthi SB, Sisley AC, Stein DM, Scalea TM (2010) Ultrasound-guided peripheral intravenous access in the intensive care unit. J Crit Care 25(3):514–519
5. Shokoohi H, Boniface K, McCarthy M, Khedir Al-tiae T, Sattarian M, Ding R, Liu YT, Pourmand A, Schoenfeld E, Scott J, Shesser R, Yadav K (2013) Ultrasound-guided peripheral intravenous access program is associated with a marked reduction in central venous catheter use in noncritically ill emergency department patients. Ann Emerg Med 61(2):198–203
6. Pandurangadu AV, Tucker JM, Brackney AR, Bahl A (2018) Ultrasound-guided intravenous catheter survival impacted by amount of catheter residing in the vein. Emerg Med J 35(9):550–555
7. Dargin JM, Rebholz CM, Lowenstein RA, Mitchell PM, Feldman JA (2010) Ultrasonography-guided peripheral intravenous catheter survival in ED patients with difficult access. Am J Emerg Med 28(1):1–7
8. Mills CN, Liebmann O, Stone MB, Frazee BW (2007) Ultrasonographically guided insertion of a 15-cm catheter into the deep brachial or basilic vein in patients with difficult intravenous access. Ann Emerg Med 50(1):68–72
9. Witting MD, Schenkel SM, Lawner BJ, Euerle BD (2010) Effects of vein width and depth on ultrasound-guided peripheral intravenous success rates. J Emerg Med 39(1):70–75
10. Tanabe H, Takahashi T, Murayama R, Yabunaka K, Oe M, Matsui Y, Arai R, Uchida M, Komiyama C, Sanada H (2016) Using ultrasonography for vessel diameter assessment to prevent infiltration. J Infus Nurs 39(2):105–111
11. Panebianco NL, Fredette JM, Szyld D, Sagalyn EB, Pines JM, Dean AJ (2009) What you see (sonographically) is what you get: vein and patient characteristics associated with successful ultrasound-guided peripheral intravenous placement in patients with difficult access. Acad Emerg Med 16(12):1298–1303
12. Bahl A, Hijazi M, Chen N-W, Chavette-Lachapelle L, Price J. Ultra long versus standard long peripheral intravenous catheters: a randomized controlled trial of ultrasound-guided catheter survival. SSRN: https://ssrn.com/abstract=3401988. Accessed 05 July 2019
13. Elia F, Ferrari G, Molino P, Converso M, De Filippi G, Milan A, Aprà F (2012) Standard-length catheters vs long catheters in ultrasound-guided peripheral vein cannulation. Am J Emerg Med 30(5):712–716
14. Blanco P (2016) Ultrasound-guided vascular cannulation in critical care patients: a practical review. Med Intensiva 40(9):560–571
15. Lamperti M, Bodenham AR, Pittiruti M, Blaivas M, Augoustides JG, Elbarbary M, Pirotte T, Karakitsos D, Ledonne J, Doniger S, Scoppettuolo G, Feller-Kopman D, Schummer W, Biffi R, Desruennes E, Melniker LA, Verghese ST (2012) International evidence-based recommendations on ultrasound-guided vascular access. Intensive Care Med 38(7):1105–1117
16. Gottlieb M, Holladay D, Peksa GD (2018) Comparison of short- vs long-axis technique for ultrasound-guided peripheral line placement: a systematic review and meta-analysis. Cureus 10(5):e2718
17. Stone MB, Moon C, Sutijono D, Blaivas M (2010) Needle tip visualization during ultrasound-guided vascular access: short-axis vs long-axis approach. Am J Emerg Med 28(3):343–347
18. Moon CH, Blehar D, Shear MA, Uyehara P, Gaspari RJ, Arnold J, Cukor J (2010) Incidence of posterior vessel wall puncture during ultrasound-guided vessel cannulation in a simulated model. Acad Emerg Med 17(10):1138–1141
19. Gottlieb M, Sundaram T, Holladay D, Nakitende D (2017) Ultrasound-guided peripheral intravenous line placement: a narrative review of evidence-based best practices. West J Emerg Med 18(6):1047–1054

8

Ultrasound-guided insertion of intra-aortic balloon counterpulsation in intensive care: description of the technique

David Rene Rodriguez Lima[1*], Ever Julián Duran[2], Ever Leonardo Rojas Díaz[2], Darío Isaías Pinilla Rojas[3], Mario Andrés Mercado Díaz[4] and Yury Forlán Bustos Martínez[5]

Abstract

Intra-aortic balloon counterpulsation (IAoBC) is a mechanical circulatory support device that has been used for more than 50 years, mainly for cardiogenic shock. Although its effect on mortality is controversial, IAoBC is still used in a wide variety of pre- and postoperative clinical settings in cardiac surgery centers. IAoBC has a complication rate of approximately 30%, mostly associated with problems during insertion and malpositioning. Thus, an insertion technique based on the use of ultrasound at the patient's bedside in the intensive care unit (ICU) is proposed.

Keywords: Ultrasound, Intra-aortic balloon counterpulsation (IAoBC), Mechanical circulatory support, Ultrasound education

Introduction

Intra-aortic balloon counterpulsation (IAoBC) is used in up to 7% of cardiac surgery patients [1]. IAoBC is used in this context to support coronary circulation and to reduce stress on the left ventricle [2, 3]. Despite the theoretical physiological advantages of IAoBC, its effect on decreasing mortality is controversial. IAoBC has been used in different groups of patients, including in those with cardiogenic shock, regardless of its etiology, refractory angina, acute myocardial infarction, refractory ventricular arrhythmias, mechanical infarct complications (acute mitral regurgitation and ventricular septal rupture), high-risk angioplasty and high-risk cardiac or noncardiac surgery, with different outcomes [1, 4].

The main complications of using IAoBC result from insertion and malpositioning. Rastan et al. [5], in abdominal tomographies, found 68.2% disagreement in balloon length related to the distance between the subclavian artery and the celiac trunk, which was associated with abdominal vessel obstruction and worse clinical outcomes.

Vascular lesions can be catastrophic and evident during IAoBC insertion; however, inadvertent dissection of the aorta or iliac artery can go unnoticed, and such dissection is suspected before death in only 20% of cases [6]. Ischemic vascular complications range from 8 to 18%, with critical lower-limb ischemia lower than 1% [7, 8].

Parissis et al. [9] showed that slowed pulse and cold feet were detected in 29.5% of the cases. Ischemia was resolved in most cases by removing the balloon and in 5.8% by thrombectomy; only one patient developed gangrene, which required amputation. Hematoma incidence ranges from 0.4 to 3.9%, and bleeding incidence ranges from 0.4 to 27.7% (mean 5.27 ± 8.5) [10].

IAoBC rupture is not frequent, but can cause a gas embolism and potential entrapment in the arterial tree. This is very rare and occurs in less than 0.5% of cases. The proposed mechanism involves mechanical disruption of the balloon against an atherosclerotic plaque or a calcified aorta and negative pressure created during deflation [11].

The use of ultrasound to perform femoral vascular access during the insertion of the IAoBC [12] and the use of transesophageal echocardiography (TEE) for positioning it [13, 14] has been described; however, since TEE is

*Correspondence: drrodriguezl@hotmail.com
[1] Emergency Medicine and Critical and Intensive Care Medicine, Hospital Universitario Mayor Méderi–Universidad Del Rosario, Bogotá, Colombia
Full list of author information is available at the end of the article

an invasive procedure, it is not routinely recommended [14, 15]. This article proposes an ultrasound-guided IAoBC insertion technique in the cardiovascular ICU. This technique is original, and similar techniques have not been previously described.

Technique

When the medical team decides to use IAoBC, the presence of any contraindication for the procedure (aortic valve disease, significant bleeding disorder or infection at the femoral puncture site) should be ruled out, and a clinical evaluation should be performed to rule out severe peripheral artery disease.

After explaining the procedure and asking the patient to sign an informed consent form, the IAoBC is inserted.

Ultrasound assessment is performed with the patient in the supine position; with a low-frequency (2 to 5 MHz) transducer, in a subxiphoid left paramedian longitudinal section, using the left hepatic lobe as a window, the abdominal aorta is represented as a pulsatile and anechogenic tubular image, supported on the vertebral bodies. From the ventral face, the celiac trunk emerges first, and then the superior mesenteric artery runs parallel to the aorta, following the aorta to the aortic bifurcation. The presence of aneurysms or dissection should not be observed, which are contraindications for the procedure (Fig. 1).

Then, with a high-frequency linear transducer (6 to 15 MHz), the femoral artery is visualized; the presence of thrombi, aneurysms, atheromas or dissection inside the femoral artery should be ruled out. The diameter of the femoral artery is measured and must be greater than

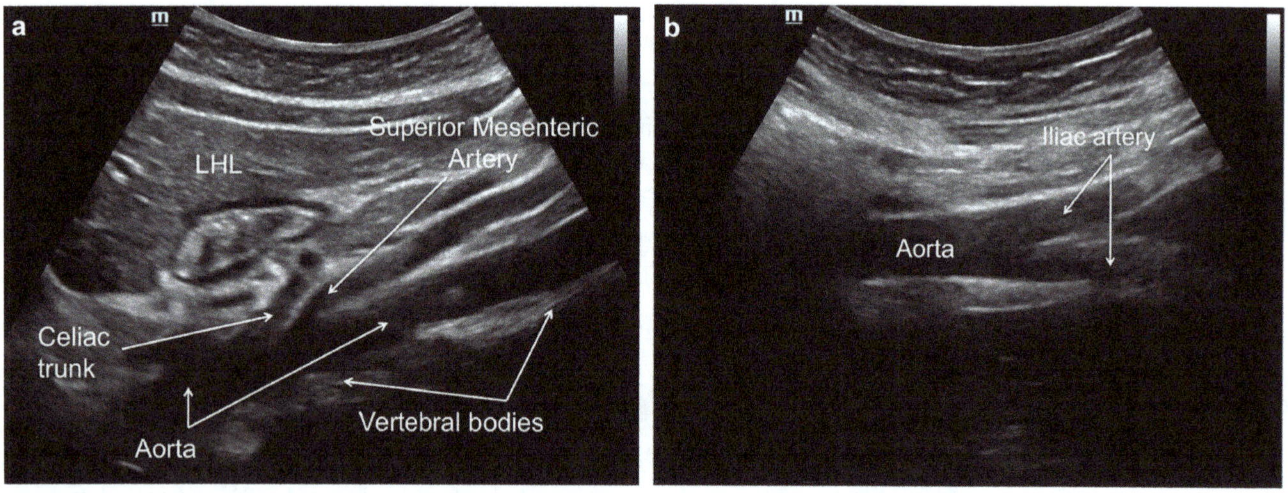

Fig. 1 **a** Subxiphoid left paramedian longitudinal section with a low-frequency convex transducer, using the left hepatic lobe (LHL) as a window, showing a pulsatile and anechogenic tubular image, supported on the vertebral bodies, corresponding to the aorta. From the ventral face, the celiac trunk emerges first, and then the superior mesenteric artery runs parallel to the aorta shortly after emerging, following the aorta to the aortic bifurcation. **b** The aorta should be followed distally until the aortic bifurcation

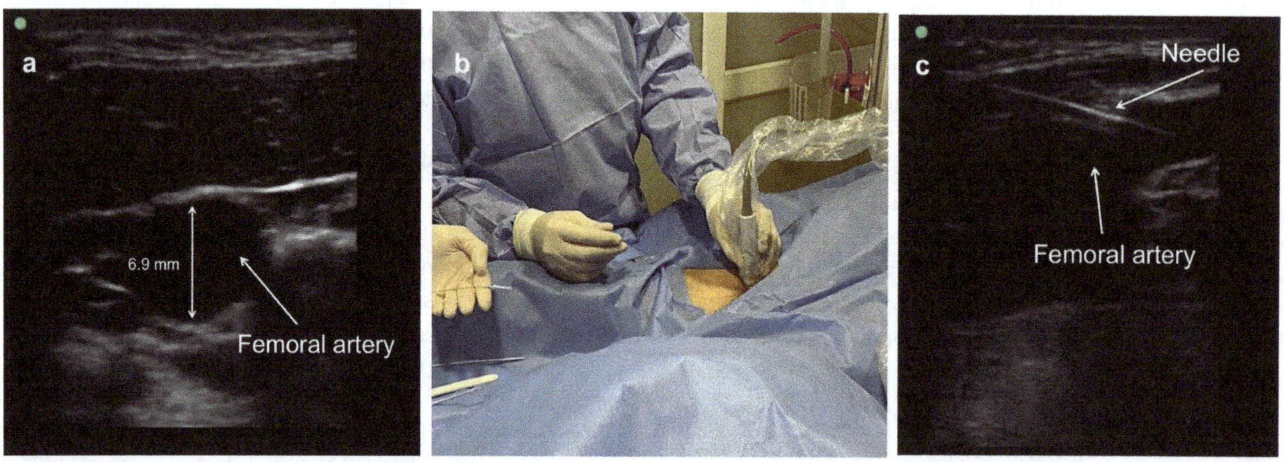

Fig. 2 **a** Short-axis visualization of the femoral artery with a high-frequency linear transducer 6.9 mm in diameter. **b** Puncture under direct visualization. **c** Long-axis visualization of the femoral artery as the needle enters the femoral artery during puncture

5 mm (mm) to allow passage of the 8-Fr balloon catheter (2.7 mm). Under sterile conditions, local anesthesia and real-time ultrasound guidance with a high-frequency linear transducer, the common femoral artery is punctured at an angle of 45 degrees or less (Fig. 2).

Then, under direct visualization, the metal guide should be advanced without resistance while assessing proper intravascular positioning with the same transducer; the metal guide is inserted 40 to 50 cm, the needle with which the puncture was made is removed, and a second operator with a low-frequency transducer views the left paramedian window again to confirm the presence of the guide in the abdominal aorta (Fig. 3).

After confirming that the guide is adequately positioned, the skin and subcutaneous cellular tissue are dilated, and the 8-Fr catheter is advanced, which is fixed.

The IAoBC is prepared by creating a vacuum in the helium compartment using a 50-mL syringe and washing the arterial canal with sterile saline. The angle of Louis is measured from the sternum to the navel, and the distance is added to the entry site of the catheter. This distance represents the length of insertion of the IAoBC, which is passed over the metal guide (Fig. 4).

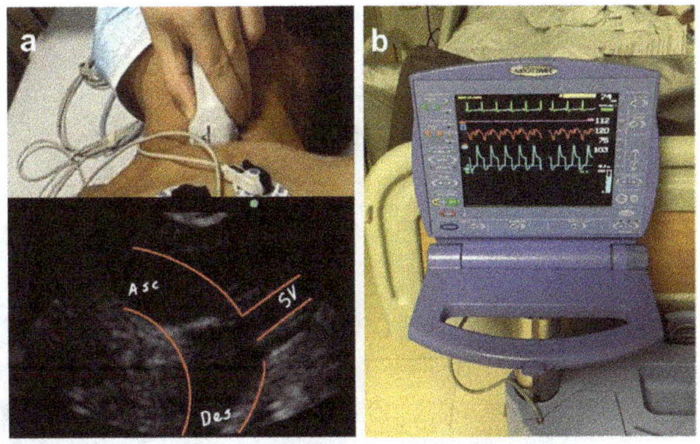

Fig. 5 **a** Supraclavicular approach with a phased array transducer, left supraclavicular window, ascending (Asc) and descending (Des) aorta and the left subclavian artery (SV). **b** IAoBC connected to the console and with adequate counterpulsation

After reaching the desired distance of insertion, a left supraclavicular window is created with a phased array transducer, confirming adequate flow and the absence of obstructions of the left subclavian artery by the IAoBC (Fig. 5a), subsequently removing the metal guide and connecting the arterial line to the helium source, starting counterpulsation (Fig. 5b).

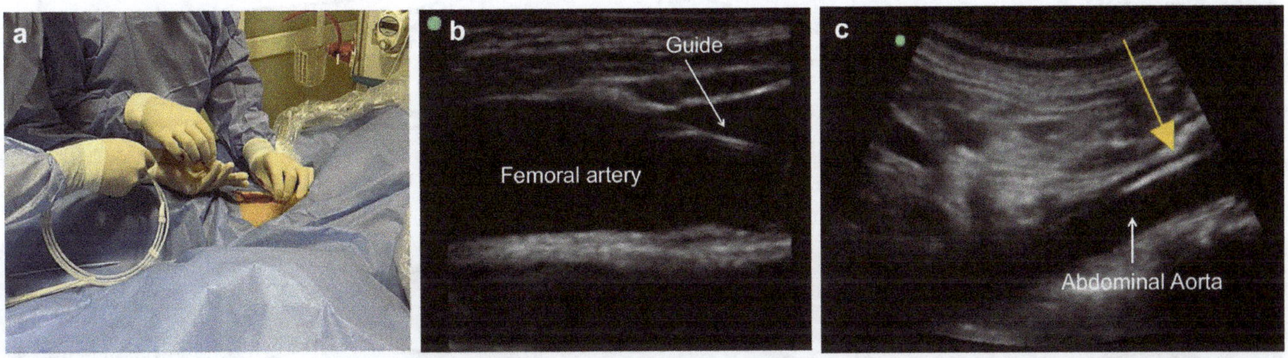

Fig. 3 **a** Passage of the metal guide through the femoral arterial puncture. **b** Visualization of the passage of the intravascular guide at the femoral artery with a high-frequency linear transducer. **c** Verification of the metal guide (yellow arrow) in the abdominal aorta with a low-frequency convex transducer

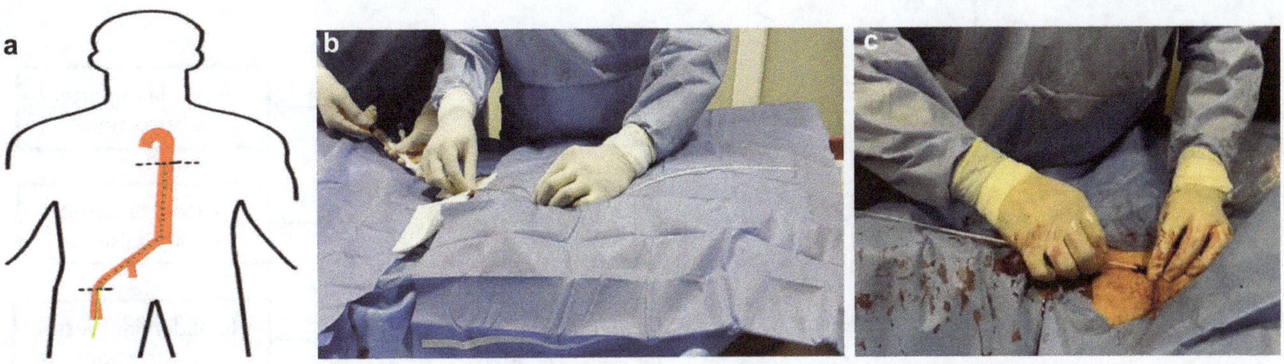

Fig. 4 **a** Distance from the second intercostal space to the right common femoral artery. **b** Measurement of the distance for inserting the IAoBC. **c** Passage of the IAoBC

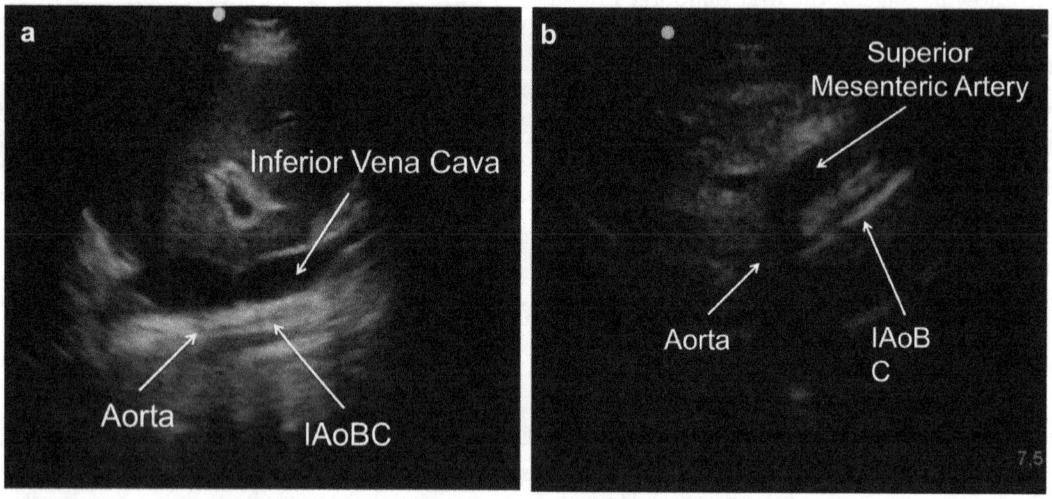

Fig. 6 **a** Right, transhepatic, longitudinal window (between the seventh and eighth intercostal space along the axillary midline) with a low-frequency transducer showing the inferior vena cava and the aorta with the functioning IAoBC. **b** Left paramedian longitudinal window to evaluate the exit of the abdominal vessels; in this case, we observe the IAoBC obstructing the superior mesenteric artery exit; thus, the IAoBC was advanced another 5 cm

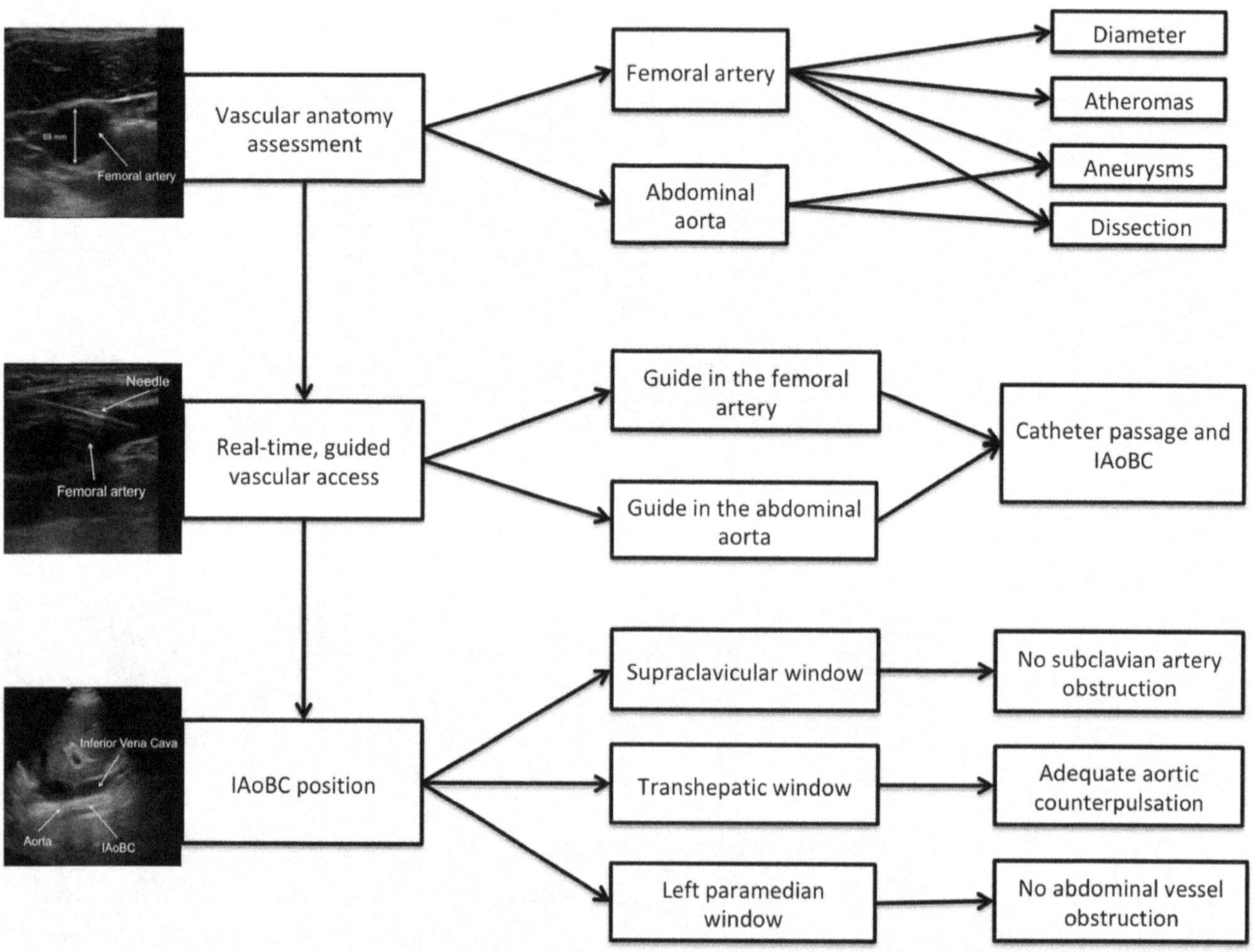

Fig. 7 Proposed technique for ultrasound-guided intra-aortic balloon counterpulsation insertion

Finally, adequate counterpulsation with a low-frequency transducer is visualized through a right transhepatic longitudinal window (between the seventh and eighth intercostal space along the axillary midline) (Fig. 6a), imaging again the left paramedian longitudinal section (Fig. 1) to assess the exit of the celiac trunk and upper mesenteric artery, verifying adequate flow and the absence of the IAoBC at this level (Fig. 6b). If all proposed windows and arterial lines can be imaged by ultrasound and adequate diastolic augmentation is confirmed, chest X-ray is not necessary to verify the position of the IAoBC. As a limitation, it remains to be determined whether the use of this technique allows the operator to improve the success rate of the procedure and reduces complications. A summary of the proposed technique for ultrasound-guided intra-aortic balloon counterpulsation insertion is shown (Fig 7).

Conclusions

An insertion technique based on the use of ultrasound is proposed, allowing safe arterial vascular access, ruling out aortic injuries that can go unnoticed and ensuring adequate positioning. It is expected that its use will reduce the rate of complications associated with the use of IAoBC.

Abbreviations

IAoBC: Intra-aortic balloon counterpulsation; ICU: Intensive care unit; TEE: Transesophageal echocardiogram.

Acknowledgements

Not applicable.

Authors' contributions

YB applied the technique described, collected images and helped write the manuscript. ED collected images and helped write the manuscript. ER collected images and helped write the manuscript. DP collected images and helped write the manuscript. MM collected data and helped write the manuscript. DR applied the technique described, collected images and helped write the manuscript. All authors read and approved the final manuscript.

Author details

[1] Emergency Medicine and Critical and Intensive Care Medicine, Hospital Universitario Mayor Méderi–Universidad Del Rosario, Bogotá, Colombia. [2] Resident, Critical and Intensive Care Medicine, Hospital Universitario Mayor Méderi –Universidad del Rosario, Bogotá, Colombia. [3] Anesthesiology and Critical and Intensive Care Medicine, Hospital Universitario Mayor Méderi–Universidad del Rosario, Bogotá, Colombia. [4] Critical and Intensive Care Medicine, Hospital Universitario Mayor Méderi–Universidad del Rosario, Bogotá, Colombia. [5] Emergency Medicine Department of Ultrasound and Simulation, Universidad del Rosario, Bogotá, Colombia.

References

1. Parissis H, Graham V, Lampridis S, Lau M, Hooks G, Mhandu PC (2016) IABP: history-evolution-pathophysiology-indications: what we need to know. J Cardiothorac Surg 11(1):122
2. Freedman RJ (1991) The intra-aortic balloon pump system: current roles and future directions. J Appl Cardiol 6(5):313–318
3. Kantrowitz A (1990) Origins of intraaortic balloon pumping. Ann Thoracic Surg 50(4):672–674
4. Moulopoulos SD, Topaz S, Kolff WJ (1962) Diastolic balloon pumping (with carbon dioxide) in the aorta—a mechanical assistance to the failing circulation. Am Heart J 63(5):669–675
5. Rastan AJ, Tillmann E, Subramanian S, Lehmkuhl L, Funkat AK, Leontyev S, Doenst T, Walther T, Gutberlet M, Mohr FW (2010) Visceral arterial compromise during intra-aortic balloon counterpulsation therapy. Circulation. 122(1):92–99
6. Isner JM, Cohen SR, Virmani R, Lawrinson W, Roberts WC (1980) Complications of the intraaortic balloon counterpulsation device: clinical and morphologic observations in 45 necropsy patients. Am J Cardiol 45(2):260–268
7. Erdogan HB, Goksedef D, Erentug V, Polat A, Bozbuga N, Mansuroglu D, Guler M, Akinci E, Yakut C (2006) In which patients should sheathless IABP be used? An analysis of vascular complications in 1211 cases. J Card Surg 21(4):342–346
8. Poirier Y, Voisine P, Plourde G, Rimac G, Perez AB, Costerousse O, Bertrand OF (2016) Efficacy and safety of preoperative intra-aortic balloon pump use in patients undergoing cardiac surgery: a systematic review and meta-analysis. Int J Cardiol 207:67–79
9. Parissis H, Leotsinidis M, Akbar MT, Apostolakis E, Dougenis D (2010) The need for intra aortic balloon pump support following open heart surgery: risk analysis and outcome. J Cardiothorac Surg 5(1):20
10. de Jong MM, Lorusso R, Al Awami F, Matteuci F, Parise O, Lozekoot P, Bonacchi M, Maessen JG, Johnson DM, Gelsomino S (2018) Vascular complications following intra-aortic balloon pump implantation: an updated review. Perfusion. 33(2):96–104
11. Rajani R, Keon WJ, Bedard P (1980) Rupture of an intra-aortic balloon. A case report. J Thoracic Cardiovasc Surg 79(2):301–302
12. Medved I (2002) Ultrasound-guided placement of intra-aortic balloon pump. Eur J Anaesthesiol 19(2):149–150
13. Nishioka T, Friedman A, Cercek B, Chaux A, Luo H, Berglund H, Kim CJ, Blanche C, Siegel RJ (1996) Usefulness of transesophageal echocardiography for positioning the intraaortic balloon pump in the operating room. Am J Cardiol 77(1):105–106
14. Klopman MA, Chen EP, Sniecinski RM (2011) Positioning an intraaortic balloon pump using intraoperative transesophageal echocardiogram guidance. Anesth Analg 113(1):40–43
15. Hahn RT, Abraham T, Adams MS, Bruce CJ, Glas KE, Lang RM, Reeves ST, Shanewise JS, Siu SC, Stewart W, Picard MH (2013) Guidelines for performing a comprehensive transesophageal echocardiographic examination: recommendations from the American society of echocardiography and the society of cardiovascular anesthesiologists. J Am Soc Echocardiogr 26(9):921–964

9

The use of an external ultrasound fixator (Probefix) on intensive care patients

M. J. Blans[1*], F. H. Bosch[1] and J. G. van der Hoeven[2]

Abstract

Background: In critical care medicine, the use of transthoracic echo (TTE) is expanding. TTE can be used to measure dynamic parameters such as cardiac output (CO). An important asset of TTE is that it is a non-invasive technique. The Probefix is an external ultrasound holder strapped to the patient which makes it possible to measure CO using TTE in a fixed position possibly making the CO measurements more accurate compared to separate TTE CO measurements. The feasibility of the use of the Probefix to measure CO before and after a passive leg raising test (PLR) was studied. Intensive care patients were included after detection of hypovolemia using Flotrac. Endpoints were the possibility to use Probefix. Also CO measurements with and without the use of Probefix, before and after a PLR were compared to the CO measurements using Flotrac. Side effects in terms of skin alterations after the use of Probefix and patient's comments on (dis)comfort were evaluated.

Results: Ten patients were included; in eight patients, sufficient recordings with the use of Probefix could be obtained. Using Bland–Altman plots, no difference was found in accuracy of measurements of CO with or without the use of Probefix before and after a PLR compared to Flotrac generated CO. There were only mild and temporary skin effects of the use of Probefix.

Conclusions: In this small feasibility study, the Probefix could be used in eight out of ten intensive care patients. The use of Probefix did not result in more or less accurate CO measurements compared to manually recorded TTE CO measurements. We suggest that larger studies on the use of Probefix in intensive care patients are needed.

Keywords: Intensive care, Cardiac ultrasound, Cardiac output, Passive leg raising test, External

Background

The use of echocardiography by intensivists is rapidly growing [1]. Transthoracic echocardiography (TTE) is performed at the bedside, provides clinically relevant information and is safe in terms of radiation. TTE can be used to estimate dynamic parameters such as cardiac output (CO) but using TTE for these kinds of dynamic measurements is not without possible flaws [2].

To detect changes in CO using TTE, successive measurements of CO are needed. To get accurate results, the CO measurements should ideally be taken at exactly the same location.

The Probefix is a non-invasive external ultrasound holder (Figs. 1, 2 and 3) which is strapped on to the patient with the use of non-traumatic straps.

When properly attached to the patient, the Probefix offers the opportunity to measure dynamic TTE parameters such as CO at exactly the same position thereby possibly increasing measurement accuracy.

To this date, there are no data on the use of the Probefix on adult intensive care patients. The Probefix has already been used in a study on adult outpatient cardiology patients [3] and another tailored holder for echocardiography was described in a study on 5 pediatric patients [4]. We designed a feasibility study to determine

*Correspondence: mblans@rijnstate.nl
[1] Department of Intensive Care, Rijnstate Hospital, PO box 9555, 6800 TA Arnhem, The Netherlands
Full list of author information is available at the end of the article

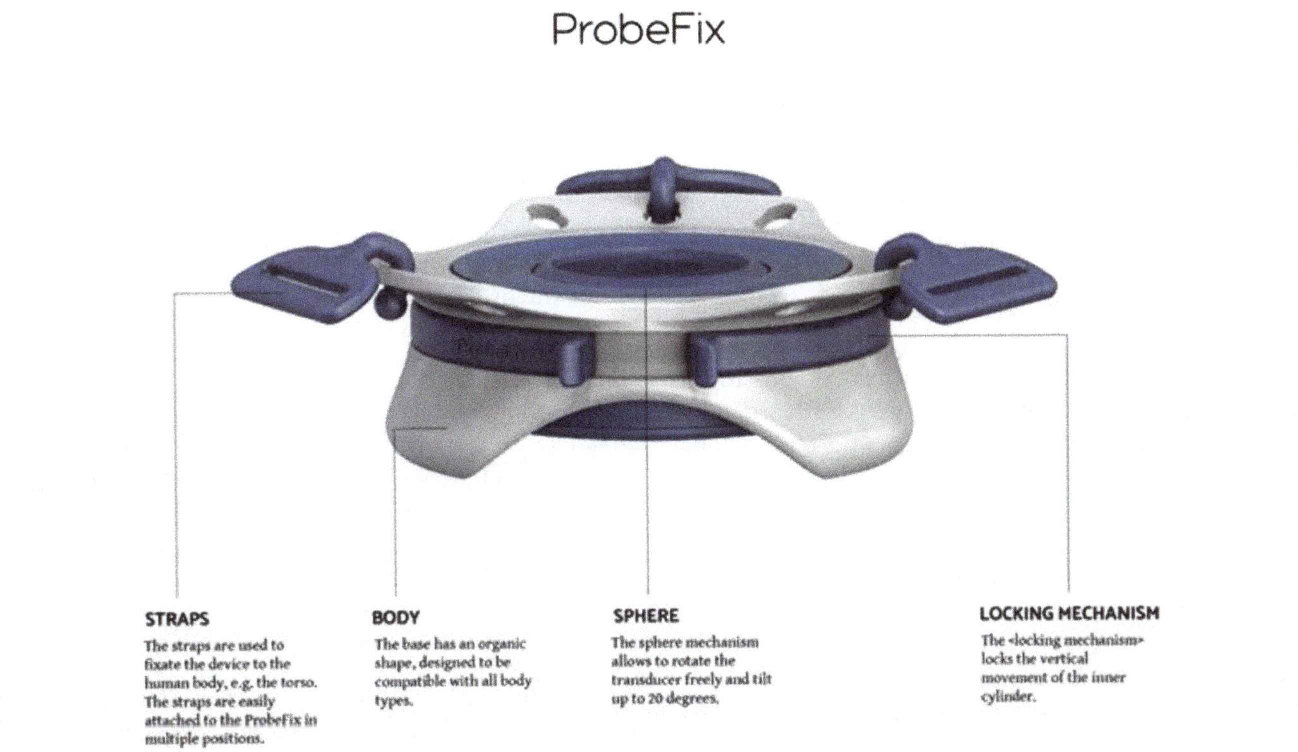

Fig. 1 Description of the Probefix

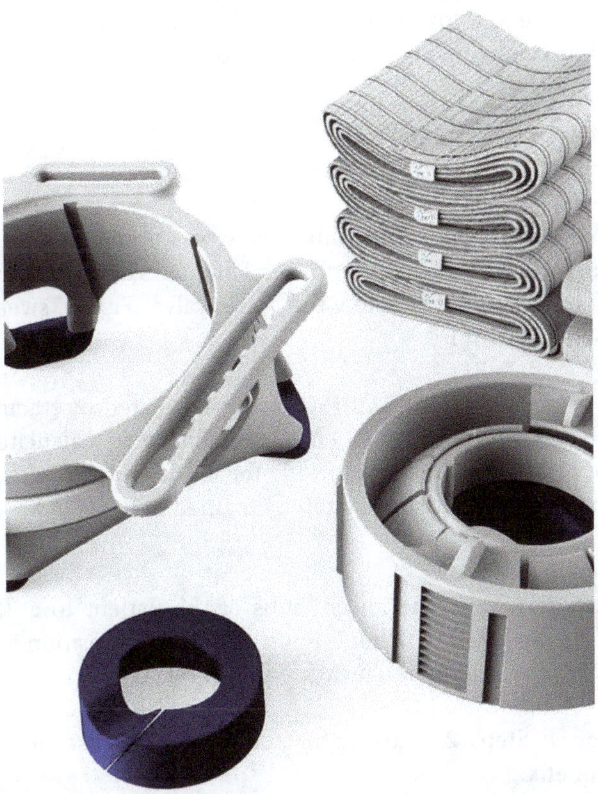

Fig. 2 Components of the Probefix

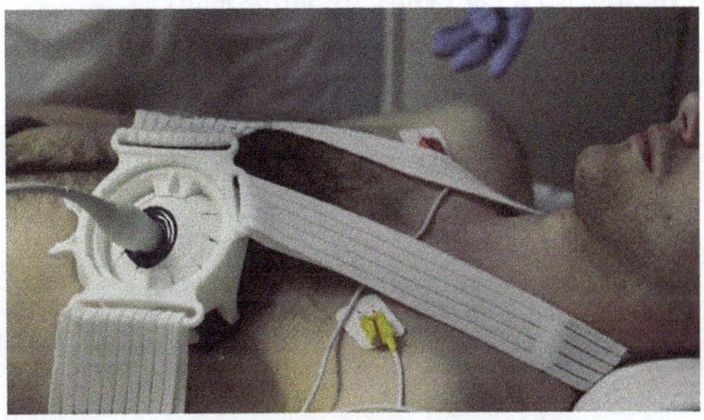

Fig. 3 Example of the fixation of the Probefix on a patient

whether the Probefix can be used on adult intensive care patients for the purpose of measuring CO. CO with TTE with and without the Probefix was measured by using CO measurements made by the Flotrac as a reference. The Flotrac is a system that monitors CO by analyzing the systolic arterial pressure wave. The arterial catheter of the Flotrac system can be placed in the radial artery and has no need for pulmonary artery catheterization or other calibration [6].

Because there is variation between CO measurements between TTE and Flotrac, it will be difficult to assess the use of the Probefix during random CO measurements. It is more interesting to know whether possible changes in CO measurements will be the same after a therapeutic intervention such as a bolus of fluid.

Besides CO, the Flotrac system monitors stroke volume and calculates the stroke volume variation (SVV). SVV is the percentage variation of stroke volume measured during a 20-s interval. Monitoring SVV can be helpful in detecting hypovolemia. When stroke volume variation is above 10%, hypovolemia is present [7]. When hypovolemia is detected with the Flotrac, a passive leg raising test (PLR) can be performed. During PLR, 150–200 mL of blood returns from the lower extremity veins to the central circulation [8]. With PLR, a reversible volume challenge is provided [9]. This is in contrast to an infusion of fluid (Fig. 4).

Methods

In this prospective pilot feasibility study, the Flotrac system was used to detect possible hypovolemia (SVV > 10%) and Flotrac CO measurements were compared with the TTE CO measurements (with and without the use of the Probefix). CO was measured before and after a PLR test.

Primary endpoints

Percentage of patients in which the Probefix can be used.

The correlation between the measurements done by Flotrac and TTE with and without Probefix.

Although no side effects are to be expected, we monitored the patients after the Probefix was removed for any skin damage. Possible skin damage was graded into three categories:

- No skin marks
- Mild skin marks (no treatment necessary)
- Severe skin marks (surgical or medical treatment necessary)

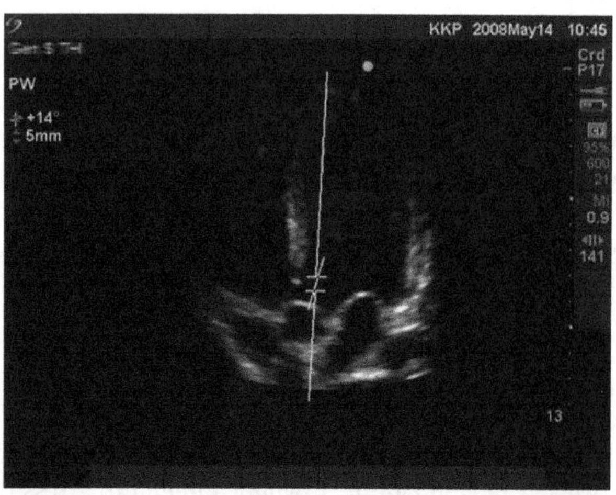

Fig. 4 Apical 5 chamber view with pulsed wave Doppler sample volume

If awake, the patients were asked whether they felt the Probefix to be unpleasant on a scale of 0–10 (0 being: I did not feel anything and 10 being very unpleasant).

Inclusion criteria

Adult intensive care patients (≥ 18 years), with hypovolemia detected with Flotrac (SVV > 10%).

Exclusion criteria

Pregnancy, atrial fibrillation or other irregular heart rhythm, pulmonary edema, PLR not possible (e.g., neurological disease, spinal trauma, restricted limb movement, deep venous thrombosis, or any other reason as indicated by the attending intensivist) or age < 18 (years).

Measurements

After detection of SVV of more than 10% by Flotrac, patients were eligible for inclusion and consent was asked. The TTE studies were done by 2 investigators (MB and FB) with Philips Affinity using the Phased Array probe; the patients were in supine position.

First in the parasternal long axis view (PLAX), the left ventricle outflow tract (LVOT) was measured in cm. Then, the following protocol was executed:

Measurements with Probefix

Step 1: The Probefix is attached to the patient.

Step 2: An apical 5 chamber view was obtained with a 2.5-MHz probe. A pulsed wave Doppler sample volume was measured just below the aortic valve (Fig. 2), sweep speed: 150 mm/s.

A velocity time integral (VTI) was calculated by tracing the envelope velocity. CO measurements were calculated by combining this result with the measurement of the opening of the aortic diameter, obtained in the PLAX.

Step 3: PLR test.

Stage 1: raise the lower limbs of the patient to a 45° while the patient's trunk is lowered in supine position.

Stage 2: after 1 min, measure the CO (Fig. 5).

Step 4: Steps 2–4 are repeated without the use of the Probefix.

Measurements without Probefix

Repeat step 2 and 3.

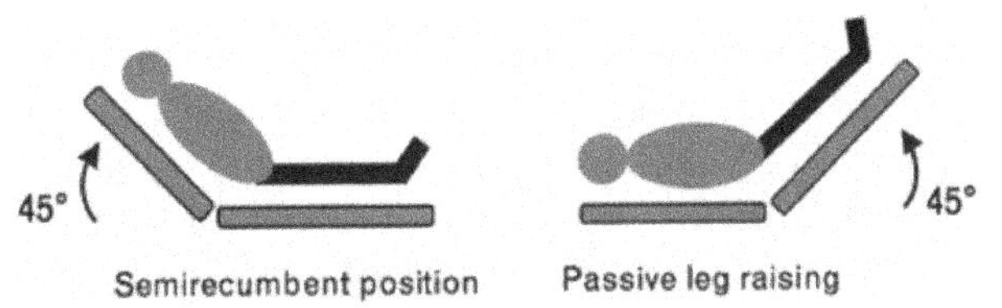

Fig. 5 The two positions in PLR

Statistical analysis

Primary study parameter(s)

1. Percentage of patients in which the Probefix can be used.
2. Scatter plots are constructed and the limits of agreement are calculated.

Secondary study parameter(s)

Possible side effects of the Probefix.

Descriptive statistics are presented as mean with standard deviation for normally distributed continuous data.

The local ethic committee approved the study (NL62664.091.17); informed consent was obtained from all participants (or their next of kin) included in the study.

Results

From May 2018 to April 2019, ten patients (six female and four male patients) were included.

In Table 1, patient characteristics are described.

In eight patients (80%), the Probefix could be used properly leading to interpretable measurements. In two patients, insufficient views with the Probefix were obtained and in these patients, there were sufficient views using the TTE probe manually; so, the problem was Probefix related and not TTE related.

One patient was breathing spontaneously, three patients were on controlled mechanical ventilation and six patients received pressure support. Mean peak inspiratory pressure was 13 cm H_2O ($\pm$6.9), mean post expiratory end pressure 6 cm H_2O ($\pm$5.1), mean tidal volume was 480 mL ($\pm$110) and mean LVOT was 2.1 cm ($\pm$0.23).

When compared to the Flotrac measurements, there was no significant difference in correlation between TTE measurements with or without the use of the Probefix

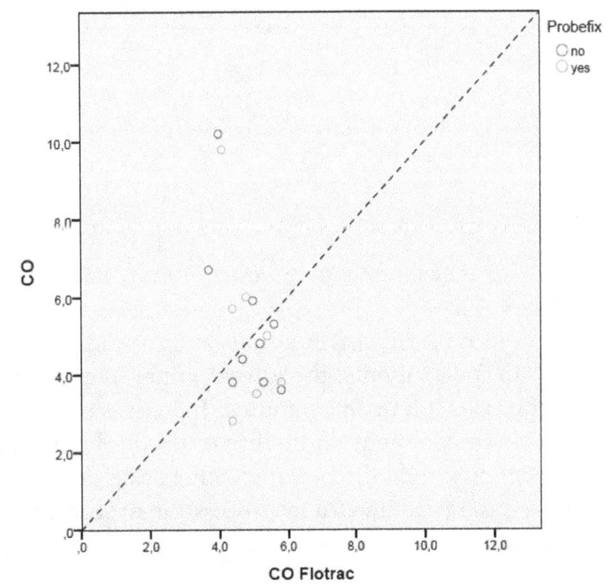

Fig. 6 Scatter plot transthoracic echo (TTE) cardiac output (CO) vs. Flotrac with (green points) and without the use of Probefix (blue points)

Table 1 Patient characteristics

	Age	M/F	BMI	Diagnosis	Mode of ventilation	Probefix feasible?
Patient 1	70	M	23.1	Out of hospital cardiac arrest	Pressure Control	Yes
Patient 2	64	F	24	Out of hospital cardiac arrest	Pressure regulated volume control	Yes
Patient 3	69	F	23.4	Pneumonia	Pressure support	Yes
Patient 4	67	F	23	Chronic bronchitis	Pressure support	Yes
Patient 5	45	F	17.7	Pneumonia	Pressure support	Yes
Patient 6	59	M	19.4	Abdominal sepsis	Pressure support	Yes
Patient 7	68	F	24.2	Interstitial lung disease	Pressure support	Yes
Patient 8	61	M	24.5	Pneumonia	Pressure support	No
Patient 9	73	M	22.8	Pneumonia	Pressure control	Yes
Patient 10	63	F	25.4	Out of hospital cardiac arrest	Pressure support	No
Mean $\pm$ SD	63.9 $\pm$ 7.9		23.5 $\pm$ 3.1			

M male, *F* female, *BMI* body mass index, *SD* standard deviation

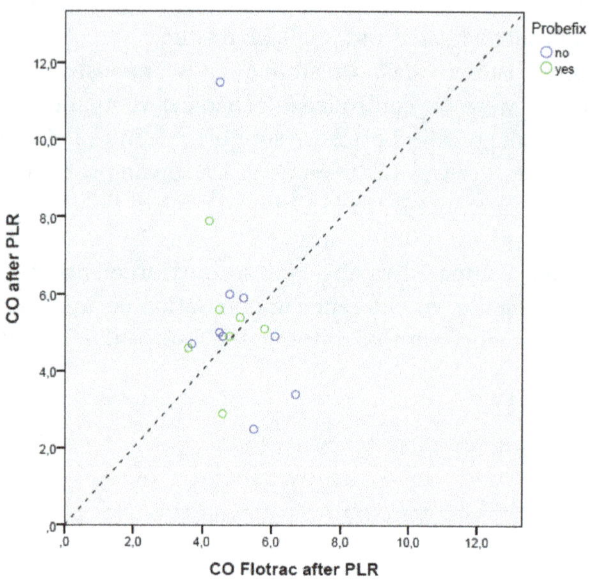

Fig. 7 Scatter plot transthoracic echo (TTE) cardiac output (CO) vs. Flotrac with (green points) and without the use of Probefix (blue points) after passive leg raising (PLR)

with the CO measurements done by Flotrac as a reference (Figs. 6, 7).

There were no serious skin lesions after the use of the Probefix. In four patients, there were minor skin marks that disappeared after some minutes. There was only one patient able to comment on the use of the Probefix and he reported only mild discomfort (2 on a scale of 10). In all patients, the time needed to process the protocol was within 15 min.

Discussion

We demonstrated in this small feasibility study that the Probefix could be used in eight of ten adult intensive care patients. All but one patient (patient 6) were medical patients. Male and female patients were included and patients were both on controlled and support mechanical ventilation. When compared to CO measurements using Flotrac, there was no statistical difference between CO measurements by TTE with or without the Probefix.

Our study is small and as far as we know the first on adult intensive care patient in which the use of Probefix is described. As mentioned before, there is already a small case study on pediatric intensive care patients but none on adult intensive care patients [5.]

The number of included patients was too small to be able to conclude whether the use of the Probefix will lead to more accurate CO measurements but the opposite was also not found.

We know that measuring CO on intensive care patients using TTE is difficult in terms of comparison to other techniques such as thermodilution techniques [2] but it is feasible when done by intensivists [10]. In this study, only one heartbeat to measure CO using TTE was used which is fewer then normally performed but the aim of this study was primarily to assess the feasibility of the Probefix, not to establish the accuracy of the TTE CO measurements. By adding a PLR test to this study, we investigated also whether the Probefix could be used for dynamic measurements and using the PLR test, the possible side effects of volume loading were diminished.

In this study, TTE measurements were compared to the measurements done by Flotrac. We acknowledge the fact that there are doubts about the usefulness of pulse pressure analysis as a monitoring tool on the intensive care [11, 12] but we think that the Flotrac measurements could be used as controls to compare the TTE measurements with and without the use of the Probefix.

No skin injuries in the studied patients were found. Whether Probefix creates pressure sores with longer attachment periods needs to be investigated. Nine of ten patients could not comment on the (dis)comfort of the Probefix due to sedative medication so on this one comment only we cannot speculate on this aspect of the use of Probefix.

There are many interesting options for the use of Probefix; eventually, its use enables continuous non-invasive CO measurements.

For this development, we need software that can translate the LVOT-VTI TTE images to real-time CO. By optimizing TTE for continuous CO monitoring, the use of more invasive techniques can be greatly diminished making this development of interest for almost every patient in the intensive care unit.

Conclusion

In this small feasibility study, it was shown that the Probefix can be used in eight out of ten adult intensive care patients for measuring CO also after a PLR test. More research is needed to further evaluate this new technique aiming at aspects such as accuracy, efficacy and costs.

Abbreviations

TTE: transthoracic echo; CO: cardiac output; PLR: passive leg raising; SVV: stroke volume variation; PLAX: parasternal long axis; VTI: velocity time integral; LVOT: left ventricle outflow tract.

Acknowledgements

Mrs. L. Roovers, PhD helped with the statistical analysis.

Authors' contributions

MJB, FHB and JGvdH designed the study, MJB and FHB included the patients and MJB, FHB and JGvdH contributed to the article. All authors read and approved the final manuscript.

Author details

[1] Department of Intensive Care, Rijnstate Hospital, PO box 9555, 6800 TA Arnhem, The Netherlands. [2] Department of Intensive Care, Radboud University Medical Center, PO box 9101, 6500 HB Nijmegen, The Netherlands.

References

1. Narasimhan M, Koenig SJ, Mayo PH (2014) Advanced echocardiography for the critical care physician: part 2. Chest 145(1):135–142
2. Wetterslev M, Moller-Sorensen H, Johansen RR, Perner A (2016) Systematic review of cardiac output measurements by echocardiography vs. thermodilution: the techniques are not interchangeable. Intensive Care Med 42(8):1223–1233
3. Salden OAE, van Everdingen WM, Spee R, Doevendans PA, Cramer MJ (2018) How I do it: feasibility of a new ultrasound probe fixator to facilitate high quality stress echocardiography. Cardiovasc Ultrasound. 16(1):6
4. Song H, Tsai SK, Liu J (2018) Tailored holder for continuous echocardiographic monitoring. Anesth Analg 126(2):435–437
5. Song H, Tsai SK, Liu J (2017) Tailored holder for continuous echocardiographic monitoring. Anesth Analg
6. Manecke GR (2005) Edwards FloTrac sensor and Vigileo monitor: easy, accurate, reliable cardiac output assessment using the arterial pulse wave. Expert Rev Med Devices 2(5):523–527
7. Biais M, Nouette-Gaulain K, Quinart A, Roullet S, Revel P, Sztark F (2009) Uncalibrated stroke volume variations are able to predict the hemodynamic effects of positive end-expiratory pressure in patients with acute lung injury or acute respiratory distress syndrome after liver transplantation. Anesthesiology 111(4):855–862
8. Rutlen DL, Wackers FJ, Zaret BL (1981) Radionuclide assessment of peripheral intravascular capacity: a technique to measure intravascular volume changes in the capacitance circulation in man. Circulation 64(1):146–152
9. Monnet X, Teboul JL (2008) Passive leg raising. Intensive Care Med 34(4):659–663
10. Villavicencio C, Leache J, Marin J, Oliva I, Rodriguez A, Bodí M et al (2019) Basic critical care echocardiography training of intensivists allows reproducible and reliable measurements of cardiac output. Ultrasound J 11(1):5
11. Vetrugno L, Costa MG, Spagnesi L, Pompei L, Chiarandini P, Gimigliano I et al (2011) Uncalibrated arterial pulse cardiac output measurements in patients with moderately abnormal left ventricular function. J Cardiothorac Vasc Anesth 25(1):53–58
12. Costa MG, Chiarandini P, Scudeller L, Vetrugno L, Pompei L, Serena G et al (2014) Uncalibrated continuous cardiac output measurement in liver transplant patients: liDCOrapid system versus pulmonary artery catheter. J Cardiothorac Vasc Anesth 28(3):540–546

Impact of an ultrasound-driven diagnostic protocol at early intensive-care stay

Julio Pontet[1,2,4*], Christian Yic[2], José L. Díaz-Gómez[3], Pablo Rodriguez[1], Igor Sviridenko[1], Diego Méndez[2], Sylvia Noveri[1], Ana Soca[1] and Mario Cancela[2]

Abstract

Background: Point-of-care ultrasound (POCUS) is a tool in increasing use, but there is still a lack of basics for its routine use and evidence of its impact in intensive care.

Objective: To measure the impact of POCUS on resource utilization, diagnostic accuracy, and clinical management in medical-surgical intensive care units (ICUs).

Methods: Prospective, controlled study, in two polyvalent ICUs. The patients were randomly assigned to POCUS or control group.

Interventions: POCUS patients received systematic ultrasound examination of optic nerve, lung/pleura, heart, abdomen, and venous system, performed at the bedside by trained intensivists. Control patients were treated by critical care specialists who do not perform ultrasound in their clinical practice.

Results: We included 80 patients, 40 per group. There were no significant differences in age, sex, APACHE II score, or admission diagnosis. POCUS group used fewer resources per patient in the first 5 days of hospitalization: chest radiography (2.6 ± 2.0 vs 4.1 ± 3.5, $P = 0.01$), additional ultrasound evaluations performed by a radiology specialist (0.6 ± 0.7 vs 1.1 ± 0.7, $P = 0.002$), and computed tomography studies (0.5 ± 0.6 vs 0.9 ± 0.7, $P = 0.007$). Time to perform any requested ultrasound evaluation after ICU admission was 2.1 ± 1.6 h versus 7.7 ± 6.7 h ($P = 0.001$). Systematic ultrasound evaluation led to better characterization of ICU admission diagnosis in 14 (35%) patients and change in clinical management in 24 (60%). POCUS group had lower fluid balance at 48 and 96 h after admission ($P = 0.01$) and spent less time mechanically ventilated (5.1 ± 5.7 days vs 8.8 ± 9.4, $P = 0.03$).

Conclusions: Systematic application of POCUS may decrease utilization of conventional diagnostic imaging resources and time of mechanical ventilation, and facilitate meticulous intravenous fluid administration in critically ill patients during the first week of stay in the ICU.

Trial registration ClinicalTrials.gov Identifier: NCT03608202.

Keywords: Clinical impact, Critical care, Diagnostic techniques and procedures, Point-of-care ultrasound, Point-of-care systems, Ultrasound protocol

*Correspondence: jpontet2003@gmail.com
[4] Larravide 2458, Montevideo, Uruguay
Full list of author information is available at the end of the article

Introduction

Ultrasonography is currently considered almost essential in the management of patients in shock, acute respiratory failure, or multiorgan dysfunction [1–4]. There is still a broad field of research aimed at generating a transformational change based on scientific evidence in critical care ultrasound [5, 6]. Given the inherent limitations for an accurate physical examination of the critically ill, imaging modalities such as chest, abdominal radiography, and computed tomography (CT) are considered more reliable, useful, and impactful in the critical care setting. However, their portability, versatility, and costs are less than ideal [1], with unnecessary delays in obtaining a diagnosis in the critically ill, and increased risk for hypoxemia or refractory arterial hypotension during transportation [3]. In contrast, ultrasound, a widely available, simpler technique that can be performed with portable equipment at the bedside, has gained progressive acceptance [4].

Recent investigations have demonstrated that multiorganic ultrasound decreases resource utilization and guides clinical management of critical ill patients while enhancing diagnostic accuracy [7–11]. Nevertheless, these previous publications lack a randomized and controlled trial methodology. We hypothesize that routine use of methodic, multisystemic ultrasound protocol in critically ill patients at admission to the intensive-care unit (ICU) reduces utilization of diagnostic resources and consultation and time to definitive diagnosis and tracheal extubation. Thus, the aims of our investigation were to analyze diagnostic and therapeutic implications of a point-of-care ultrasound (POCUS)-driven protocol during the first 5 days of ICU admission.

Materials and methods

Study design

Our prospective, randomized, controlled study was conducted at two major referral hospitals, Asociación Española Primera de Socorros Mutuos and Hospital Pasteur, Administración de Servicios de Salud del Estado. Patients admitted to a 12-bed medical-surgical ICU and 8-bed stepdown unit in those institutions were included in the study. The study protocol was approved by the Institutional Ethics Committee, and informed consent was obtained prior to each patient's enrollment.

Patients

We screened patients between February 1, 2017 and May 31, 2017, admitted to the ICUs. Inclusion criteria to the study were: (1) 18 years of age or older; (2) mechanical ventilation (MV) required at ICU admission. Patients with more than 24 h of hospitalization and those considered with low likelihood of survival by the treating intensivist at ICU admission were excluded.

Clinical data

We collected pertinent clinical data, including Acute Physiology and Chronic Health Evaluation, second version (APACHE II) score at admission, reason for admission to the ICU, and other relevant physiologic data.

The Distensibility index of inferior vena cava (%) was utilized as the primary measure for fluid responsiveness based on a previous investigation [12] (Table 1). In addition, we routinely used invasive MAP monitoring, capillary filling, hourly diuresis, central venous saturation, arteriovenous CO_2 difference, and plasma lactate measurement alongside measure of cardiac output and LVEF as supportive parameters of the clinical-decision making of administering intravenous fluids to patients suffering from shock.

Intervention

Two groups were compared; the study group received routine evaluation with an ultrasound-driven protocol (POCUS group), while a control group received conventional management according to the pre-established protocols in the ICU (in sepsis, pneumonia, postoperative care, heart failure and myocardial ischemia, trauma, COPD, etc.).

Patients were randomly assigned by permuted blocks to either the POCUS group or the control group.

The POCUS protocol is shown in Table 1; the following variables were evaluated: confirmation of initial diagnosis; change in initial diagnosis; new unsuspected finding; lack of change in initial diagnosis, inability to rule out a condition, and no changes in treatment; association with wrong diagnosis; and association with subsequent pharmacologic, medical, procedural, or surgical measures. In addition, these resource- and outcome-related variables were analyzed for comparison between the two groups: number of additional radiologic, ultrasound, and CT studies; number and type of procedures or interventions ordered; time to for ultrasound evaluation; duration of MV; length of stay in the ICU; and mortality rate.

POCUS studies were conducted with Logiq-e (General Electric Healthcare Japan Corporation) system with digital image storage capacity. Clinical data were saved in the SPSS Statistics 23 program (International Business Machines Corp.).

Statistical analysis

With a sample size of 40 patients per group for an annual population of 400 patients admitted to each ICU, we estimated a margin of error of 14% (95% CI). The qualitative

Table 1 POCUS protocol

Type of ultrasound	Instruments questions	Theoretic considerations
Optical behavior	Diameter optic nerve: right eye (mm); left eye (mm)	A diameter > 5.7 is a noninvasive indication of intracranial hypertension
Neck anatomy	Visualization of great vessels (jugular vein, carotid artery): normal or abnormal	Detection of patency (thrombosis) and anatomical variants or abnormalities
Pulmonary	Lung ultrasound score, 0–36 points	Score increases as pulmonary water increases; indicates pulmonary edema
Pleural	Presence of pleural occupation and estimation of pleural effusion (mL)	Confirmation of diagnosis, volume evaluation and follow-up
Echocardiography overall function	Estimation of left-ventricular systolic function by LVEF (%) and right-ventricular systolic function by TAPSE (mm)	LVEF > 50% and TAPSE > 15 mm is considered normal
Prediction of volume responsiveness	Distensibility index of inferior vena cava (%)	An index > 12% indicates response to intravenous fluid challenges
Estimation of CO	CO (L/min) estimated by left ventricular outflow tract by velocity time integral and diameter	Normal values, 4–6 L/min
Abdominal screening	FAST protocol for presence or absence of intraperitoneal free fluid	Presence of free fluid is abnormal
Biliary	Presence of lithiasis or dilated biliary tract	Biliary tract pathology may be an incidental finding or the cause of critical illness
Renal	Presence of urinary lithiasis or dilated urinary tract	Urinary tract pathology may be an incidental finding or the cause of critical illness
Ultrasound-guided invasive procedures	Venous or arterial access, pleural or abdominal drainage	Ultrasound-guided invasive procedures are more secure, with fewer adverse effects

CO cardiac output, *FAST* focused assessment with sonography in trauma, *IH* intracranial hypertension, *LVEF* left-ventricular ejection fraction, *POCUS* point-of-care ultrasound, *TAPSE* tricuspid annular plane systolic excursion

variables were records as percentages and the quantitative as mean ± standard deviation. For the comparison of mean between groups, either the Student's *t* test for independent groups or Mann–Whitney test was applied according to the case; and binaries in contingency tables by χ^2 or Fisher's exact test. A *P* value < 0.05 was considered significant in all tests.

Results

Patient demographics

We included 80 patients, 40 in each group. In the POCUS group, 24 were men (61%) and 16 were women (39%); similarly, in the control group, there were 25 men (62%) and 15 women (38%). There were no statistical differences between the groups regarding age, sex, APACHE II score at 24 h after admission, or reason for admission to ICU (Table 2).

Clinical information or decision-making following POCUS

The POCUS protocol was performed in 15–30 min in all cases.

In the POCUS group, 48 clinical decisions were made in 36 of 40 patients (90%). Furthermore, 35% of these observations were related to the diagnostic category, and either due to new or changed diagnosis. Modifications in pharmacologic therapy occurred in 24 patients (60%), and invasive maneuvers or procedures were necessary in 9 (23%) (Table 3).

Utilization of additional diagnostic testing

Overall, there was lower utilization of resources per patient during the first 5 days of ICU stay in the POCUS group compared with the control group (Table 4): lower number of chest radiography requested (2.6 ± 2.0 vs 4.1 ± 3.5, respectively, $P = 0.01$); lower utilization of additional ultrasound ICU imaging per radiology specialist (0.6 ± 0.7 vs 1.1 ± 0.7, respectively, $P = 0.002$); and fewer CT scans performed (0.5 ± 0.6 vs 0.9 ± 0.7, respectively, $P = 0.007$).

Analysis of delay times

We measured time from admission to first ultrasound (delay time). The delay in performing diagnostic ultrasound was significantly reduced in the POCUS group versus control (2.1 ± 1.6 h vs 7.7 ± 6.7, $P = 0.001$). In the control group, all diagnostic ultrasound evaluations were performed by radiology specialists available via telephone.

Table 2 Demographic data and diagnosis at admission in each group

Groups ($N=80$)	POCUS ($n=40$)	Control ($n=40$)	P value
Age, median ± SD, y	60 ± 15	57 ± 15	0.99
Sex, no. (%), male	24 (60.0)	23 (57.5%)	0.99
APACHE II, median ± SD	27 ± 9	26 ± 7	0.99
Diagnosis at admission, no. (%)			0.99
Respiratory sepsis	6 (15.0)	4 (10.0)	
Severe community-acquired pneumonia	5 (12.5)	3 (7.5)	
Decompensated heart failure	5 (12.5)	4 (10.0)	
Peritoneal sepsis	4 (10.0)	4 (10.0)	
Pulmonary tuberculosis	2 (5.0)	1 (2.5)	
Guillain–Barré syndrome	2 (5.0)	1 (2.5)	
Sepsis unknown origin	1 (2.5)	0 (0.0)	
Third-degree AV block	1 (2.5)	2 (5.0)	
Stroke	3 (7.5)	3 (7.5)	
COPD exacerbation	2 (5.0)	5 (12.5)	
Acute myocardial infarction	2 (5.0)	2 (5.0)	
Severe trauma	2 (5.0)	3 (7.5)	
Suicide attempt	2 (5.0)	3 (7.5)	
Acute bacterial meningitis	1 (2.5)	0 (0.0)	
Pulmonary embolism	1 (2.5)	1 (2.5)	
Thyrotoxicosis	1 (2.5)	0 (0.0)	
Enteric sepsis	0 (0.0)	2 (5.0)	
Acute encephalitis	0 (0.0)	1 (2.5)	
Status epilepticus	0 (0.0)	1 (2.5)	

APACHE II Acute Physiology and Chronic Health Evaluation II, *AV* atrioventricular, *COPD* chronic obstructive pulmonary disease, *POCUS* point-of-care ultrasound

Table 3 Description of changes in clinical information or decisions led by ultrasound

Modification in diagnosis and therapeutic decisions led by US	No. changes	No. patients
Related to clinical decision-making, total	48	36
New or unidentified diagnosis: Pneumonia, 2; significant pleural effusion, 5; pneumothorax, 1; significant pericardial effusion, 1; cholecystitis, 1	10	8
Clinical diagnosis: Pneumonia to respiratory distress due to biliary sepsis, 1; pneumonia to heart failure, 2; asthma to pneumonia, 1	4	4
Pharmacological therapy: Fluid challenges, 6; start diuretics, 5; dobutamine, 5; noradrenaline, 2; antibiotics, 5; alteplase, 1	24	16
Invasive procedures: Thoracic drainage, 5; emergency bronchoscopy, 2; laparotomy, 1; suprapubic bladder catheterization, 1	9	7
Alveolar recruitment maneuver, 1	1	1
No changes	0	4

US ultrasound

Clinical outcomes

Fluid management

The POCUS-driven decision of fluid management in each patient was left at treating intensivist discretion. Similarly, clinical decisions on fluid, inotropic, or vasopressor therapy, and adjustments to MV were made based on POCUS assessment. Fluid balance (FB) was much lower in the POCUS group than in the control at 48 and 96 h after ICU admission (− 1600 ± 2750 mL vs − 400 ± 2130 mL, $P=0.03$, and − 3200 ± 3510 mL vs − 890 ± 3900 mL, $P=0.006$, respectively). There was a significant positive linear correlation between left-ventricular ejection fraction (LVEF) and FB at 48 (Pearson correlation $r=0.57$, $P=0.002$) (Fig. 1) and 96 h ($r=0.58$, $P=0.03$).

Table 4 Comparison of resource utilization, length of stay and mortality in ultrasound-driven evaluation versus conventional management in ICU

Variable	POCUS group (mean ± SD)	Control group (mean ± SD)	*P* value
Chest radiography[a]	2.6 ± 2.0	4.1 ± 3.5	0.01
US requested outside of ICU[a]	0.6 ± 0.7	1.1 ± 0.7	0.002
Computed tomography[a]	0.5 ± 0.6	0.9 ± 0.7	0.007
Mechanical ventilation, days	5.1 ± .7	8.8 ± 9.4	0.03
Length of stay in ICU, d	9 ± 8	13 ± 10	0.05
Mortality, no. (%)	7 (17)	6 (15)	>0.99

Echo echocardiography, *ICU* intensive-care unit, *US* ultrasound

[a] During the first 5 days of intensive-care unit stay

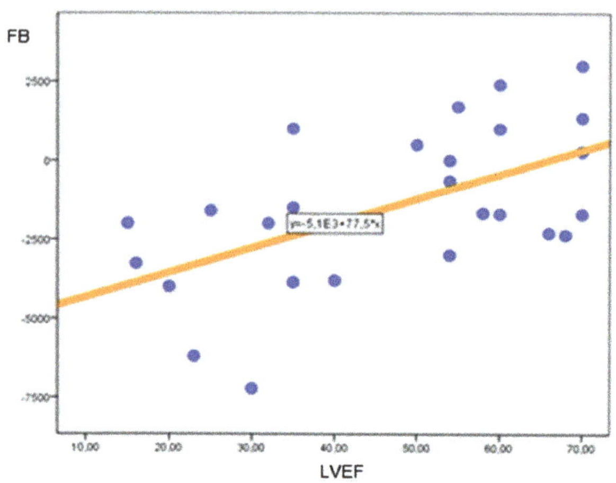

Fig. 1 Linear correlation between fluid balance at 48 h and left-ventricular ejection fraction. Pearson correlation $r = 0.57$, $P = 0.002$. *FB* fluid balance, *LVEF* left-ventricular ejection fraction

Duration of MV

The POCUS group showed a lower duration of MV than the control (5.1 ± 5.7 days vs 8.8 ± 9.4 days, $P = 0.03$) (Table 4). There was no significant correlation between the time spent on MV and FB, or between the time spent on MV and LVEF.

Length of stay in ICU and mortality

Mortality rates did not differ between POCUS and control groups. Of note, there was a tendency for decreased ICU length of stay with POCUS (Table 4).

Discussion

We demonstrated the direct impact of a routine POCUS-driven protocol in patients during the early phase after admission to medical–surgical ICUs. A systematic application of POCUS resulted in decreased utilization of conventional diagnostic imaging resources and time of MV, and facilitated a judicious intravenous fluid administration in critically ill patients during the first week of ICU hospitalization. Application of routine POCUS appears to be safe if utilized by appropriately trained intensivist as no complications were directly associated with POCUS use in the study group.

Previous investigations [2, 5] applying particular ICU-sound protocol led to more accurate admission diagnosis in 25.6% to 24.9%. They had an observational design, but are comparable to the 22% accuracy rate of new or corrected diagnoses in our study. Moreover, the majority of our patient population suffered from sepsis. Manno et al. [2] proposed that septic patients may be the most favored subgroup of patients receiving a POCUS protocol because of the myriad of information and therapies that can be tailored to each individual patient.

The main effect of routine utilization of our POCUS protocol was the clinical decision-making, more specifically in pharmacologic management adjustments in shock patients (60%) and ordering of ultrasound-guided procedures (23%). In our study, we found that 23% of our population required ultrasound-guided invasive procedures, which is similar to the 21.6% reported by the Manno group [2]. Vignon et al. [13] described a change in therapeutic management of patients in 51% of the cases, and Bernier-Jean et al. [5] in 44%.

Management of intravascular volume status can be a difficult decision at the bedside. Meticulous fluid management in treating shock patients with heart disease is desirable. In our case, the most common clinical decision was related to fluid management. Similar findings have been described in an observational study [13], but we emphasize the randomized-controlled design of our study. Nonetheless, our direct comparison of timely ultrasound-driven versus conventional management allows us to represent the current practice in the majority of medical centers due to lack of routine utilization of ultrasound by intensivists. Furthermore, positive fluid responsiveness test does not indicated necessity of further fluid administration, our clinical-decision making was determined by the echocardiography measurements (LVEF, IVC distensibility index) in addition to systemic perfusion surrogates (central venous saturation, arteriovenous CO2 difference, and plasma lactate measurements). Finally, in cases of heart failure, we guided restriction of fluids by signs of pulmonary and systemic congestion. However, we acknowledge tolerance to fluids must be assessed with diastolic function parameters and may be in addition to lung ultrasonography [14–16].

Our POCUS protocol led to a significantly lower utilization of chest radiography, ultrasound performed by non-intensivist specialists, and CT scans (up to 56% reduction in CT requests). We found a reduction of radiology evaluation utilization from 4.1 in the control group to 2.6 in the POCUS group (63% reduction). This finding differs from other groups reporting 22% to 26% reduction in radiography utilization [17, 18]. Possible explanations include intensivist discretion versus specific protocol, considerable critical care ultrasound expertise by attending intensivist at time of the study, and more availability of fully capable ultrasound devices. Of note, the American College of Radiology expert panel recommended daily radiology for each intubated patient [17]. The direct clinical implications of our findings were associated with lower radiation exposure, less intra-hospital transportation of unstable patients, and inherent economic savings with more sophisticated evaluations, including in improved imaging suites workflow and reduced necessity for personnel to transport patients [19–21].

We found a significant correlation between cardiac function (left systolic ventricle function measured by LVEF index) and a negative FB in the first 5 days of ICU management. This might indicate that judicious fluid management and decisions in administration of diuretic agents are facilitated with real-time utilization of POCUS since ICU admission. We did not find a significant correlation between time spent on MV and FB or between duration of MV and LVEF. This can possibly be explained by the heterogeneity of our population. However, there was correlation between lower LVEF and negative FB, since patients with low LVEF are likely to receive less fluids and more diuretics.

We acknowledge several limitations in the current investigation. First, our small patient population avoids finding significant differences in meaningful clinical outcomes, such as mortality. Second, we analyzed only the first 5 days of ICU stay. However, as patients stay longer in the ICU, additional confounding factors not necessarily related with admission diagnosis can affect the outcomes (late-onset, ventilator-associated pneumonia). Mortality was similar between both groups, but it should be noted that future studies with larger patient populations having a shorter time of MV as found in the POCUS group could potentially determine a decrease in mortality related to MV complications. Third, we did not find a significant correlation between normal or high ejection fraction and pulmonary B profile in our study that can imply possible tolerance to fluid administration. However, patients with CHF and preserved EF can be only characterized with advanced echocardiography parameters of diastolic function. We recognize that the lack of diastolic function assessment is another limitation of this study. However, we aimed to evaluate a practical approach for assessment of ventricular function and fluid responsiveness, so we propose further investigation of the correlation between normal or high ejection fraction and pulmonary B profile in addition to diastolic function assessment in septic shock patients.

Finally, the absence of a reposition protocol guided by pre-established ultrasound should be endorsed in multicentric studies.

Conclusions

A systematically applied POCUS protocol upon admission to the ICU can guide diagnostic and therapeutic decisions in critically ill patients. This potentially leads to greater resourcefulness and shorter duration of MV. Definitive associations, such as ultrasound-driven fluid resuscitation and improved outcomes, remain to be proven in larger multicenter studies. Diastolic function assessment can improve overall evaluation of fluid tolerance to the fluid management of septic shock patients.

Acknowledgements

Stella Calvo, MD for his technical help in the elaboration of the manuscript.

Preliminary results and abstract presented at 13th WINFOCUS World Congress, Argentina, September 2017, and received the Golden Probe Award as Best Poster Presentation.

Authors' contributions

JP and CY have made substantial contributions to the conception and design of the work, the acquisition, analysis, and interpretation of data, and have drafted the work. JLD have made contributions to the analysis and interpretation of data and substantively revised it. PR, IS, and DM have made contributions to the acquisition and analysis of data. SN, AS, and MC have made contributions to the analysis and interpretation of data and substantively revised it. All authors read and approved the final manuscript.

Author details

[1] Intensive Care Unit, Hospital Pasteur, Administración de Servicios de Salud del Estado, Montevideo, Uruguay. [2] Intensive Care Unit, Asociación Española Primera de Socorros Mutuos, Montevideo, Uruguay. [3] Department of Critical Care Medicine, Mayo Clinic, Jacksonville, USA. [4] Larravide 2458, Montevideo, Uruguay.

References

1. Frankel HL, Kirkpatrick AW, Elbarbary M et al (2015) Guidelines for the appropriate use of bedside general and cardiac ultrasonography in the evaluation of critically ill patients—part I: general ultrasonography. Crit Care Med 43:2479–2502
2. Manno E, Navarra M, Faccio L et al (2012) Deep impact of ultrasound in the intensive care unit: the "ICU-sound" protocol. Anesthesiology 117:801–809
3. Moore CL, Copel JA (2011) Point-of-care ultrasonography. N Engl J Med 364:749–757
4. Narasimhan M, Koenig SJ, Mayo PH (2016) A whole-body approach to point of care ultrasound. Chest 150:772–776
5. Bernier-Jean A, Albert M, Shiloh AL, Eisen LA, Williamson D, Beaulieu Y (2017) The diagnostic and therapeutic impact of point-of-care ultrasonography in the intensive care unit. J Intensive Care Med. 32:197–203
6. Bossone E, DiGiovine B, Watts S et al (2002) Range and prevalence of cardiac abnormalities in patients hospitalized in a medical ICU. Chest 122:1370–1376
7. Kristensen MS, Teoh WH, Graumann O, Laursen CB (2014) Ultrasonography for clinical decision-making and intervention in airway management: from the mouth to the lungs and pleurae. Insights Imaging. 5:253–279
8. Laursen CB, Sloth E, Lassen AT et al (2014) Point-of-care ultrasonography in patients admitted with respiratory symptoms: a single-blind, randomised controlled trial. Lancet Respir Med. 2:638–646

9. Oks M, Cleven KL, Cardenas-Garcia J et al (2014) The effect of point-of-care ultrasonography on imaging studies in the medical ICU: a comparative study. Chest 146:1574–1577
10. Pontet J, Yic C, Diaz-Gomez J, et al. Ultrasonografía En Medicina de Urgencias, Terapia Intensiva Y Anestesia. 1st ed: Montevideo; 2016
11. Volpicelli G, Lamorte A, Tullio M et al (2013) Point-of-care multiorgan ultrasonography for the evaluation of undifferentiated hypotension in the emergency department. Intensive Care Med 39:1290–1298
12. Feissel M, Michard F, Faller JP, Teboul JL (2004) The respiratory variation in inferior cava diameter as a guide to fluid therapy. Intensive Care Med 30(9):1834–1837
13. Vignon P, Frank MB, Lesage J et al (2004) Hand-held echocardiography with Doppler capability for the assessment of critically-ill patients: is it reliable? Intensive Care Med 30:718–723
14. Geri G, Vignon P, Aubry A, Fedou AL, Charron C, Silva S, Repessé X, Vieillard-Baron A (2019) Cardiovascular clusters in septic shock combining clinical and echocardiographic parameters: a post hoc analysis. Intensive Care Med 45(5):657–667
15. Nair S, Sauthoff H (2019) Assessing extravascular lung water with ultrasound: a tool to individualize fluid management? J Intensive Care Med. https://doi.org/10.1177/0885066619855000 **(Epub ahead of print)**
16. Orme RM, Oram MP, McKinstry CE (2009) Impact of echocardiography on patient management in the intensive care unit: an audit of district general hospital practice. Br J Anaesth 102:340–344
17. Expert Panel on Thoracic Imaging, McComb BL, Chung JH et al (2016) ACR appropriateness criteria routine chest radiography. J Thorac Imaging. 31:W13–15
18. Krinsley JS (2003) Test-ordering strategy in the intensive care unit. J Intensive Care Med. 18:330–339
19. Expert Round Table on Echocardiography in ICU (2014) International consensus statement on training standards for advanced critical care echocardiography. Intensive Care Med 40:654–666
20. Kue R, Brown P, Ness C, Scheulen J (2011) Adverse clinical events during intrahospital transport by a specialized team: a preliminary report. Am J Crit Care. 20:153–161 **(quiz 162)**
21. Smith I, Fleming S, Cernaianu A (1990) Mishaps during transport from the intensive care unit. Crit Care Med 18:278–281

11

ABCDE of prehospital ultrasonography

Rein Ketelaars[1,2*], Gabby Reijnders[3], Geert-Jan van Geffen[1,2], Gert Jan Scheffer[1] and Nico Hoogerwerf[1,2]

Abstract

Prehospital point-of-care ultrasound used by nonradiologists in emergency medicine is gaining ground. It is feasible on-scene and during aeromedical transport and allows health-care professionals to detect or rule out potential harmful conditions. Consequently, it impacts decision-making in prioritizing care, selecting the best treatment, and the most suitable transport mode and destination. This increasing relevance of prehospital ultrasonography is due to advancements in ultrasound devices and related technology, and to a growing number of applications. This narrative review aims to present an overview of prehospital ultrasonography literature. The focus is on civilian emergency (trauma and non-trauma) setting. Current and potential future applications are discussed, structured according to the airway, breathing, circulation, disability, and environment/exposure (ABCDE) approach. Aside from diagnostic implementation and specific protocols, procedural guidance, therapeutic ultrasound, and challenges are reviewed.

Keywords: Prehospital, Ultrasonography, Diagnostic imaging, Emergency medical services, Air ambulances, Emergency medicine, Review

Introduction

Point-of-care ultrasound (PoCUS) refers to a sign or symptom-based ultrasonography (US) examination either at the bedside or wherever patients are being treated [1]. The use of PoCUS by nonradiologists is being adopted in prehospital emergency care. It may help health-care professionals of emergency medical services (EMS) to diagnose or rule out potential life-threatening or otherwise harmful conditions [2–4]. Prehospital point-of-care ultrasonography (PHUS) may have an impact on decision-making in prioritizing initial treatment and choosing the most appropriate hospital and mode of transportation [5, 6]. Besides deploying PHUS for diagnostic purposes, it is used for procedural and therapeutic interventions.

Although the use of PHUS is increasing, its added value is still under debate. In 2010, Jørgensen was unable to conclude that PHUS improves treatment of trauma patients [5]. Five years later, O'Dochartaigh found only moderate evidence to support the use of PHUS in physician-staffed prehospital systems [6]. A recent Cochrane review concluded that, at best, abdominal US has no negative impact on mortality and morbidity, although it might reduce ordered computed tomography (CT)-scans [7]. Rudolph et al. found that PHUS may improve patient management with respect to diagnosis, treatment, and hospital referral [8]. However, they were unable to assess the effect of PHUS on patient outcomes based on the current body of evidence.

The image quality, size, and weight of portable ultrasound devices are improving. Costs for equipment are decreasing, while the number of indications for PHUS is increasing. The result is an exponentially growing body of publications, including some narrative reviews, with varying perspectives [9–11].

This narrative review is based on relevant papers selected from an extensive search in the Ovid MEDLINE® database. We added additional papers found in the references and from the authors' personal libraries.

The aim is to present an overview of the literature on PHUS in a civilian emergency (trauma and non-trauma) setting. The first part deals with current PHUS applications structured according to the familiar airway,

*Correspondence: Rein.Ketelaars@radboudumc.nl

[1] Radboud Institute for Health Sciences, Department of Anesthesiology, Pain, and Palliative Medicine, Radboud university medical center, Geert Grooteplein-Zuid 10, 6525 GA Nijmegen, The Netherlands

Full list of author information is available at the end of the article

breathing, circulation, disability, and exposure/environment (ABCDE) approach [12]. The second part will discuss interventions, procedures, challenges, and potential future applications.

PHUS in general

The use of PHUS provides diagnostic and therapeutic benefit, and it does not delay patient management [3, 8, 13–15]. It has been found to be feasible to enhance clinical assessment in a variety of out-of-hospital settings [15]. Price was among the first to show that ultrasonography (US) is also feasible during helicopter transport and that focused assessment with sonography for trauma (FAST) can be rapidly performed in-flight and has no influence on aircraft avionics [16].

Physicians and paramedics without being educated as a radiologist can be trained effectively to perform PoCUS. Lyon et al. demonstrated that prehospital critical care providers could learn to detect the sonographic sliding lung sign with a high level of sensitivity (97%) and specificity (94%) and retain their skill over time [17]. Forty physicians participated in a 4-h hands-on training and demonstrated significant improvements in the ability to perform US examinations [18]. Although the initial learning curve for FAST is steep, it starts to flatten after 30–100 scans [19]. Probably even more training and experience is required for advanced applications such as transcranial Doppler for ischemic stroke or specific triage protocols.

With the right education and mentorship, paramedics can obtain ultrasound images of sufficient quality to positively identify significant pathologies in critically ill patients [20]. A recent Canadian study found that PHUS performed by both physicians and non-physicians supported interventions in both trauma and medical patients [21].

The reported diagnostic accuracy of PHUS varies widely. Some reported a sensitivity of 85–90% and a specificity of 96–100% for chest, abdominal, and cardiac US. Positive predictive value (PPV) and negative predictive value (NPV) were 100 and 95.5% [3, 13]. Diagnostic accuracy during transportation also varies. For PHUS during transfer by ground ambulance and PHUS on-scene, Brun reported a sensitivity of 94.7 and 95.2%, respectively [22]. In-flight ultrasound examinations of the lung, abdomen, and pericardium yielded a sensitivity of only 50–64.7% when compared to pathology that required an intervention, rather than to all positive findings [23]. Others found a sensitivity of 78.6% for in-flight extended FAST (eFAST) compared to CT scan [24]. Because of the high specificity, the activation of a trauma surgery team is justified for positive PHUS findings [23].

Despite the range in diagnostic accuracy, PHUS is still highly reliable compared to clinical assessment [3, 5]. In 169 non-trauma patients, PHUS improved the diagnostic accuracy based on traditional clinical examination to 67% compared to the final in-hospital diagnosis. Diagnostic accuracy was improved in 90% of patients in whom the initial diagnosis was uncertain (n = 115) [25]. Blaivas found that PHUS improved the certainty of the diagnosis in 68% of 25 mainly non-trauma patients [26].

PHUS potentially impacts life-saving procedures, priorities in the care for one or many patients, and the most appropriate destination. Indications exist that PHUS benefits outcome, but evidence is still lacking [5]. Nevertheless, O'Dochartaigh and Jørgensen noted that PHUS impacted and streamlined in-hospital treatment [5, 6]. The impact was not quantified, but O'Dochartaigh suggested that PHUS-supported interventions were more frequent in the more severely injured patients.

Diagnostic applications

A—Airway

First-attempt success rates of prehospital rapid sequence intubations vary between 46 and 85% [27]. An attempt fails when the endotracheal tube (ETT) cannot be placed between the vocal cords in the trachea or is inadvertently placed in the esophagus. It is of paramount importance to acknowledge esophageal intubation as soon as possible.

The use of tracheal and cricothyroid ultrasound can be very useful to confirm correct ETT placement. This was first described in neonates by Slovis in 1986 [28]. Fourteen years later, Dreschler was the first to also visualize the esophagus and to detect esophageal intubation in five out of five cadaver models [29]. A recent review showed a pooled sensitivity and specificity of, respectively, 98 and 94% of transtracheal US in emergency intubations [30]. Therefore, the confirmation of correct ETT position by PoCUS in the prehospital setting is likely to be beneficial [12, 31, 32]. Although capnography is considered the gold standard to confirm a correct tube position, it does not discriminate between endotracheal and endobronchial intubation [33]. Furthermore, in a prehospital setting, chest radiography is impossible, and auscultation is not always feasible. Therefore, PHUS might be a valuable tool to assess the airway [34].

Zadel et al. confirmed endotracheal tube position by the detection of bilateral lung sliding and bilateral diaphragmatic excursion in 124 out-of-hospital patients [32]. Esophageal intubation occurred in 13 patients (10.5%), of which only 30% was detected visually or by auscultation before waveform capnography was recorded. Both sensitivity and specificity of PHUS for a correct tube position was 100%. The performance of PHUS took a median of 30 s (sd = 8–120 s). A prospective study in pediatrics preferred the assessment of bilateral diaphragmatic excursions to confirm proper ETT placement [35]. Therefore, the assessment of lung sliding and diaphragmatic excursions is of value in the absence of chest radiography or capnography.

B—Chest, pulmonary

The cause of acute dyspnea is not immediately apparent, especially in the prehospital setting. Caregivers must differentiate between a cardiac or a pulmonary cause. In an emergency department (ED) study, Kajimoto proposed a quick method to integrate (1) lung ultrasound, (2) cardiac ultrasound, and (3) measurements of the inferior vena cava (LCI) [36]. Lung ultrasound is performed in eight chest areas (four anterior and four lateral). Cardiac ultrasound estimates the global left ventricular function and mitral or tricuspid valve regurgitation. Subsequently, collapsibility of the inferior vena cava is determined. The LCI integrated examination will take only up to 3 min. The sensitivity and specificity were 94.3 and 91.9% for acute heart failure syndromes, compared to the traditional methods of differentiating between pulmonary and cardiac causes including electrocardiogram, chest X-ray, and B-type natriuretic peptide (BNP).

A similar *triple scan* consisting of basic echocardiography, lung ultrasound, and assessment of inferior vena cava collapsibility was proposed by Mantuani et al. [37]. They included 57 patients with acute dyspnea caused by acute decompensated heart failure (ADHF), chronic obstructive pulmonary disease (COPD), and pneumonia. After the triple scan, the accuracy of the diagnosis, based on history and physical examination, increased from 53 to 77%. Sensitivity and specificity of the triple scan for ADHF were 100 and 84%.

Lichtenstein's bedside lung ultrasound in emergency (BLUE) protocol allows rapid diagnosis of acute respiratory failure and can be completed in under 3 min [38, 39]. Four standardized points on either side of the chest are assessed for ten signs indicative of normal lung surface, pleural effusions, lung consolidations, alveolar–interstitial syndrome, and pneumothorax. For simplicity, echocardiography is not included. Distinct profiles are recognized for the main causes of respiratory distress: pneumonia, congestive heart failure, COPD, asthma, pulmonary embolism, and pneumothorax as summarized in Table 1. It has a diagnostic accuracy of > 90% [40].

The LCI, *triple scan*, and BLUE protocol all might be relevant and valuable in the prehospital setting because of simplicity and nominal time investment. With the help of these protocols, the EMS caregiver can accurately differentiate between causes and direct treatment and avoid unnecessary or harmful interventions.

Besides the diagnosis of dyspnea, lung US may be used to support prehospital continuous positive airway pressure (CPAP) treatment [41]. In 20 ADHF patients, a physician-staffed EMS sonographically assessed 15 chest wall regions before and after CPAP treatment compared to standard treatment. The number of B-lines (explained in Table 1 and shown in Figs. 1, 2) was significantly lower in the CPAP group, and their respiratory and hemodynamic variables improved after CPAP. The number of B-lines correlates with the amount of extravascular lung water (EVLW) and NT-proBNP levels and thus with the severity of ADHF. They develop at a pulmonary artery occlusion pressure (PAOP) > 18 mmHg [42].

In high-altitude medicine, Wimalasena described the value of lung US in the early detection of high-altitude pulmonary edema (HAPE) before symptoms appear, and in differentiating HAPE from other causes of dyspnea such as pneumonia or pneumothorax [43]. The number of B-lines, indicating an increased amount of EVLW, is inversely correlated with the oxygen saturation and both values improve on (early) treatment [44].

B—Chest, traumatic

Pneumothorax

Using PoCUS for detecting pneumothorax is feasible, fast, without any radiation, has a steep learning curve and high diagnostic accuracy, and it allows for dynamic and repeated examinations [45, 46].

A pneumothorax is characterized by the abolition of lung sliding, the absence of B-lines, and the appearance of the A-line sign [39]. Lung sliding is the representation of the visceral and parietal pleura sliding against each other during respiration. B-lines are the result of the accumulation of fluid in the pulmonary interstitium. Therefore, the presence of B-lines on PoCUS rules out a pneumothorax. Horizontal A-lines are reflections of the pleural line caused by gas below the parietal pleura either within or outside of the lung. These signs are explained further in Table 1; adapted from Lichtenstein's paper on the BLUE and FALLS protocol [39]. A normal lung US image is shown in Figs. 1, 2, and 3. Images of pneumothorax are shown in Figs. 4, 5, and Additional file 1: Video 1.

An important implication of detecting or excluding pneumothorax is the subsequent decision to perform (or withhold) a tube thoracostomy. An evaluation of prehospital chest US in 281 patients revealed that the acute medical management changed in 21%. The intention to introduce a tube thoracostomy was abandoned in 4% (n = 10) and the transport destination changed in another 4% [4]. Similarly, Mazur found that chest US examinations (n = 60) performed in preparation for air transport helped them prevent four (8%) chest tube thoracostomies [47].

Table 1 BLUE protocol profiles. Lichtenstein [39]

P#	Profile name	Location	Appearance	Implication/diagnosis
1	A-profile	Anterior chest wall	Lung sliding—visualization of the movement of the visceral pleura against the parietal pleura with respiration A-lines—an indication of the presence of air below the parietal pleura[a]	Normal lung surface
2	B-profile		Lung sliding Lung rockets—a pattern of three vertical B-lines caused by edema in the interlobular septa[b]	Pulmonary edema
3	B′-profile		No lung sliding—in the B′ profile lung sliding is abolished by the deposition of fibrin caused by pneumonia Lung rockets	Pneumonia
4	A/B-profile		Unilateral lung rockets—indicative for a (unilateral) pneumonia and does not correspond with generalized pulmonary edema	Pneumonia
5	C-profile	Anterior chest wall	Anterior lung consolidation—anteriorly located, therefore unlike to be caused by hemodynamic pulmonary edema or embolism	Pneumonia
6	A-profile without DVT[c]		Lung sliding A-lines[a] No DVT	Normal
	A-no-V-PLAPS profile	Posterolateral chest wall	Lung sliding A-lines[a] No DVT PLAPS[e]—posterolateral alveolar and/or pleural syndrome—pulmonary consolidation and pleural effusion	Pneumonia
7	A-profile with DVT[c]		Lung sliding A-lines[a] DVT	Pulmonary embolism
8	A′-profile	Anterior chest wall	No lung sliding—lung sliding abolished by separation of the visceral pleura from the parietal pleura A-lines—an indication of the presence of air below the parietal pleura[a]	Pneumothorax when the mandatory 'lung point'[d] is visualized
9	A-profile without DVT and no PLAPS (nude profile)		Lung sliding A-lines[a] No DVT No PLAPS	Asthma or COPD

The bedside lung ultrasound in emergency (BLUE) protocol defines nine profiles. They are defined by their sonographic appearance and are associated with the different diagnoses as described in the right-most column

[a] A-lines = Horizontal repetition of the pleural line appearing below the pleural line at multiples of the skin–pleural line distance. Their appearance is an indication of air below the parietal pleura, either in or outside of the lung. They are particularly apparent in the absence of B-lines potentially obscuring the A-lines

[b] B-lines = A long, well-defined, hyperechoic comet tail artifact arising from the pleural line that obliterates the A-lines

[c] DVT= Deep venous thrombosis. Has to be separately found or excluded at the lower extremities

[d] Lung point = The location where the visceral pleura is only partially in contact with the parietal pleura. With respirations, the A′ profile (without lung rockets) is intermittently replaced with the A-profile (lung rockets are possible). The lung point is a pathognomonic sign for the diagnosis of pneumothorax! See Additional file 1: Video 1

[e] PLAPS= Posterolateral alveolar and/or pleural syndrome (posterolateral consolidations or pleural effusions)

Detection of pneumothorax during flight

In some EMS systems, patients are evaluated and treated while in-flight in a helicopter or fixed-wing aircraft. In prehospital and flight medicine, lung US was found to be feasible and safe [16, 24, 48]. For instance, M-mode (Figs. 3, 5) ultrasonography was used to successfully evaluate a pleural interface model on board a helicopter while stationary, with rotor rotation before take-off, and at level flight [49]. Madill reported the case of a blast injury patient in whom an in-flight chest US examination identified an untreated pneumothorax. This directed the decision to perform a successful in-flight thoracentesis and tube thoracostomy [50]. In 2013, Roline was reported to be the first to evaluate in-flight chest US in a helicopter emergency medical service (HEMS) operation [51]. They performed 41 chest US examinations in 71 patients. Expert sonographers reviewed the images and reached substantial agreement with the providers. Image quality was good or poor in 54 and 46%, respectively. Challenges consisted of the

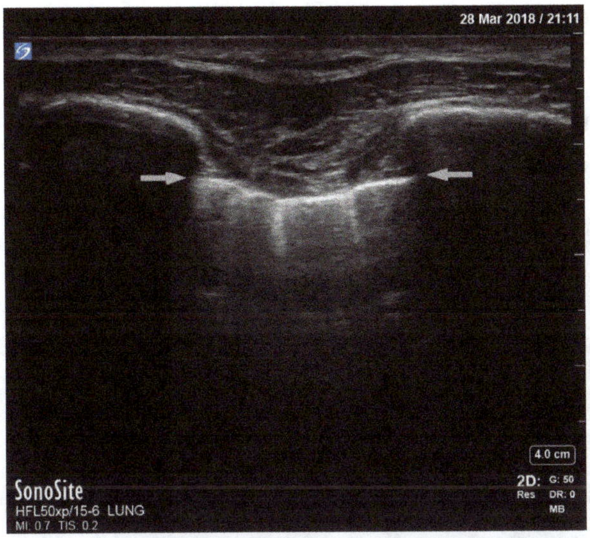

Fig. 1 Normal lung. A normal lung ultrasound image acquired with a 15–6 MHz linear transducer. The ribs are visible with their anechoic shadows on both sides of the image. The pleural line is shown in between the ribs, indicated with two horizontal arrows. Emanating down from the pleural line are comet tails. B-lines (not visible here) also start at the pleural line, but extend all the way down to edge of the image

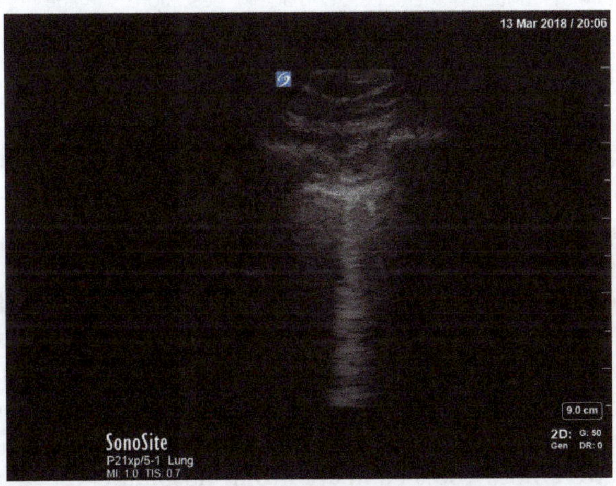

Fig. 2 Normal lung + B-line. A normal lung ultrasound image acquired with a 5–1 MHz phased-array cardiac transducer. In the middle of the image, one B-line is seen. This is also seen in healthy subjects and a single B-line is without meaning

lack of time, limited aircraft space, and, less frequently, the presence of pacer pads. They concluded that in-flight chest US is feasible, has a steep learning curve, and that additional training is needed to improve image quality. Quick et al. found that the diagnostic accuracy of in-flight US for pneumothorax is nearly similar to US in the ED: 91 and 96%, respectively [52].

These reports suggest that PHUS augment the diagnostic capabilities of prehospital aeromedical providers, also when in-flight, and might lead to better outcomes.

Hemothorax

No studies with substantial data on the diagnostic performance of PHUS and hemothorax are available. Ketelaars described that PHUS detected one hemothorax in seven cases specifically assessed for hemothorax with 100% accuracy [4]. In a 2007 *best evidence topic report* the authors concluded that ultrasound is a sensitive, specific, and accurate method to detect the presence of hemothorax in trauma patients [53]. A more recent meta-analysis of hospital studies revealed a pooled sensitivity and specificity of 67 and 99% of PoCUS for hemothorax. For radiography, these were 54 and 99% [54]. Therefore, PoCUS for hemothorax may be valuable in both in-hospital and prehospital settings. Future studies might demonstrate the added value of early, prehospital, detection of hemothorax although an early chest tube thoracostomy is rarely required [55]. Still, PHUS yields valuable information to include in the prearrival notification to the receiving trauma center.

Diaphragmatic rupture

Diaphragmatic rupture occurs in up to 5% of blunt abdominal trauma patients and may be present despite a negative FAST scan [56]. Ultrasonographic signs may be poor movement (on M-mode) or elevation of the diaphragm, a liver sliding sign (at the right chest wall), subphrenic effusion, or the presence of an intrathoracic spleen or liver [57–59]. In addition, Gangahar introduced *Rip's absent organ sign* as an indirect marker: nonvisualization of the spleen or heart caused by displacement of abdominal contents anteriorly to these organs [60, 61].

B—Gastric tube

The only indication for a gastric tube (GT) in the prehospital setting is to relieve gastric distention that is often caused or aggravated by bag-valve-mask ventilation. Traditionally, correct positioning is verified by injecting air in the tube while listening for air bubbles, or by aspiration of gastric contents. These methods are unreliable, especially in the noisy prehospital environment, and the recommended pH measurements and chest X-rays are not feasible [62]. Chenaitia et al. estimated the diagnostic accuracy of PHUS confirming GT placement in 130 prehospital intubated patients, compared to in-hospital chest X-ray. They positioned the probe subxiphoidal in the transverse plane, oriented toward the left hypochondrium to visualize the GT tip in the gastric antrum. Examination time was limited to 1 min. Sensitivity and

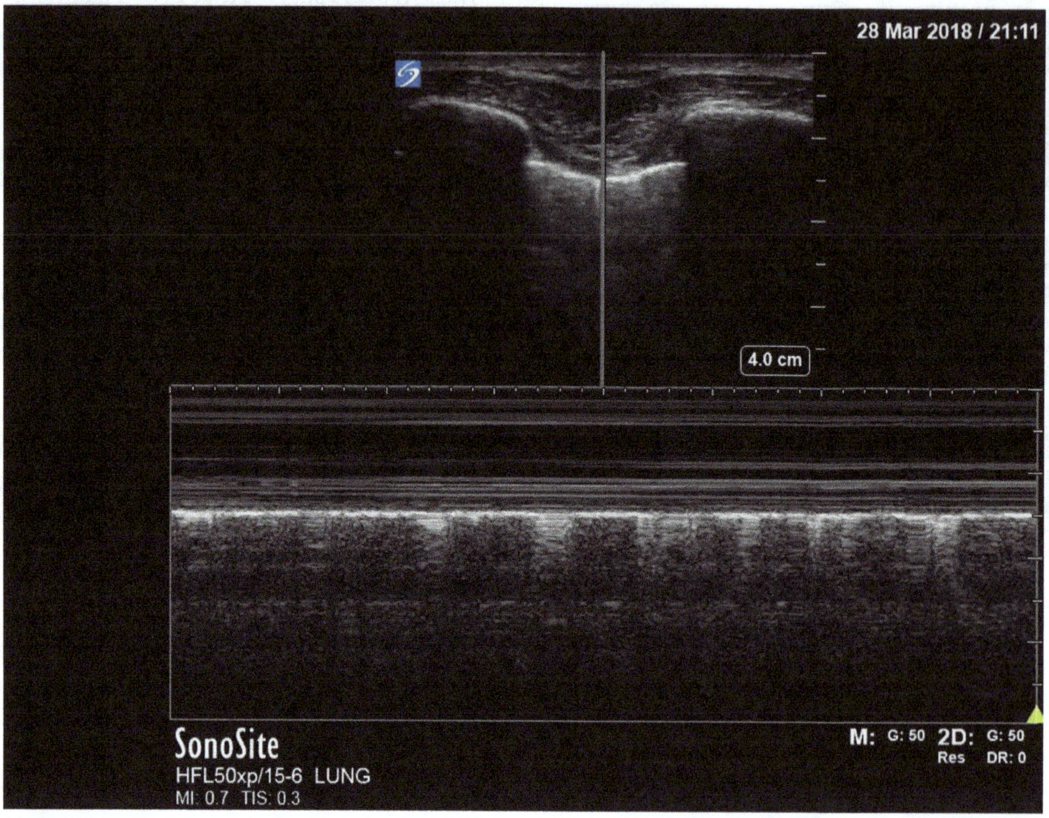

Fig. 3 Normal lung—M-mode ultrasound image. The ultrasound reflections on the vertical line in the upper part of the image are sequentially displayed from left to right in the lower part as time progresses. It allows to capture the motion of the upper 2D image in the stationary image below. A normal M-mode image of the chest wall and pleura is displayed here. The stationary chest wall produces straight horizontal lines above the pleural line. The lung sliding and movement of the artifacts below produces a grainy image. This is called the seashore sign

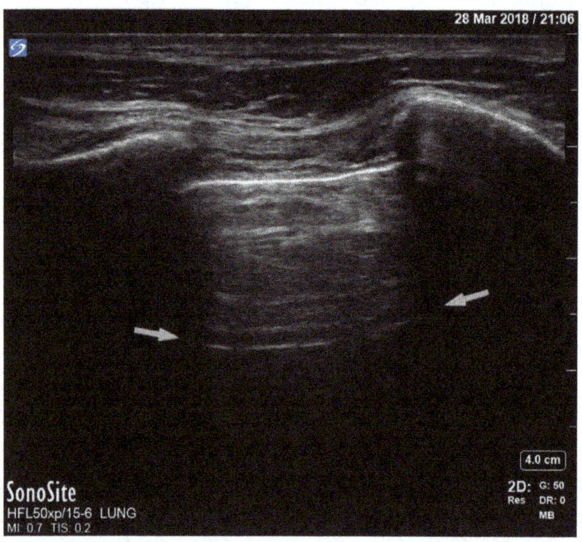

Fig. 4 Pneumothorax + A-line. A-lines are reflections of the pleural line caused by gas below the parietal pleura. An A-line is indicated by the arrows. The A is for "air" either within or outside of the lung. In case of a pneumothorax, there are no B-lines (Fig. 2) that may obscure the A-lines making them stand out more clearly

specificity were 98.3 and 100%. PPV and NPV were 100 and 85.7% [63].

In a follow-up study they added an esophageal view at the anterior neck during and after GT insertion. In case the GT was visualized in the esophagus but not in the stomach, 50 ml of air was inserted. An intragastric position of the tip was visualized or assumed when gastric air entry was observed as *dynamic fogging*: an expanding volume of hyperechoic 'fog'. Sensitivity and specificity were both 100% compared to in-hospital chest X-ray [64]. When US is only performed after GT insertion, it is as fast as the traditional air insufflation and aspiration method.

C—Circulation-cardiac arrest

Current European resuscitation guidelines state that there is no doubt that focused cardiac ultrasound (FoCUS)—using specific protocols for US evaluation—has the potential to detect reversible causes of cardiac arrest [12]. FoCUS can help distinguish the PEA type, identify the cause of the arrest, choose a suitable

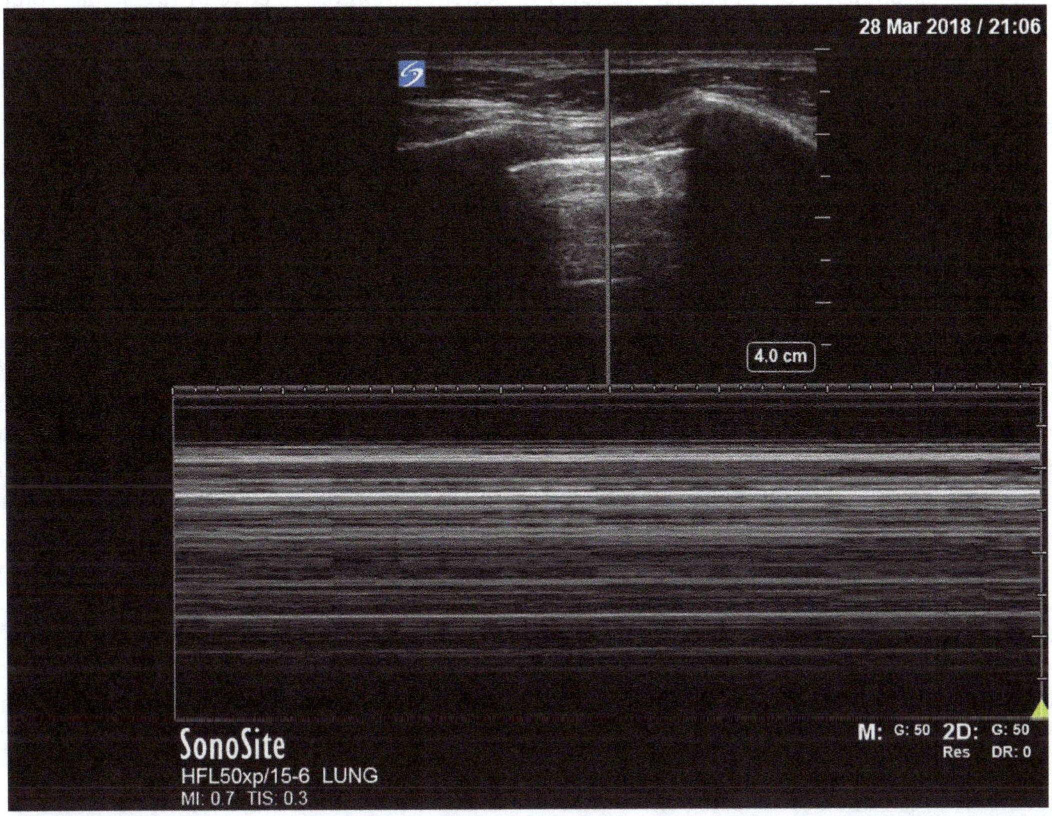

Fig. 5 Pneumothorax—M-mode ultrasound image. There is no visible movement above or below the pleural line. Because all tissue and artifacts are stationary, the M-mode image appears as horizontal straight lines throughout the image. This is called a barcode sign or stratosphere sign

treatment, and make the right decision on cardiopulmonary resuscitation (CPR) termination [65]. In 75% of the patients with pulseless electrical activity (PEA), FoCUS showed coordinated cardiac motion (pseudo-PEA) in a prehospital peri-resuscitation care study [66]. Pseudo-PEA is strongly associated with increased survival compared to a true PEA. Treatable causes were reduced ventricular function (59%), pericardial tamponade (9.8%), a significantly dilated right ventricle (7.8%), and hypovolemia (3.9%) [66]. A return of spontaneous circulation (ROSC) was indeed achieved after pericardiocentesis. Three of five tamponade patients survived to hospital admission.

Similarly, cardiac motion in PEA patients in the ED is positively associated with ROSC. Salen found that in 8 of 11 (73%) patients with sonographic cardiac activity, ROSC was achieved but in none of 23 without cardiac activity [67]. A retrospective analysis of 318 pulseless trauma patients revealed that the survival of pulseless traumatic arrest patients without sonographic cardiac activity is rare [68]. In non-trauma ED patients, cardiac standstill on FoCUS during CPR correlated with death with a PPV of 97.1% and an NPV of 57.1% [69]. However, the timing and the duration of the FoCUS examination could be very important.

Termination of resuscitation (TOR) may be considered in out-of-hospital cardiac arrest patients when these four criteria are met: no ROSC before transport, no shock delivered, no bystander CPR, and an unwitnessed arrest [70]. Goto developed a similar TOR rule: no prehospital ROSC, non-shockable initial rhythm, and unwitnessed by bystanders. Their rule is a > 99% predictor of death within 1 month after out-of-hospital cardiac arrest (OHCA) [71]. Cardiac standstill on initial FoCUS may predict non-ROSC and could be used in the decision for the termination of treatment [67, 72]. However, a 2016 study in non-traumatic OHCA patients undergoing serial FoCUS confirmed ROSC could occur within 10 min after initial cardiac standstill [73]. However, after a cardiac standstill of 10 min or longer, no ROSC occurred. These findings suggest that PHUS might play an important role here: consider TOR after 10 min of sonographic cardiac standstill?

In addition to uncovering treatable causes of cardiac arrest, FoCUS is invaluable in confirming mechanical ventricular capture (as opposed to electrical capture) during transcutaneous cardiac pacing [74].

C—Shock

Although the cause of shock may not be apparent, FoCUS might guide therapy such as intravenous fluid administration, inotropic therapy, and the choice of destination hospital. FoCUS directly altered treatment in 51% of the cardiac arrest and peri-resuscitation patients in Breitkreutz's prehospital study [66]. This implies that every hemodynamically unstable patient could potentially benefit from PHUS.

Non-traumatic shock

To evaluate critically ill patients with acute circulatory failure, Lichtenstein devised the fluid administration limited by lung sonography (FALLS)-protocol aimed at reducing the mortality from septic shock [39]. It aims to sequentially rule out (1) obstructive, (2) cardiogenic, and (3) hypovolemic shock for expediting the diagnosis of distributive (usually septic) shock, displayed in Fig. 6. When other causes of shock are eliminated and distributive shock (sepsis) remains, fluid therapy and vasopressors are indicated. Fluid therapy is guided by repeated chest ultrasound based on the appearance of the so-called B-profile as defined in the BLUE protocol (Table 1).

The rapid ultrasound in shock (RUSH) examination involves a three-part assessment simplified as (1) the pump, (2) the tank, and (3) the pipes [75]. *The pump* refers to an evaluation of the pericardial sac, left ventricular contractility, and the relative size of the right ventricle to the left ventricle. *The tank* refers to the determination of effective intravascular volume status by measuring the inferior vena cava (IVC) and assessment of the lung, pleural and abdominal cavity. *The pipes* refer to scanning for an aneurysm or dissection of the thoracic and abdominal aorta, and deep venous thrombosis.

Both the FALLS and RUSH protocol combine familiar US scans proven to be feasible in the prehospital setting. Although we are unaware of any reports, these protocols are potentially valuable in prehospital care.

Traumatic shock

In traumatic shock, the (extended) FAST protocol may be used to detect a hemoperitoneum. A US image of a normal hepatorenal recess and one with a hemoperitoneum are displayed in Figs. 7, 8. In abdominal trauma, its sensitivity and specificity are comparable between in-hospital and prehospital: 100 and 97.5% in-hospital and 90 and 99% prehospital, respectively [2]. The feasibility and efficiency of the extended FAST were also comparable, with no significant difference in US duration [22].

In shocked blunt abdominal trauma patients, expeditious PoCUS should take a minimum amount of time. Clarke found that mortality increases by 1% for every 3-min delay of a necessary intervention [76, 77]. Unfortunately, false-negative results do occur and they do most frequently in scans performed early in the disease process [22, 78]. Therefore, when FAST is negative it is recommended to repeat the examination every 15 min [2, 77]. Repeated abdominal US scans may lead to a 50% reduction of false negatives [79]. However, a hemorrhage in the retroperitoneum or any solid organ injuries cannot be detected reliably with FAST. So, a negative FAST

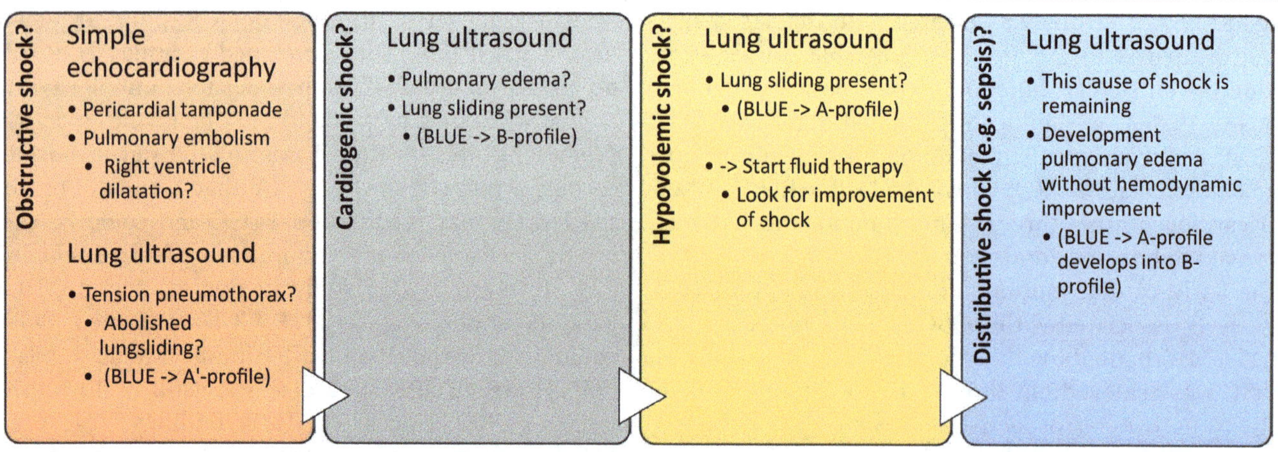

Fig. 6 FALLS protocol. This diagram is an adaptation of the work by Dr. Lichtenstein [39]. Firstly, this diagram shows the type of shock the focus is on. Secondly, the type of ultrasound examination is shown. Thirdly, possible diagnoses to consider are shown including their appearance in terms of the BLUE protocol. Every cause of shock is sequentially excluded for expediting the diagnosis of distributive (septic) shock. *FALLS* fluid administration limited by lung sonography, *BLUE* bedside lung ultrasound in emergency, BLUE and the A, B, and A' profile are explained in Table 1, items 1, 2, and 8, respectively

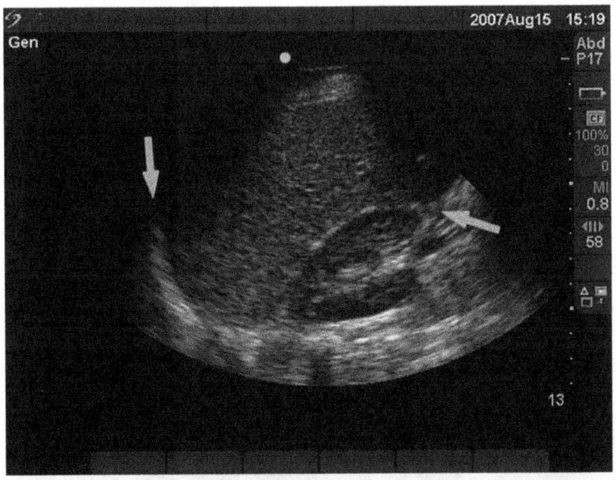

Fig. 7 Normal hepatorenal recess. A normal ultrasound image of the hepatorenal recess (Morison's pouch). A phased-array cardiac transducer was used with the abdominal settings. The left arrow indicates the diaphragm. The right arrow indicates the hepatorenal recess. The liver is shown above this line and the right kidney below

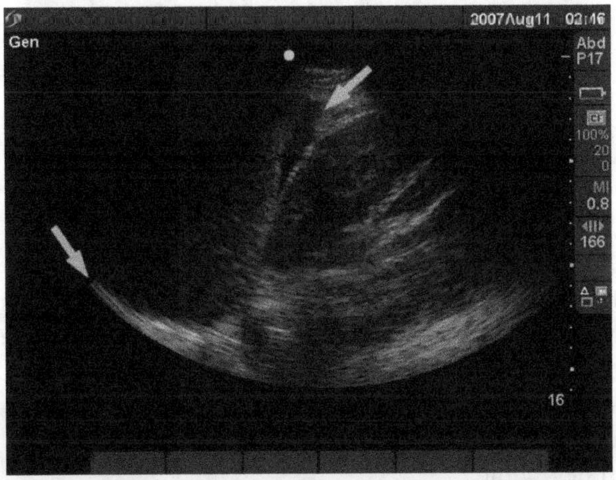

Fig. 8 Hemoperitoneum at the splenorenal recess. An ultrasound image of the splenorenal recess (Koller's pouch). A phased-array cardiac transducer was used with the abdominal settings. The left arrow indicates the diaphragm. The right arrow indicates the splenorenal recess with a hypoechoic collection between the spleen (left) and the left kidney (right). This is the image of free intraperitoneal fluid and is very suggestive for intraperitoneal hemorrhage when encountered in a trauma victim

does not compensate for a high suspicion of abdominal hemorrhage.

A (non) traumatic pneumoperitoneum is almost invariably caused by gastrointestinal perforation. When detected prehospitally, this might steer early treatment and transportation. Sensitivity and specificity of abdominal US for pneumoperitoneum is 85–90% and 100%. In experienced hands it can be as good as CT; an amount as small as 1 ml of free air can be detected [80–82]. Thus, it appears plausible to use PHUS also for this indication.

In their meta-analysis, Stengel et al. concluded that US for blunt abdominal trauma does not decrease the laparotomy rate or mortality. Nevertheless, the number of ordered CT scans decreased by 50%. However, this might reflect a false sense of security due to the low sensitivity of abdominal ultrasound for both free fluid and organ lacerations [7]. Montoya also reported that US led to fewer CT scans. In addition, however, they found a decreased time to appropriate interventions, shortened hospital stay, and decreased use of healthcare resources [78].

C—Abdominal aortic aneurysm

US is feasible and suitable to assess for an aneurysm of the abdominal aorta in symptomatic patients. An ED study showed a sensitivity and specificity of 100 and 98% [83]. Prehospitally this is also feasible, reported Heegaard et al. Trained ambulance paramedics performed PHUS scans of the abdominal aorta in 20 symptomatic patients. A blinded expert also judged the images and agreed 100% with the paramedics' judgment [84].

D—Central nervous system

Stroke—transcranial US

Reducing the interval between ischemic stroke and intravenous thrombolysis is associated with reduced mortality, reduced symptomatic intracranial hemorrhage, and higher rates of independent ambulation at discharge and discharge to home [85, 86]. Unfortunately, prehospital delays lead to missed opportunities to initiate treatment within the preferred 90 min after the onset of symptoms [87]. For instance, in an American study, only 38% of patients arrived within 2 h of the onset of their symptoms [88].

Early prehospital detection of ischemic stroke may be beneficial to a favorable outcome. Prehospital caregivers could allocate patients to the most appropriate hospital, provide a prearrival notification, and initiate stroke-specific therapies such as sonothrombolysis and neuroprotective strategies [87, 89, 90]. Intravenous thrombolysis, however, is only administered safely after a CT or magnetic resonance imaging (MRI) scan excludes an intracranial hemorrhage.

Herzberg et al. evaluated the diagnostic accuracy of prehospital neurological examination supported by transcranial color-coded sonography (TCCS) [89]. The TCCS consisted of color-mode visualization and flow measurements in the proximal M-1 segment of both middle cerebral arteries (MCA) to find an occlusion. When desired, they scanned the anterior and posterior cerebral arteries or administered an intravenous ultrasound contrast agent (UCA). Sensitivity and specificity were 95 and 48%; PPV and NPV were 82 and 77% for the prehospital diagnosis of 'any stroke' compared to in-hospital CT angiography (CTA) and magnetic resonance angiography (MRA). With appropriate training, telemedicine, and UCAs, these results might still improve [89].

In their prehospital study, Schlachetzki found that 36% of the physicians used microbubbles as a UCA to save time or to increase the diagnostic confidence when temporal window anatomy did not allow an optimal visualization of the MCAs. The sensitivity and specificity of ultrasound for MCA occlusions were 90 and 98%. PPV and NPV were 90 and 98% [90].

Besides arterial occlusions, vasospasm due to aneurysmal subarachnoid hemorrhage may be detected by transcranial US. However, its diagnostic accuracy varies widely depending on the vessel, the diagnostic criteria, and timing [91]. Anecdotal evidence exists on other intracranial pathologies which may be detected by PHUS such as intracranial hematomas and ventricular system enlargement [92, 93].

The biggest limitation of the application of transcranial US is the ability to obtain US images through the temporal window (Fig. 9). This is the thinnest part of the temporal bone that allows penetration of the US beam at a suitable angle and distance in relation to basal portions of the major cerebral arteries and the circle of Willis. This procedure may be very demanding and requires training and experience. Therefore, transcranial US might not be suitable for every ultrasound-equipped (H)EMS service.

The therapeutic applications of transcranial US in ischemic stroke are discussed in the *interventions* section of this paper.

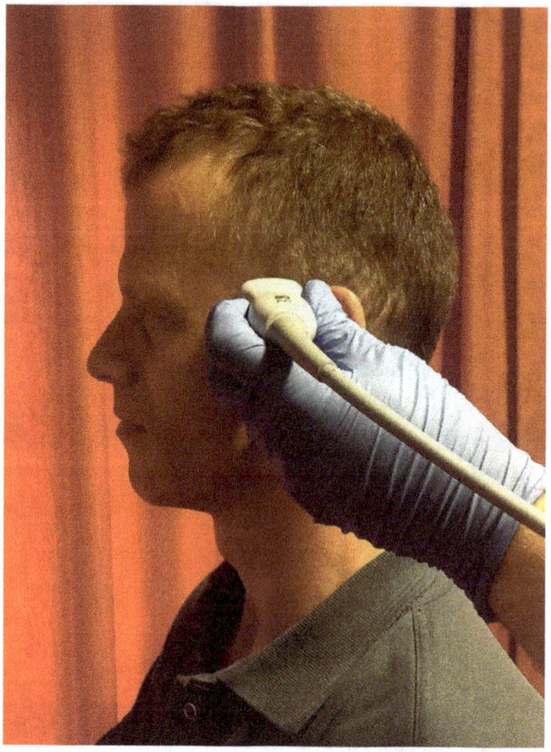

Fig. 9 Ultrasound transducer positioned at the temporal window. The ultrasound transducer is positioned at the site where the temporal bone is thinnest and the ultrasound beam is least obstructed penetrating the skull (Reproduced with permission from Rob Stoffels and Yvonne Houben)

ONSD

Both optic disc edema detected by fundoscopy and an increased optic nerve sheath diameter (ONSD) are indications of increased intracranial pressure (ICP) [94]. The ONSD can easily be measured using US, although the use of a UCA might enhance the recognition of relevant anatomy [95]. ONSD measurements, using a cutoff value of 5.0 mm, have a sensitivity and specificity of 100 and 95% in predicting an elevated ICP compared to CT [96]. Moretti et al. compared US to invasive ICP measurements. Using a cutoff value of 5.2 mm, they found a sensitivity and specificity of 93.1 and 73.9% for an ICP $\geq$ 20 mmHg [97]. More recently, Maissan et al. measured the ONSD in ICP-monitored traumatic brain injury (TBI) patients before, during, and after routine suctioning of the endotracheal tube leading to a transient ICP rise. With a cutoff value of 5.0 mm they found the sensitivity and specificity to be 94 and 98% for a rise in ICP [98].

Like US in ischemic stroke, the benefit of prehospital ONSD measurements might be to start neuroprotective strategies, to determine the need for neurosurgical care, or to provide a prearrival notification. However, the evidence on prehospital feasibility and benefit is still negligible.

E—Injuries

Fractures

Dulchavsky concluded that non-physicians in the ED (cast technicians) can reliably diagnose orthopedic injury with an accuracy of 94% after a brief PoCUS training. This was more reliable for fractures of the humerus, forearm, femur, and lower leg than for hand and foot fractures, and tendon injuries [99].

Bozorgi et al. evaluated US in 108 ED patients with 158 fractures in the extremities. The overall sensitivity was 68.3%. Sensitivity for femoral fractures and humeral fractures was 100 and 76.2%, respectively. The detection of intra-articular fractures was the most difficult with a sensitivity of only 48% [100].

In the civilian prehospital setting, PHUS for fractures is probably feasible. It is useful for (long) bone fractures in the upper and lower arm, and leg. Advantages in the prehospital setting could be early reduction and splinting, triage, and selecting the best destination provided with a specific prearrival notification.

Foreign objects

In the wilderness environment, Paziana described two cases where PHUS was successfully used to aid in the removal of foreign objects from soft tissue [101]. PHUS may determine the exact location and depth of a foreign object despite that some are radiolucent. The location and size of the incision can be determined, and the removal may take place under direct US visualization.

Ocular ultrasonography

Besides ONSD measurements, ocular US appears useful and feasible in the prehospital setting. It is useful to diagnose penetrating globe injury, foreign body retention, retinal detachment, vitreous detachment, central retinal artery occlusion, lens dislocation, retrobulbar hematoma, and retinal and vitreous hemorrhage [102, 103]. The eye can be accurately assessed without the need to open the eyelid in case of swelling. An austere environment case report described PHUS helping to diagnose a retinal detachment after a facial gunshot wound. Immediate evacuation was arranged to facilitate appropriate follow-up care [104].

Interventions

Here, many diagnostic applications of PHUS have been discussed. Besides its diagnostic applications, PHUS has been shown to be potentially valuable in guiding interventions or as a therapeutic intervention in its own right.

Interventions—airway

Emergency percutaneous cricothyroidotomy may be unsuccessful or produce a tear in the posterior tracheal wall. Siddiqui et al. compared anatomical orientation by either digital palpation or US for performing a percutaneous cricothyroidotomy with the Portex® device. In cadavers in which palpation of the cricothyroid ligament is difficult, US increased the probability of a correct device insertion by 5.6 times and reduced the incidence of laryngeal and tracheal injury from 100 to 33%. A possible disadvantage of US may be the prolonged time to airway insertion [105].

In the emergency prehospital setting, the open cricothyroidotomy is the preferred approach in invasive airway management. Whether a US-guided percutaneous technique should be used in an emergency at all is a matter of debate. Nevertheless, Curtis et al. found a US-guided bougie-assisted open cricothyroidotomy to be a rapid and reliable technique. Cricothyroidotomy was successful in 20 of 21 cadavers, with a median time to completion of 26.2 s [106].

Interventions—breathing

Medical patients with severe symptomatic pleural effusion might require early pleural aspiration in the prehospital setting. Pleural US is useful in the diagnosis and localization of fluid. US-guided thoracentesis is a safer and more effective method to relieve symptoms than a blind approach [107, 108].

Interventions—circulation

To guide interventions, PHUS is most frequently used for (central) venous access. It was the second most used PHUS application overall (after assessment of blunt abdominal trauma) in an Australian retrieval team [47]. Intraosseous access is the most appropriate approach in time critical emergencies. However, for less urgent but difficult to obtain peripheral intravenous access, US guidance is faster and more effective than traditional catheter insertion [109].

Symptomatic pericardial effusion might need prompt treatment in the prehospital setting. US-guided pericardiocentesis under continuous visualization using a multi-angled needle guide was found to be effective, safe, and easy to perform [110].

First described in 1954, resuscitative endovascular balloon occlusion of the aorta (REBOA) is a technique to stabilize patients suffering hemodynamic shock by temporarily interrupting blood flow to non-compressible hemorrhage in the chest, abdomen, or pelvis [111, 112]. In animal studies, REBOA resulted in a 74% mortality risk reduction [113]. After 40 min of occlusion, however, the risks start outweighing the benefits [113, 114]. In 2014, the London HEMS was the first to report a prehospital performed REBOA in a patient with a pelvic fracture resulting in successful hemorrhage control [115].

Chaudery found that the use of US improved the correct placement of REBOA catheters, shortened the time until correct placement, and improved the participants' confidence in catheter placement of Zone III (infrarenal aorta) REBOA catheters in 20 porcine cadavers [116].

These developments are promising for future prehospital US-guided REBOA hemorrhage control. However, future research is needed on prehospital feasibility, variations in body habitus, and zone I (intrathoracic aorta) placement.

Interventions—disability

In the aforementioned *disability* section, we highlighted the value of TCCS in diagnosing ischemic stroke. A therapeutic application of ultrasound in ischemic stroke patients is continuous transcranial Doppler (TCD) to enhance the thrombolytic activity of tissue plasminogen activator (t-PA) [117]. In a phase II multicenter randomized trial (CLOTBUST), transducers were applied over the temporal bone in a head frame. The investigators applied TCD (or placebo TCD) on maximum power output continuously for 2 h and simultaneously started intravenous t-PA treatment in all patients. Two hours after starting thrombolysis, recanalization or almost full recovery was observed in 49% in the continuous TCD group versus 30% in the control group. However, clinical recovery after 24 h and outcome after 3 months was similar [117]. In 2014, another analysis of the CLOTBUST trial, including more subjects, revealed 38.6% complete recanalization in the sonothrombolysis group and 17.1% in the intravenous t-PA group [118]. A phase III trial is underway [119]. Tsivgoulis concluded in a meta-analysis that high-frequency ultrasound (both TCD and TCCS) combined with t-PA was associated with a higher likelihood of complete recanalization (pooled OR = 2.99) than t-PA alone [120]. They found no increased risk of symptomatic intracerebral hemorrhage.

Probably, transcranial US combined with microbubbles but without t-PA is effective as well [121, 122]. Microbubbles consist of an injectable aqueous suspension of small (1.5–4.7 μm) bubbles of a high molecular-weight gas that is used as a US contrast agent to improve the visualization of blood vessels [123]. In a meta-analysis, Saqqur indeed concluded that sonothrombolysis with or without microbubbles or t-PA was effective and safe [124]. These findings allow the exploration of early prehospital initiation of sonothrombolysis in suspected ischemic stroke without needing a CT or MRI scan. Hölscher already suggested that PHUS could serve to 'precondition' the culprit clot to increase its therapeutic sensitivity to t-PA or neuro intervention while providing neuroprotection for tissue at risk [121].

Interventions—regional anesthesia

US-guided regional anesthesia is a common technique for providing perioperative pain relief for elective surgical procedures of the extremities. These techniques can also be employed in the prehospital setting to provide effective analgesia for extremity injuries and avoid the side effects associated with the administration of systemic analgesics. For instance, ultrasound-guided femoral nerve blocks effectively provide pain relief in hip fractures [125]. Also, PHUS might facilitate already successful prehospital fascia iliaca compartment blocks [126]. Similarly, Lippert et al. suggested the added value of US-guided nerve blocks to improve pain control in disaster settings [127].

The transversus abdominis plane (TAP) block is an effective technique for pain relief in pelvic fractures and because of its ease and safety it may be applicable in the prehospital setting [128]. Blocking the nerves that supply the anterior abdominal wall relaxes the abdominal wall muscles that will subsequently reduce the traction on the ischium and pubis. The 'flank bulge sign' is a direct consequence of this relaxation [129].

Disaster triage

In a multiple casualty incident (MCI), resources are limited. Triage systems are used to determine treatment priority of the injured patients based on history and physical examination. PoCUS was reported to be valuable in the

Table 2 The CAVEAT protocol. Stawicki et al. [135]

Urgency	Step	Examination	Focus on	Looking for
CAVEAT protocol				
Primary assessment (mandatory)	1	Evaluation of the pleura	Chest	Pneumothorax
	2	Complete FAST examination	Abdomen Costophrenic recesses	Hemoperitoneum Hemothorax
	3	Inferior Vena Cava assessment	Collapsibility index	Volume depletion
Secondary assessment (optional)	4	Upper- and lower extremities	Long bones; regions of pain, tenderness, or deformity	Major fractures eligible for more accurate reduction and stabilization Fractures to prioritize utilization of radiographic resources, or achieve even more accurate triage

CAVEAT sonographic evaluation of the chest, abdomen, vena cava, extremities for acute triage, *FAST* focused assessment with sonography for trauma

This table shows the suggested order of examinations in the CAVEAT protocol. Specific components may depend on the operators' skill level and on the individual patient's injuries

triage process during several earthquake disasters [130–134]. Stawicki proposed a protocol that integrates some common PoCUS applications to evaluate the chest, abdomen, vena cava, and extremities as an adjunct to acute triage (CAVEAT) and to be executed during the secondary survey [135]. The protocol will take approximately 5 min longer than a traditional FAST scan. It is explained in more detail in Table 2. Although the merits of its component parts have been described extensively, the benefit of the protocol is yet to be established.

Future applications

Sonothrombolysis

As we have discussed in the *interventions* section, early prehospital sonothrombolysis in ischemic stroke patients might be safe and effective. The CLOTBUST investigators have developed a hands-free headframe containing 18 ultrasound transducers positioned at the temporal occipital bone windows to deliver operator-independent ultrasound energy directly to the culprit clot. It was successfully applied to and well tolerated by 15 volunteers and is currently evaluated in stroke patients [136]. It may facilitate and enhance early thrombolysis because of its portability and that no formal ultrasound training is needed.

Telemedicine

With improving data communication technologies, telemedicine is a promising technique for remotely evaluating ultrasound clips acquired by less experienced operators. They might even be coached in real time supported by remotely operating the ultrasound device settings in complex scenarios [137]. Kolbe introduced a PoCUS curriculum in a one-room medical clinic in rural Nicaragua. Despite limited resources, after the first introduction the ultrasound instructors used telemedicine to remotely view the ultrasound images in real time [138]. In 2016, Kirkpatrick demonstrated the feasibility of remotely telementoring ultrasound-naïve firefighters using trauma ultrasound for free fluid detection on a phantom [137]. Remote telementored ultrasound was feasible to coach untrained and inexperienced nurse practitioners to assess patients for pneumothorax immediately after removal of their tube thoracostomy [139]. Rubin demonstrated the feasibility of remote review and interpretation of TCD and carotid ultrasound data in healthy volunteers dubbed "teleneurosonology" [140].

Integrating telemedicine concepts in PoCUS-enhanced disaster triage might be promising and feasible in the light of progressing technological advancements.

Wearable US

Mierzwa developed a flat and flexible 5 MHz US probe designed to wear on a fingertip to aid in US-guided vascular access, for instance. The device can be configured as a linear or curvilinear transducer array and it can be mounted directly onto the body as an adhesive patch or wearable device. They speculate on many applications such as point-of-care imaging, combat casualty care, ultrasound therapy, and patient monitoring [141]. A specific prehospital application might also be a US patch for continuous cardiac visualization during cardiopulmonary resuscitation.

Assessment of intraosseous needle position

Tsung demonstrated the feasibility of US to determine the location of an intraosseous needle in six resuscitation cases. He argues that every intraosseous access should be verified with color Doppler because a correct position cannot be accurately confirmed by the aspiration of blood, blood on the stylet tip, the needle being firmly in place, or the absence of soft tissue extravasation [142].

Predicting outcomes in resuscitative thoracotomy (RT)

In some countries, a prehospital or ED resuscitative thoracotomy (RT) is performed on patients with a penetrating (sometimes also blunt) thoracic injury decompensating into cardiac arrest. The goal is to treat a cardiac tamponade or major injuries of the heart, control intrathoracic bleeding, clamp the thoracic aorta, or perform direct cardiac massage or defibrillation. The RT is an invasive and last-resort treatment. Inaba found that FoCUS was a predictor of futile care in these patients [143]. In 187 RT patients, only 6 survived and 3 were eligible organ donors. All survivors and organ donors had visible cardiac motion before RT was performed. If no cardiac motion or pericardial effusion on US was observed, the survival was zero. Thus, utilizing US would have avoided a considerable number of RTs that were ultimately futile [143]. Because of these findings, PHUS would be a valuable addition to prehospital RT protocols.

US-guided cannulation for extracorporeal life support (ECLS)

Lamhaut concluded in 2013 that prehospital implementation of ECLS by non-surgeons was safe and feasible [144]. Four years later their group described a case of ECLS cannulation in the Louvre museum in Paris in which they used a hybrid surgical/Seldinger technique [145, 146]. Another future PHUS application might be US-guided percutaneous ECLS cannulation that may be easier, faster, and less invasive. It could be complemented by (contrast enhanced) echocardiography to verify correct placement of the venous catheter tip [147, 148].

Challenges of prehospital ultrasonography

PHUS is subject to specific challenges in the prehospital environment: ambient lighting, confined space, extremes of temperature, precipitation, dressings, splints, and rapid transport times [3, 6].

Diagnostic ultrasound is generally considered harmless. However, it may heat up tissue depending on these factors: exposure duration, the acoustic output, and tissue characteristics. For instance, some unique properties of the eye such as high absorption of ultrasound and the absence of cooling blood supply may cause the lens to heat up faster than other tissues [149, 150]. Therefore, this has to be considered in ocular ultrasound or ONSD measurements.

PHUS is used by nonradiologists mainly to answer simple yes/no questions and to guide treatment decisions. Sensitivity for solid organ injuries is low and small quantities of blood early in the post-injury phase may be missed. Traumatic aortic pathology cannot be detected by chest or abdominal US; therefore, PHUS is not a valid replacement for CT angiography in patients subjected to high-energy thoracic trauma [78]. False negatives will occur; therefore, negative findings should not indicate a final exclusion of diagnoses [3]. Thus, for some indications, the sensible choice might be to use PHUS only as a 'rule-in' tool not to be falsely reassured by (false) negative test results.

Another concern of PHUS is the potential delay in treatment. In general, a slight delay might occur when PHUS is performed on-scene. However, delays are nonexistent when performed in parallel with other procedures, while in-flight, or during ground ambulance transport. Busch found the median PHUS duration to be 2.5 min (range 1–3) [13]. For a range of PHUS examinations, Hoyer measured a mean of 1 min 54 s, decreasing to 56 s during the 3-year study period [3]. In their review, Jørgensen et al. reported a delay of 0–6 min. Examination time depends on the protocol and the results: positive findings will reduce the examination time [5].

Although a slight delay may occur, this might easily be outweighed by the advantage of improved diagnostic and therapeutic accuracy, and the potential time gains by transporting the patient directly to the most appropriate hospital.

Conclusions

We have provided a comprehensive summary of the literature on prehospital applications of diagnostic and therapeutic ultrasound structured according to the ABCDE approach. Also, we have highlighted in-hospital PoCUS procedures that appear useful and plausible for prehospital use, current challenges in PHUS, and potential future applications. It may be commendable to revise this review in the near future when, undoubtedly, additional useful PHUS applications will have emerged.

Improvements in portability, quality, and price of handheld ultrasound systems add to the accessibility and its feasibility for prehospital use. PHUS improves the diagnostic capabilities of prehospital health-care providers and might improve treatment decisions, prearrival notifications, and transport mode and destination. As new PoCUS techniques and applications are being researched, new protocols are being tested for diagnostics, procedural guidance, and therapeutic use.

However, prehospital caregivers should unabatedly be aware of the limitations of PHUS. The time investment will not always pay off and diagnostic accuracy is not perfect. Diagnostic accuracy is quite dependent on training and experience of the providers.

The diagnostic and therapeutic possibilities of PoCUS are increasing. With promising techniques, such as sonothrombolysis in ischemic stroke, we are bringing the hospital-level medical care to prehospital patients to an ever-increasing extent [119].

Additional file

Additional file 1: Video 1. Lung point.

Abbreviations

ABCDE: airway, breathing, circulation, disability, exposure/environment; ADHF: acute decompensated heart disease; BLUE: bedside lung ultrasound in emergency; BNP: B-type natriuretic peptide; CAVEAT: chest, abdomen, vena cava, and extremities as an adjunct to acute triage; COPD: chronic obstructive pulmonary disease; CPAP: continuous positive airway pressure; CPR: cardiopulmonary resuscitation; CT: computed tomography; CTA: CT angiography; ECLS: extracorporeal life support; ED: emergency department; eFAST: extended FAST; EMS: emergency medical service; ETT: endotracheal tube; EVLW: extravascular lung water; FALLS: fluid administration limited by lung sonography; FAST: focused assessment with sonography for trauma; FoCUS: focused cardiac ultrasound; GT: gastric tube; HAPE: high-altitude pulmonary edema; HEMS: helicopter emergency medical service; ICP: intracranial pressure; IVC: inferior vena cava; LCI: lung ultrasound; cardiac ultrasound; inferior vena cava measurements; MCA: middle cerebral artery; MCI: multiple casualty incident/mass casualty incident; M-mode: motion mode; MRA: magnetic resonance angiography; MRI: magnetic resonance imaging; NPV: negative predictive value; OHCA: out-of-hospital cardiac arrest; ONSD: optic nerve sheath diameter; PAOP: pulmonary artery occlusion pressure; PEA: pulseless electrical activity; PHUS: prehospital ultrasound; PoCUS: point-of-care ultrasound; PPV: positive predictive value; REBOA: resuscitative endovascular balloon occlusion of the aorta; ROSC: return of spontaneous circulation; RT: resuscitative thoracotomy; RUSH: rapid ultrasound in shock; TAP: transversus abdominis plane (block); TBI: traumatic brain injury; TCCS: transcranial color-coded sonography; TCD: transcranial Doppler; TOR: termination of resuscitation; UCA: ultrasound contrast agent; US: ultrasound.

Authors' contributions

All authors contributed substantially to the manuscript and all agree with this definitive version. RK and GR were responsible for conceiving the paper and have collected all the source papers, analyzed all abstracts and full articles, and written the manuscript. RK, GR, and NH formulated the literature search strategies. All authors have contributed to the design, the writing, and revising of the manuscript drafts. All authors read and approved the final manuscript.

Authors' information
RK, GJvG, and NH are anesthesiologists and experienced HEMS physicians at the Lifeliner 3 station at the Volkel Air Force Base, The Netherlands. GR is employed as a resident in intensive care medicine with a special interest in anesthesiology and prehospital emergency medicine. GJS is an anesthesiologist and chair of the anesthesiology department.

Author details
[1] Radboud Institute for Health Sciences, Department of Anesthesiology, Pain, and Palliative Medicine, Radboud university medical center, Geert Grooteplein-Zuid 10, 6525 GA Nijmegen, The Netherlands. [2] Radboud Institute for Health Sciences, Helicopter Emergency Medical Service Lifeliner 3, Radboud university medical center, Geert Grooteplein-Zuid 10, 6525 GA Nijmegen, The Netherlands. [3] Department of Intensive Care, Catharina Hospital, Michelangelolaan 2, 5623 EJ Eindhoven, The Netherlands.

Acknowledgements
We would like to thank Rob Stoffels and Yvonne Houben for their demonstration of transcranial sonography.

References

1. Moore CL, Copel JA (2011) Point-of-care ultrasonography. N Engl J Med 364(8):749–757
2. Walcher F, Weinlich M, Conrad G, Schweigkofler U, Breitkreutz R, Kirschning T, Marzi I (2006) Prehospital ultrasound imaging improves management of abdominal trauma. Br J Surg 93(2):238–242
3. Hoyer HX, Vogl S, Schiemann U, Haug A, Stolpe E, Michalski T (2010) Prehospital ultrasound in emergency medicine: incidence, feasibility, indications and diagnoses. Eur J Emerg Med 17(5):254–259
4. Ketelaars R, Hoogerwerf N, Scheffer GJ (2013) Prehospital chest ultrasound by a Dutch helicopter emergency medical service. J Emerg Med 44(4):811–817
5. Jorgensen H, Jensen CH, Dirks J (2010) Does prehospital ultrasound improve treatment of the trauma patient? A systematic review. Eur J Emerg Med 17(5):249–253
6. O'Dochartaigh D, Douma M (2015) Prehospital ultrasound of the abdomen and thorax changes trauma patient management: a systematic review. Injury 46(11):2093–2102
7. Stengel D, Rademacher G, Ekkernkamp A, Guthoff C, Mutze S (2015) Emergency ultrasound-based algorithms for diagnosing blunt abdominal trauma. Cochrane Database Syst Rev 9:CD004446
8. Rudolph SS, Sorensen MK, Svane C, Hesselfeldt R, Steinmetz J (2014) Effect of prehospital ultrasound on clinical outcomes of non-trauma patients—a systematic review. Resuscitation 85(1):21–30
9. El Sayed MJ, Zaghrini E (2013) Prehospital emergency ultrasound: a review of current clinical applications, challenges, and future implications. Emerg Med Int 2013:531674
10. Sun J-T, Huang C-Y, Huang Y-S, Sim S-S, Chong K-M, Wang H-P, Lien W-C (2014) Prehospital ultrasound. J Med Ultrasound 22(2):71–77
11. Nelson BP, Sanghvi A (2016) Out of hospital point of care ultrasound: current use models and future directions. Eur J Trauma Emerg Surg 42(2):139–150
12. Soar J, Nolan JP, Bottiger BW, Perkins GD, Lott C, Carli P, Pellis T, Sandroni C, Skrifvars MB, Smith GB, Sunde K, Deakin CD (2015) Adult advanced life support section C. European Resuscitation Council Guidelines for Resuscitation Section 3. Adult advanced life support. Resuscitation 2015(95):100–147
13. Busch M (2006) Portable ultrasound in pre-hospital emergencies: a feasibility study. Acta Anaesthesiol Scand 50(6):754–758
14. Kirkpatrick AW, Breeck K, Wong J, Hamilton DR, McBeth PB, Sawadsky B, Betzner MJ (2005) The potential of handheld trauma sonography in the air medical transport of the trauma victim. Air Med J 24(1):34–39
15. Nelson BP, Melnick ER, Li J (2011) Portable ultrasound for remote environments, part I: feasibility of field deployment. J Emerg Med 40(2):190–197
16. Price DD, Wilson SR, Murphy TG (2000) Trauma ultrasound feasibility during helicopter transport. Air Med J 19(4):144–146
17. Lyon M, Walton P, Bhalla V, Shiver SA (2012) Ultrasound detection of the sliding lung sign by prehospital critical care providers. Am J Emerg Med 30(3):485–488
18. Krogh CL, Steinmetz J, Rudolph SS, Hesselfeldt R, Lippert FK, Berlac PA, Rasmussen LS (2016) Effect of ultrasound training of physicians working in the prehospital setting. Scand J Trauma Resusc Emerg Med 24:99
19. Gracias VH, Frankel HL, Gupta R, Malcynski J, Gandhi R, Collazzo L, Nisenbaum H, Schwab CW (2001) Defining the learning curve for the Focused Abdominal Sonogram for Trauma (FAST) examination: implications for credentialing. Am Surg 67(4):364–368
20. Brooke M, Walton J, Scutt D (2010) Paramedic application of ultrasound in the management of patients in the prehospital setting: a review of the literature. Emerg Med J 27(9):702–707
21. O'Dochartaigh D, Douma M, MacKenzie M (2017) Five-year retrospective review of physician and non-physician performed ultrasound in a Canadian Critical Care Helicopter Emergency Medical Service. Prehosp Emerg Care 21(1):24–31
22. Brun PM, Bessereau J, Chenaitia H, Pradel AL, Deniel C, Garbaye G, Melaine R, Bylicki O, Lablanche C (2014) Stay and play eFAST or scoop and run eFAST? That is the question! Am J Emerg Med 32(2):166–170
23. Press GM, Miller SK, Hassan IA, Alade KH, Camp E, Junco DD, Holcomb JB (2014) Prospective evaluation of prehospital trauma ultrasound during aeromedical transport. J Emerg Med 47(6):638–645
24. Yates JG, Baylous D (2017) Aeromedical ultrasound: the evaluation of point-of-care ultrasound during helicopter transport. Air Med J 36(3):110–115
25. Lapostolle F, Petrovic T, Lenoir G, Catineau J, Galinski M, Metzger J, Chanzy E, Adnet F (2006) Usefulness of hand-held ultrasound devices in out-of-hospital diagnosis performed by emergency physicians. Am J Emerg Med 24(2):237–242
26. Blaivas M, Kuhn W, Reynolds B, Brannam L (2005) Change in differential diagnosis and patient management with the use of portable ultrasound in a remote setting. Wilderness Environ Med 16(1):38–41
27. Peters J, van Wageningen B, Hendriks I, Eijk R, Edwards M, Hoogerwerf N, Biert J (2015) First-pass intubation success rate during rapid sequence induction of prehospital anaesthesia by physicians versus paramedics. Eur J Emerg Med 22(6):391–394
28. Slovis TL, Poland RL (1986) Endotracheal tubes in neonates: sonographic positioning. Radiology 160(1):262–263
29. Drescher MJ, Conard FU, Schamban NE (2000) Identification and description of esophageal intubation using ultrasound. Acad Emerg Med 7(6):722–725
30. Das SK, Choupoo NS, Haldar R, Lahkar A (2015) Transtracheal ultrasound for verification of endotracheal tube placement: a systematic review and meta-analysis. Can J Anaesth 62(4):413–423
31. Grmec S (2002) Comparison of three different methods to confirm tracheal tube placement in emergency intubation. Intensive Care Med 28(6):701–704

32. Zadel S, Strnad M, Prosen G, Mekis D (2015) Point of care ultrasound for orotracheal tube placement assessment in out-of hospital setting. Resuscitation 87:1–6
33. Li J (2001) Capnography alone is imperfect for endotracheal tube placement confirmation during emergency intubation. J Emerg Med 20(3):223–229
34. Hunt RC, Bryan DM, Brinkley VS, Whitley TW, Benson NH (1991) Inability to assess breath sounds during air medical transport by helicopter. JAMA 265(15):1982–1984
35. Kerrey BT, Geis GL, Quinn AM, Hornung RW, Ruddy RM (2009) A prospective comparison of diaphragmatic ultrasound and chest radiography to determine endotracheal tube position in a pediatric emergency department. Pediatrics 123(6):e1039–e1044
36. Kajimoto K, Madeen K, Nakayama T, Tsudo H, Kuroda T, Abe T (2012) Rapid evaluation by lung-cardiac-inferior vena cava (LCI) integrated ultrasound for differentiating heart failure from pulmonary disease as the cause of acute dyspnea in the emergency setting. Cardiovasc Ultrasound 10(1):49
37. Mantuani D, Frazee BW, Fahimi J, Nagdev A (2016) Point-of-care multi-organ ultrasound improves diagnostic accuracy in adults presenting to the emergency department with acute dyspnea. West J Emerg Med 17(1):46–53
38. Lichtenstein D (2009) Lung ultrasound in acute respiratory failure an introduction to the BLUE-protocol. Minerva Anestesiol 75(5):313–317
39. Lichtenstein DA (2015) BLUE-protocol and FALLS-protocol: two applications of lung ultrasound in the critically ill. Chest 147(6):1659–1670
40. Lichtenstein DA, Meziere GA (2008) Relevance of lung ultrasound in the diagnosis of acute respiratory failure: the BLUE protocol. Chest 134(1):117–125
41. Strnad M, Prosen G, Borovnik Lesjak V (2016) Bedside lung ultrasound for monitoring the effectiveness of prehospital treatment with continuous positive airway pressure in acute decompensated heart failure. Eur J Emerg Med 23(1):50–55
42. Lichtenstein DA, Meziere GA, Lagoueyte JF, Biderman P, Goldstein I, Gepner A (2009) A-lines and B-lines: lung ultrasound as a bedside tool for predicting pulmonary artery occlusion pressure in the critically ill. Chest 136(4):1014–1020
43. Wimalasena Y, Windsor J, Edsell M (2013) Using ultrasound lung comets in the diagnosis of high altitude pulmonary edema: fact or fiction? Wilderness Environ Med 24(2):159–164
44. Fagenholz PJ, Gutman JA, Murray AF, Noble VE, Thomas SH, Harris NS (2007) Chest ultrasonography for the diagnosis and monitoring of high-altitude pulmonary edema. Chest 131(4):1013–1018
45. Lichtenstein DA, Meziere G, Lascols N, Biderman P, Courret JP, Gepner A, Goldstein I, Tenoudji-Cohen M (2005) Ultrasound diagnosis of occult pneumothorax. Crit Care Med 33(6):1231–1238
46. Schaal JV, Pasquier P, Renner J, Dubost C, Merat S (2014) Ultrasounds for prehospital recognition of tension pneumothorax. Injury 45(6):1019
47. Mazur SM, Pearce A, Alfred S, Sharley P (2007) Use of point-of-care ultrasound by a critical care retrieval team. Emerg Med Australas 19(6):547–552
48. Lichtenstein D, Courret JP (1998) Feasibility of ultrasound in the helicopter. Intensive Care Med 24(10):1119
49. Lyon M, Shiver SA, Walton P (2012) M-mode ultrasound for the detection of pneumothorax during helicopter transport. Am J Emerg Med 30(8):1577–1580
50. Madill JJ (2010) In-flight thoracic ultrasound detection of pneumothorax in combat. J Emerg Med 39(2):194–197
51. Roline CE, Heegaard WG, Moore JC, Joing SA, Hildebrandt DA, Biros MH, Caroon LV, Plummer DW, Reardon RF (2013) Feasibility of bedside thoracic ultrasound in the helicopter emergency medical services setting. Air Med J 32(3):153–157
52. Quick JA, Uhlich RM, Ahmad S, Barnes SL, Coughenour JP (2016) In-flight ultrasound identification of pneumothorax. Emerg Radiol 23(1):3–7
53. McEwan K, Thompson P (2007) Ultrasound to detect haemothorax after chest injury. Emerg Med J 24(8):581–582
54. Rahimi-Movaghar V, Yousefifard M, Ghelichkhani P, Baikpour M, Tafakhori A, Asady H, Faridaalaee G, Hosseini M, Safari S (2016) Application of ultrasonography and radiography in detection of hemothorax; a systematic review and meta-analysis. Emergency 4(3):116–126
55. Wells BJ, Roberts DJ, Grondin S, Navsaria PH, Kirkpatrick AW, Dunham MB, Ball CG (2015) To drain or not to drain? Predictors of tube thoracostomy insertion and outcomes associated with drainage of traumatic hemothoraces. Injury 46(9):1743–1748
56. Blaivas M, Brannam L, Hawkins M, Lyon M, Sriram K (2004) Bedside emergency ultrasonographic diagnosis of diaphragmatic rupture in blunt abdominal trauma. Am J Emerg Med 22(7):601–604
57. Kim HH, Shin YR, Kim KJ, Hwang SS, Ha HK, Byun JY, Choi KH, Shinn KS (1997) Blunt traumatic rupture of the diaphragm: sonographic diagnosis. J Ultrasound Med 16(9):593–598
58. Rattan KN, Magu S, Agrawal K, Ratan S (2005) Traumatic diaphragmatic herniation. Indian J Pediatr 72(11):985–986
59. Kirkpatrick AW, Ball CG, Nicolaou S, Ledgerwood A, Lucas CE (2006) Ultrasound detection of right-sided diaphragmatic injury; the "liver sliding" sign. Am J Emerg Med 24(2):251–252
60. Gangahar R, Doshi D (2010) FAST scan in the diagnosis of acute diaphragmatic rupture. Am J Emerg Med 28(3):387-e1
61. Brun PM, Bessereau J, Levy D, Billeres X, Fournier N, Kerbaul F (2014) Prehospital ultrasound thoracic examination to improve decision making, triage, and care in blunt trauma. Am J Emerg Med 32(7):817-e1
62. Walker LJ (2005) Methods to correct placement of a nasogastric tube: beware of the pitfalls. Age Ageing 34(6):655
63. Chenaitia H, Brun PM, Querellou E, Leyral J, Bessereau J, Aime C, Bouaziz R, Georges A, Louis F, France WG (2012) Ultrasound to confirm gastric tube placement in prehospital management. Resuscitation 83(4):447–451
64. Brun PM, Chenaitia H, Lablanche C, Pradel AL, Deniel C, Bessereau J, Melaine R (2014) 2-point ultrasonography to confirm correct position of the gastric tube in prehospital setting. Mil Med 179(9):959–963
65. Zengin S, Yavuz E, Al B, Cindoruk S, Altunbas G, Gumusboga H, Yildirim C (2016) Benefits of cardiac sonography performed by a non-expert sonographer in patients with non-traumatic cardiopulmonary arrest. Resuscitation 102:105–109
66. Breitkreutz R, Price S, Steiger HV, Seeger FH, Ilper H, Ackermann H, Rudolph M, Uddin S, Weigand MA, Muller E, Walcher F, Emergency Ultrasound Working Group of the Johann Wolfgang Goethe-University Hospital FaM (2010) Focused echocardiographic evaluation in life support and peri-resuscitation of emergency patients: a prospective trial. Resuscitation 81(11):1527–1533
67. Salen P, Melniker L, Chooljian C, Rose JS, Alteveer J, Reed J, Heller M (2005) Does the presence or absence of sonographically identified cardiac activity predict resuscitation outcomes of cardiac arrest patients? Am J Emerg Med 23(4):459–462
68. Cureton EL, Yeung LY, Kwan RO, Miraflor EJ, Sadjadi J, Price DD, Victorino GP (2012) The heart of the matter: utility of ultrasound of cardiac activity during traumatic arrest. J Trauma Acute Care Surg 73(1):102–110
69. Aichinger G, Zechner PM, Prause G, Sacherer F, Wildner G, Anderson CL, Pocivalnik M, Wiesspeiner U, Fox JC (2012) Cardiac movement identified on prehospital echocardiography predicts outcome in cardiac arrest patients. Prehosp Emerg Care 16(2):251–255
70. Morrison LJ, Verbeek PR, Vermeulen MJ, Kiss A, Allan KS, Nesbitt L, Stiell I (2007) Derivation and evaluation of a termination of resuscitation clinical prediction rule for advanced life support providers. Resuscitation 74(2):266–275
71. Goto Y, Maeda T, Goto YN (2013) Termination-of-resuscitation rule for emergency department physicians treating out-of-hospital cardiac arrest patients: an observational cohort study. Crit Care 17(5):R235
72. Blaivas M, Fox JC (2001) Outcome in cardiac arrest patients found to have cardiac standstill on the bedside emergency department echocardiogram. Acad Emerg Med 8(6):616–621
73. Kim HB, Suh JY, Choi JH, Cho YS (2016) Can serial focussed echocardiographic evaluation in life support (FEEL) predict resuscitation outcome or termination of resuscitation (TOR)? A pilot study. Resuscitation 101:21–26
74. Holger JS, Lamon RP, Minnegan HJ, Gornick CC (2003) Use of ultrasound to determine ventricular capture in transcutaneous pacing. Am J Emerg Med 21(3):227–229
75. Perera P, Mailhot T, Riley D, Mandavia D (2010) The RUSH exam: Rapid Ultrasound in SHock in the evaluation of the critically ill. Emerg Med Clin North Am 28(1):29–56

76. Clarke JR, Trooskin SZ, Doshi PJ, Greenwald L, Mode CJ (2002) Time to laparotomy for intra-abdominal bleeding from trauma does affect survival for delays up to 90 minutes. J Trauma 52(3):420–425
77. Ruesseler M, Kirschning T, Breitkreutz R, Marzi I, Walcher F (2009) Prehospital and emergency department ultrasound in blunt abdominal trauma. Eur J Trauma Emerg Surg 35(4):341
78. Montoya J, Stawicki SP, Evans DC, Bahner DP, Sparks S, Sharpe RP, Cipolla J (2016) From FAST to E-FAST: an overview of the evolution of ultrasound-based traumatic injury assessment. Eur J Trauma Emerg Surg 42(2):119–126
79. Nunes LW, Simmons S, Hallowell MJ, Kinback R, Trooskin S, Kozar R (2001) Diagnostic performance of trauma US in identifying abdominal or pelvic free fluid and serious abdominal or pelvic injury. Acad Radiol 8(2):128–136
80. Seitz K, Reising KD (1982) Ultrasound detection of free air in the abdominal cavity. Ultraschall Med 3(1):4–6
81. Moriwaki Y, Sugiyama M, Toyoda H, Kosuge T, Arata S, Iwashita M, Tahara Y, Suzuki N (2009) Ultrasonography for the diagnosis of intraperitoneal free air in chest-abdominal-pelvic blunt trauma and critical acute abdominal pain. Arch Surg 144(2):137–141 **(discussion 42)**
82. Nazerian P, Tozzetti C, Vanni S, Bartolucci M, Gualtieri S, Trausi F, Vittorini M, Catini E, Cibinel GA, Grifoni S (2015) Accuracy of abdominal ultrasound for the diagnosis of pneumoperitoneum in patients with acute abdominal pain: a pilot study. Crit Ultrasound J 7(1):15
83. Tayal VS, Graf CD, Gibbs MA (2003) Prospective study of accuracy and outcome of emergency ultrasound for abdominal aortic aneurysm over two years. Acad Emerg Med 10(8):867–871
84. Heegaard W, Hildebrandt D, Spear D, Chason K, Nelson B, Ho J (2010) Prehospital ultrasound by paramedics: results of field trial. Acad Emerg Med 17(6):624–630
85. Saver JL, Fonarow GC, Smith EE, Reeves MJ, Grau-Sepulveda MV, Pan W, Olson DM, Hernandez AF, Peterson ED, Schwamm LH (2013) Time to treatment with intravenous tissue plasminogen activator and outcome from acute ischemic stroke. JAMA 309(23):2480–2488
86. Emberson J, Lees KR, Lyden P, Blackwell L, Albers G, Bluhmki E, Brott T, Cohen G, Davis S, Donnan G, Grotta J, Howard G, Kaste M, Koga M, von Kummer R, Lansberg M, Lindley RI, Murray G, Olivot JM, Parsons M, Tilley B, Toni D, Toyoda K, Wahlgren N, Wardlaw J, Whiteley W, del Zoppo GJ, Baigent C, Sandercock P, Hacke W, Stroke Thrombolysis Trialists' Collaborative G (2014) Effect of treatment delay, age, and stroke severity on the effects of intravenous thrombolysis with alteplase for acute ischaemic stroke: a meta-analysis of individual patient data from randomised trials. Lancet 384(9958):1929–1935
87. Ragoschke-Schumm A, Walter S, Haass A, Balucani C, Lesmeister M, Nasreldein A, Sarlon L, Bachhuber A, Licina T, Grunwald IQ, Fassbender K (2014) Translation of the 'time is brain' concept into clinical practice: focus on prehospital stroke management. Int J Stroke. 9(3):333–340
88. Lichtman JH, Watanabe E, Allen NB, Jones SB, Dostal J, Goldstein LB (2009) Hospital arrival time and intravenous t-PA use in US Academic Medical Centers, 2001–2004. Stroke 40(12):3845–3850
89. Herzberg M, Boy S, Holscher T, Ertl M, Zimmermann M, Ittner KP, Pemmerl J, Pels H, Bogdahn U, Schlachetzki F (2014) Prehospital stroke diagnostics based on neurological examination and transcranial ultrasound. Crit Ultrasound J 6(1):3
90. Schlachetzki F, Herzberg M, Holscher T, Ertl M, Zimmermann M, Ittner KP, Pels H, Bogdahn U, Boy S (2012) Transcranial ultrasound from diagnosis to early stroke treatment: part 2: prehospital neurosonography in patients with acute stroke: the Regensburg stroke mobile project. Cerebrovasc Dis 33(3):262–271
91. Lysakowski C, Walder B, Costanza MC, Tramer MR (2001) Transcranial Doppler versus angiography in patients with vasospasm due to a ruptured cerebral aneurysm: a systematic review. Stroke 32(10):2292–2298
92. Chenaitia H, Squarcioni C, Marie BP, Emgan Q, Tomislav P (2011) Transcranial sonography in prehospital setting. Am J Emerg Med 29(9):1231–1233
93. Behnke S, Becker G (2002) Sonographic imaging of the brain parenchyma. Eur J Ultrasound 16(1–2):73–80
94. Moretti R, Pizzi B (2011) Ultrasonography of the optic nerve in neurocritically ill patients. Acta Anaesthesiol Scand 55(6):644–652
95. Bergauer A, Prosen G, Flis V, Seruga T, Brvar M, Kobilica N (2012) Contrast enhanced ultrasound imaging of the optic nerve sheath diameter—what are we really measuring? Crit Ultrasound J 4(Suppl 1):A2
96. Blaivas M, Theodoro D, Sierzenski PR (2003) Elevated intracranial pressure detected by bedside emergency ultrasonography of the optic nerve sheath. Acad Emerg Med 10(4):376–381
97. Moretti R, Pizzi B, Cassini F, Vivaldi N (2009) Reliability of optic nerve ultrasound for the evaluation of patients with spontaneous intracranial hemorrhage. Neurocrit Care 11(3):406–410
98. Maissan IM, Dirven PJ, Haitsma IK, Hoeks SE, Gommers D, Stolker RJ (2015) Ultrasonographic measured optic nerve sheath diameter as an accurate and quick monitor for changes in intracranial pressure. J Neurosurg 123(3):743–747
99. Dulchavsky SA, Henry SE, Moed BR, Diebel LN, Marshburn T, Hamilton DR, Logan J, Kirkpatrick AW, Williams DR (2002) Advanced ultrasonic diagnosis of extremity trauma: the FASTER examination. J Trauma 53(1):28–32
100. Bozorgi F, Shayesteh Azar M, Montazer SH, Chabra A, Heidari SF, Khalilian A (2017) Ability of ultrasonography in detection of different extremity bone fractures; a case series study. Emergency 5(1):e15
101. Paziana K, Fields JM, Rotte M, Au A, Ku B (2012) Soft tissue foreign body removal technique using portable ultrasonography. Wilderness Environ Med 23(4):343–348
102. Kilker BA, Holst JM, Hoffmann B (2014) Bedside ocular ultrasound in the emergency department. Eur J Emerg Med 21(4):246–253
103. Blaivas M, Theodoro D, Sierzenski PR (2002) A study of bedside ocular ultrasonography in the emergency department. Acad Emerg Med 9(8):791–799
104. Whitfield DA, Portouw SJ (2012) Retinal detachment due to facial gunshot wound: the utility of ultrasonography in a medically austere environment. J Emerg Med 42(6):678–681
105. Siddiqui N, Arzola C, Friedman Z, Guerina L, You-Ten KE (2015) Ultrasound improves cricothyrotomy success in cadavers with poorly defined neck anatomy: a randomized control trial. Anesthesiology 123(5):1033–1041
106. Curtis K, Ahern M, Dawson M, Mallin M (2012) Ultrasound-guided, Bougie-assisted cricothyroidotomy: a description of a novel technique in cadaveric models. Acad Emerg Med 19(7):876–879
107. Jones PW, Moyers JP, Rogers JT, Rodriguez RM, Lee YC, Light RW (2003) Ultrasound-guided thoracentesis: is it a safer method? Chest 123(2):418–423
108. Soni NJ, Franco R, Velez MI, Schnobrich D, Dancel R, Restrepo MI, Mayo PH (2015) Ultrasound in the diagnosis and management of pleural effusions. J Hosp Med 10(12):811–816
109. Costantino TG, Parikh AK, Satz WA, Fojtik JP (2005) Ultrasonography-guided peripheral intravenous access versus traditional approaches in patients with difficult intravenous access. Ann Emerg Med 46(5):456–461
110. Maggiolini S, Gentile G, Farina A, De Carlini CC, Lenatti L, Meles E, Achilli F, Tempesta A, Brucato A, Imazio M (2016) Safety, efficacy, and complications of pericardiocentesis by real-time echo-monitored procedure. Am J Cardiol 117(8):1369–1374
111. Hughes CW (1954) Use of an intra-aortic balloon catheter tamponade for controlling intra-abdominal hemorrhage in man. Surgery 36(1):65–68
112. Qasim Z, Brenner M, Menaker J, Scalea T (2015) Resuscitative endovascular balloon occlusion of the aorta. Resuscitation 96:275–279
113. Chaudery M, Clark J, Wilson MH, Bew D, Yang GZ, Darzi A (2015) Traumatic intra-abdominal hemorrhage control: has current technology tipped the balance toward a role for prehospital intervention? J Trauma Acute Care Surg 78(1):153–163
114. Avaro JP, Mardelle V, Roch A, Gil C, de Biasi C, Oliver M, Fusai T, Thomas P (2011) Forty-minute endovascular aortic occlusion increases survival in an experimental model of uncontrolled hemorrhagic shock caused by abdominal trauma. J Trauma 71(3):720–725 **(discussion 5-6)**
115. London's Air Ambulance. World's first pre-hospital REBOA performed. 2014. https://londonsairambulance.co.uk/our-service/news/2014/06/we-perform-worlds-first-pre-hospital-reboa. Accessed 14 Nov 2017
116. Chaudery M, Clark J, Morrison JJ, Wilson MH, Bew D, Darzi A (2016) Can contrast-enhanced ultrasonography improve Zone III REBOA placement for prehospital care? J Trauma Acute Care Surg 80(1):89–94

117. Alexandrov AV, Molina CA, Grotta JC, Garami Z, Ford SR, Alvarez-Sabin J, Montaner J, Saqqur M, Demchuk AM, Moye LA, Hill MD, Wojner AW, Investigators C (2004) Ultrasound-enhanced systemic thrombolysis for acute ischemic stroke. N Engl J Med 351(21):2170–2178
118. Barlinn K, Tsivgoulis G, Barreto AD, Alleman J, Molina CA, Mikulik R, Saqqur M, Demchuk AM, Schellinger PD, Howard G, Alexandrov AV (2014) Outcomes following sonothrombolysis in severe acute ischemic stroke: subgroup analysis of the CLOTBUST trial. Int J Stroke 9(8):1006–1010
119. Schellinger PD, Alexandrov AV, Barreto AD, Demchuk AM, Tsivgoulis G, Kohrmann M, Alleman J, Howard V, Howard G, Alexandrov AW, Brandt G, Molina CA, Investigators C (2015) Combined lysis of thrombus with ultrasound and systemic tissue plasminogen activator for emergent revascularization in acute ischemic stroke (CLOTBUST-ER): design and methodology of a multinational phase 3 trial. Int J Stroke 10(7):1141–1148
120. Tsivgoulis G, Eggers J, Ribo M, Perren F, Saqqur M, Rubiera M, Sergentanis TN, Vadikolias K, Larrue V, Molina CA, Alexandrov AV (2010) Safety and efficacy of ultrasound-enhanced thrombolysis: a comprehensive review and meta-analysis of randomized and nonrandomized studies. Stroke 41(2):280–287
121. Holscher T, Dunford JV, Schlachetzki F, Boy S, Hemmen T, Meyer BC, Serra J, Powers J, Voie A (2013) Prehospital stroke diagnosis and treatment in ambulances and helicopters-a concept paper. Am J Emerg Med 31(4):743–747
122. Porter TR, Xie F, Lof J, Powers J, Vignon F, Shi W, White M (2017) The thrombolytic effect of diagnostic ultrasound-induced microbubble cavitation in acute carotid thromboembolism. Invest Radiol 52(8):477–481
123. Mehta KS, Lee JJ, Taha AA, Avgerinos E, Chaer RA (2017) Vascular applications of contrast-enhanced ultrasound imaging. J Vasc Surg 66(1):266–274
124. Saqqur M, Tsivgoulis G, Nicoli F, Skoloudik D, Sharma VK, Larrue V, Eggers J, Perren F, Charalampidis P, Storie D, Shuaib A, Alexandrov AV (2014) The role of sonolysis and sonothrombolysis in acute ischemic stroke: a systematic review and meta-analysis of randomized controlled trials and case-control studies. J Neuroimaging 24(3):209–220
125. Dickman E, Pushkar I, Likourezos A, Todd K, Hwang U, Akhter S, Morrison S (2016) Ultrasound-guided nerve blocks for intracapsular and extracapsular hip fractures. Am J Emerg Med 34(3):586–589
126. Dochez E, van Geffen GJ, Bruhn J, Hoogerwerf N, van de Pas H, Scheffer G (2014) Prehospital administered fascia iliaca compartment block by emergency medical service nurses, a feasibility study. Scand J Trauma Resusc Emerg Med 22:38
127. Lippert SC, Nagdev A, Stone MB, Herring A, Norris R (2013) Pain control in disaster settings: a role for ultrasound-guided nerve blocks. Ann Emerg Med 61(6):690–696
128. Schaeffer E, Millot I, Landy C, Nadaud J, Favier JC, Plancade D (2014) Another use of continuous transversus abdominis plane (TAP) block in trauma patient: pelvic ring fractures. Pain Med 15(1):166–167
129. Grady MV, Cummings KC 3rd (2008) The "flank bulge" sign of a successful transversus abdominis plane block. Reg Anesth Pain Med 33(4):387
130. Sarkisian AE, Khondkarian RA, Amirbekian NM, Bagdasarian NB, Khojayan RL, Oganesian YT (1991) Sonographic screening of mass casualties for abdominal and renal injuries following the 1988 Armenian earthquake. J Trauma 31(2):247–250
131. Sztajnkrycer MD, Baez AA, Luke A (2006) FAST ultrasound as an adjunct to triage using the START mass casualty triage system: a preliminary descriptive system. Prehosp Emerg Care 10(1):96–102
132. Dan D, Mingsong L, Jie T, Xiaobo W, Zhong C, Yan L, Xiaojin L, Ming C (2010) Ultrasonographic applications after mass casualty incident caused by Wenchuan earthquake. J Trauma 68(6):1417–1420
133. Shorter M, Macias DJ (2012) Portable handheld ultrasound in austere environments: use in the Haiti disaster. Prehosp Disaster Med 27(2):172–177
134. Zhang S, Zhu D, Wan Z, Cao Y (2014) Utility of point-of-care ultrasound in acute management triage of earthquake injury. Am J Emerg Med 32(1):92–95
135. Stawicki SP, Howard JM, Pryor JP, Bahner DP, Whitmill ML, Dean AJ (2010) Portable ultrasonography in mass casualty incidents: The CAVEAT examination. World J Orthop 1(1):10–19
136. Barlinn K, Barreto AD, Sisson A, Liebeskind DS, Schafer ME, Alleman J, Zhao L, Shen L, Cava LF, Rahbar MH, Grotta JC, Alexandrov AV (2013) CLOTBUST-hands free: initial safety testing of a novel operator-independent ultrasound device in stroke-free volunteers. Stroke 44(6):1641–1646
137. Kirkpatrick AW, McKee I, McKee JL, Ma I, McBeth PB, Roberts DJ, Wurster CL, Parfitt R, Ball CG, Oberg S, Sevcik W, Hamilton DR (2016) Remote just-in-time telementored trauma ultrasound: a double-factorial randomized controlled trial examining fluid detection and remote knobology control through an ultrasound graphic user interface display. Am J Surg 211(5):894–902
138. Kolbe N, Killu K, Coba V, Neri L, Garcia KM, McCulloch M, Spreafico A, Dulchavsky S (2015) Point of care ultrasound (POCUS) telemedicine project in rural Nicaragua and its impact on patient management. J Ultrasound 18(2):179–185
139. Biegler N, McBeth PB, Tiruta C, Hamilton DR, Xiao Z, Crawford I, Tevez-Molina M, Miletic N, Ball CG, Pian L, Kirkpatrick AW (2013) The feasibility of nurse practitioner-performed, telementored lung telesonography with remote physician guidance—'a remote virtual mentor'. Crit Ultrasound J 5(1):5
140. Rubin MN, Barrett KM, Freeman WD, Lee Iannotti JK, Channer DD, Rabinstein AA, Demaerschalk BM (2015) Teleneurosonology: a novel application of transcranial and carotid ultrasound. J Stroke Cerebrovasc Dis 24(3):562–565
141. Mierzwa AP, Huang SP, Nguyen KT, Culjat MO, Singh RS (2016) Wearable ultrasound array for point-of-care imaging and patient monitoring. Stud Health Technol Inform 220:241–244
142. Tsung JW, Blaivas M, Stone MB (2009) Feasibility of point-of-care colour Doppler ultrasound confirmation of intraosseous needle placement during resuscitation. Resuscitation 80(6):665–668
143. Inaba K, Chouliaras K, Zakaluzny S, Swadron S, Mailhot T, Seif D, Teixeira P, Sivrikoz E, Ives C, Barmparas G, Koronakis N, Demetriades D (2015) FAST ultrasound examination as a predictor of outcomes after resuscitative thoracotomy: a prospective evaluation. Ann Surg 262(3):512–518 **(discussion 6-8)**
144. Lamhaut L, Jouffroy R, Soldan M, Phillipe P, Deluze T, Jaffry M, Dagron C, Vivien B, Spaulding C, An K, Carli P (2013) Safety and feasibility of prehospital extra corporeal life support implementation by non-surgeons for out-of-hospital refractory cardiac arrest. Resuscitation 84(11):1525–1529
145. Lamhaut L, Hutin A, Deutsch J, Raphalen JH, Jouffroy R, Orsini JP, Baud F, Carli P (2017) Extracorporeal cardiopulmonary resuscitation (ECPR) in the prehospital setting: an illustrative case of ECPR performed in the Louvre museum. Prehosp Emerg Care. 21(3):386–389
146. Hutin A, Corrocher R, Loosli F, Mantz B, Lamhaut L. How physicians perform prehospital ECMO on the streets of Paris. 2017. http://www.jems.com/articles/print/volume-42/issue-12/features/how-physicians-perform-prehospital-ecmo-on-the-streets-of-paris.html. Accessed 11 Dec 2017
147. Vezzani A, Brusasco C, Palermo S, Launo C, Mergoni M, Corradi F (2010) Ultrasound localization of central vein catheter and detection of postprocedural pneumothorax: an alternative to chest radiography. Crit Care Med 38(2):533–538
148. Wen M, Stock K, Heemann U, Aussieker M, Kuchle C (2014) Agitated saline bubble-enhanced transthoracic echocardiography: a novel method to visualize the position of central venous catheter. Crit Care Med 42(3):e231–e233
149. King RL, Liu Y, Harris GR (2017) Quantification of temperature rise within the lens of the porcine eye caused by ultrasound insonation. Ultrasound Med Biol 43(2):476–481
150. Herman BA, Harris GR (1999) Theoretical study of steady-state temperature rise within the eye due to ultrasound insonation. IEEE Trans Ultrason Ferroelectr Freq Control 46(6):1566–1574

12

Temporary transvenous pacing guided by the combined use of ultrasound and intracavitary electrocardiography: a feasible and safe technique

Pablo Blanco*

Abstract

Temporary transvenous pacing is a crucial procedure in emergency and critical care medicine. While fluoroscopy guidance is considered the gold-standard to place the temporary pacing electrode catheter (EC), its use is usually limited by equipment availability and time. By contrast, ultrasound (US) guidance is a useful alternative, since it is widely available at the bedside, does not emit ionizing radiation and provides optimal times to active pacing with fewer complications. However, many times, in spite of visualizing the EC in the right ventricle using US, the pacing capture and sensing are not optimal, and thus, having an easily applicable method for best assessing this issue is desirable, especially if it could be combined with US without difficulties. With the purpose of illustrating the points made previously, the combined US-intracavitary electrocardiography technique is described in detail in this paper.

Keywords: Transthoracic echocardiography, Cardiac pacing, Ultrasonography, Electrocardiography, Point-of-care

Introduction

Temporary transvenous pacing (TVP) is a lifesaving procedure which is mainly indicated in patients with symptomatic bradyarrhythmias as well as in patients with specific tachyarrhythmias (i.e., overdrive pacing) [1–4].

Temporary transvenous pacing consists in inserting a temporary pacing electrode catheter (EC) into the right ventricle and then applying an electric stimulus with the goal of restoring effective cardiac depolarization and heart contraction, resulting in the delivery of an adequate heart rate and cardiac output [3].

Several complications can result from this critical procedure such as failure to secure venous access, failure to place the lead correctly, sepsis, puncture of arteries, lungs or myocardium and life-threatening arrhythmias [5]. Giving these facts, a safe method to monitor the EC insertion is desirable [3].

*Correspondence: ohtusabes@gmail.com
Intensive Care Physician, Intensive Care Unit, Clínica Cruz Azul, 2651, 60 St., 7630 Necochea, Argentina

The placement of the EC can be achieved in several ways, including a blind technique as well as a couple of guided techniques, such as intracavitary electrocardiography (ECG) [6, 7], ultrasonographic-guided insertion (US) [8–10] and fluoroscopy [9, 10]. Since the blind technique is neither safe nor effective most of the times, and considering that fluoroscopy is not usually available at the bedside or patients are commonly unstable to be transferred to the radiology department, ECG and/or real-time ultrasonographic (US) guidance are generally chosen to assist in the procedure at the patient's bedside. The combination of guided techniques for the placement of the EC is a valid and useful strategy, with the intention of making the procedure easy, safe, and effective. This is the case of the combination of US guidance with intracavitary ECG, which is easy to perform, may lead to a reduction in the time to active pacing and may avoid complications.

Regarding the selection of the route of insertion, this may be guided by several factors, such as the presence of hypovolemia, anticoagulation status, or adequate anatomy. As a general rule, the right-sided veins are preferred over the left because permanent systems are usually inserted on the left side and because it is often technically easier from the right side [5]. In general, the right internal jugular vein provides the most direct route to the right ventricle and it is associated with lowest rate of loss of ventricular capture and thus is the recommended route for using in practice [5]. Right subclavian/axillary route follows the right IJV and is preferred in patients with hypovolemia, given the ability of these vessels to remain patent even in patients with volume depletion. Femoral access can be performed with ease; however, it can be more difficult to advance the electrodes to the right ventricle, limits patient mobility, has a higher risk of venous thromboembolism, and offers the least stable wire position [11]. Of note, securing a venous access is not a minor issue, with a high failure rate reported among studies (average 15%, range 6–40%) [5]. Ultrasound-guided insertion of the introducer sheath, which is in fact a central venous canulation, has proven to improve canulation success and reduce complications related to the procedure [12]. Thus, all introducer sheaths should be placed under ultrasound guidance, unless there is no time to prepare the ultrasound equipment, such as in extreme situations (e.g., cardiopulmonary resuscitation), or eventually when ultrasound cannot be used for technical reasons (e.g., subcutaneous emphysema).

The combined technique (ultrasound and intracavitary ECG) will be described after discussing some aspects of both techniques when used in isolation.

Feasibility of ultrasound guidance in placing the electrocatheter

Aguilera et al. [8] reported the transthoracic echocardiography (TTE)-guided insertion of the EC in nine patients in the ED. The EC was successfully observed by TTE in eight patients, allowing also to detect mispositioning of the EC and its adequate repositioning in three patients. Right IJV was used in six patients, while right subclavian vein was used in three. US-guided insertion of the introducer was not reported. The total time to pacemaker insertion was 4–13 min in this study.

The study carried out by Pinneri et al. [9] compared the placement of EC using TTE guidance ($n=53$, with EC inserted through the internal jugular vein) versus fluoroscopy ($n=53$, with EC inserted through the femoral vein). Although some of the differences between the two groups may be accounted for by the site of insertion and the guidance method, in the presence of an adequate acoustic window, the TTE guidance allows for a reliable temporary pacing with short procedural times, showing lower costs, avoiding the use of ionizing radiation and adding the advantage to perform the procedure at the bedside.

More recently, Ferri et al. [10] compared the insertion of the EC via the echo-guided approach (jugular vein) in 113 patients vs fluoroscopy ($n=90$) via the femoral vein. In this study, the echo-guided approach reduced the median time to active pacing (22 vs 43 min), showed less complications (lower infections rates and puncture-related hematomas) and reduced the time to implantation of the definitive pacemaker.

In cases of inadequate cardiac windows, the use of transesophageal echocardiography (TEE) guidance has been anecdotally described [13]; however, this technique is invasive and it is not yet widely available in the emergency and critical care settings.

Intracavitary ECG-guidance in placing the EC

While this technique is well-described in the literature, it is scarcely utilized in many EDs and ICUs. Although time to active pacing using this technique is not described in literature according to author´s knowledge, in practice, this is a reliable method to safely insert the EC in the RV and ensure a correct capture and sensing of the device [6, 7]. Although expected ECG patterns are observed based on the EC position, it is sometimes difficult to know where the EC is actually placed. For example, when it is placed in the coronary sinus, inferior vena cava or in RV perforations. Also, recording the intracavitary ECG as the EC is advanced is time-consuming in practice and not the best option when pacing urges, so having in practice a direct visualization of the EC passing through the tricuspid valve into the RV may save the time spent in recording these lead positions.

Simultaneous use of ultrasound and intracavitary ECG: the technique

After inserting the introducer sheath into the internal jugular (right internal jugular vein preferred as noted above) or subclavian/axillary vein both under US guidance, a 5-7F-bipolar EC (balloon-tipped floating catheter is preferred) is advanced by an operator while a second operator performs the transthoracic echocardiogram (TTE) exam. The EC is seen as a bright linear hyperechoic structure. The most important echocardiographic views to observe the EC are the subcostal four-chamber and the apical four-chamber, which are normally required to monitor the position of the EC while it is advanced into the right ventricle (RV). Both views allow practitioners to follow the EC into the right atrium (RA) and its progression through the tricuspid valve (TV) up to the preferred lead position into the RV apex (Fig. 1 and Additional file 1: Videos S1, Additional file 2: Videos S2). Other alternative EC

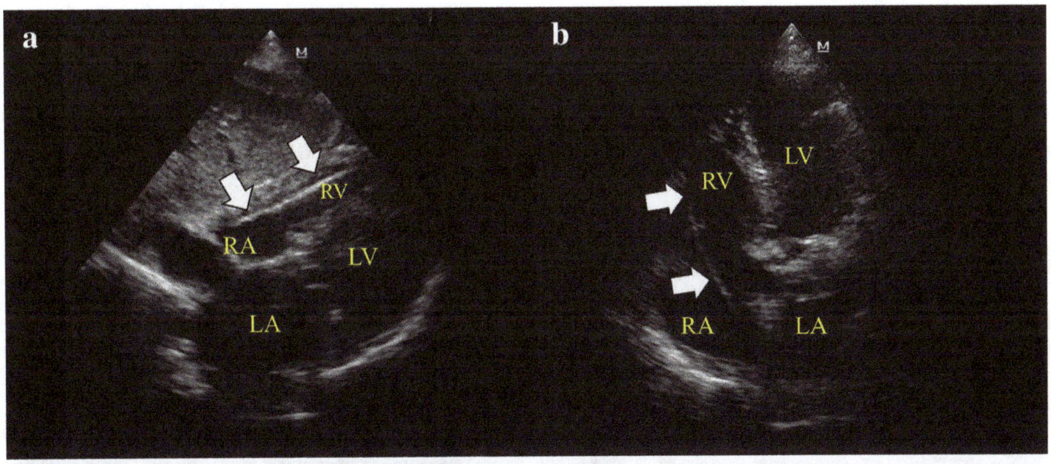

Fig. 1 Subcostal 4-chamber view (**a**) and apical 4-chamber view (**b**) demonstrating the temporary pacing electrode catheter (EC, arrows) into the right ventricle (RV). *RV* right ventricle, *RA* right atrium, *LV* left ventricle, *LA* left atrium

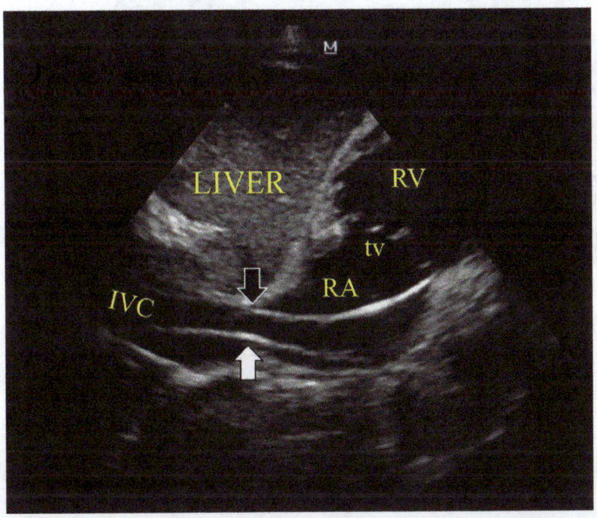

Fig. 2 Subcostal inferior vena cava (IVC) view demonstrating the EC entering (white arrow) and getting out (black arrow) the IVC in direction of the right heart chambers. *RA* right atrium, *tv* tricuspid valve, *RV* right ventricle

positions, although somewhat unstable, are the interventricular septum, RV free wall, and RV outflow tract (RVOT). The inferior vena cava (IVC) view should be checked when, despite advancement of the EC, there is no apparent EC progression into the RV (Fig. 2 and Additional file 1: Videos S3). Due to the anatomic continuity between the superior vena cava and IVC, the EC inadvertently passing into the IVC is the most frequent incorrect placement observed in practice. Short-axis views (subcostal and/or parasternal) at the level of the great vessels are useful to detect the EC passing through the TV and a RVOT and, also importantly, to exclude an accidental misplacement into the pulmonary artery.

Although the lead is positioned into the RV by TTE, ultrasound usually does not provide complete certainty as to whether the tip of the EC is free-floating or in close contact with the endocardium of the RV wall, which is a critical requirement for the device to achieve an appropriate sensing and capture. One study showed that only 62% of the ECs seen in the RV have an adequate capture [8]. To assess this issue, an intracavitary ECG (Figs. 3 and 4 and Additional file 1: Videos S1) is then performed at this moment. To do so, a cable with one alligator clip (also called a "crocodile clip" outside of the United States) on each end is needed: one alligator clip is connected to the negative or distal pole from the end of the EC; the second alligator clip is attached to any of the precordial leads on the ECG machine; ECG limb leads are connected to the patient in the usual fashion [7]. Intracavitary ECG (recording the V lead that has the alligator clip attached) may allow to recognize the position of the EC as it is advanced from the superior vena cava up to the desired heart position. To demonstrate that the EC is in contact with the RV endocardium and not free-floating, an intracavitary ECG must show a subepicardial injury pattern, which is usually obtained at a lead depth of approximately 35–40 cm. If this injury pattern is not evident, minimal adjustments of the EC (backing off or advancing it a few centimeters) generally allow to achieve it without difficulty. Further EC advancement beyond 40–45 cm may result in coiling and also atypical lead positions instead of showing a RV subepicardial injury pattern [4, 5]. As a rule, the definite and optimal

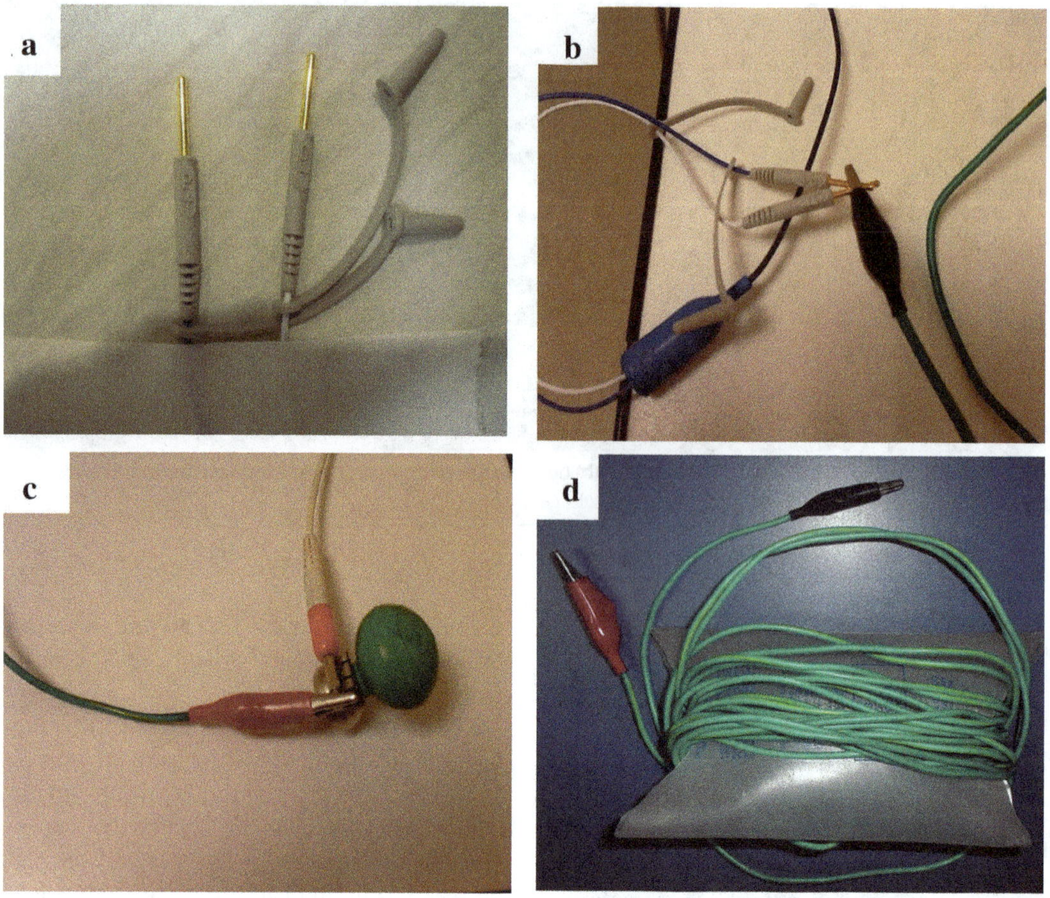

Fig. 3 Intracavitary electrocardiogram (ECG) technique attaching the electrodes of the EC (**a**, **b**) to a precordial lead (V1 in this case, **c** by a cable with an alligator clip on each end (**d**). Of note, while the alligator clip is attached to a precordial lead as seen by its suction cup, this is in fact registering the cardiac electrical activity from an intracavitary view, thus it is indistinct whether or not it is placed on the patient's chest; ECG limb leads are placed in the usual fashion

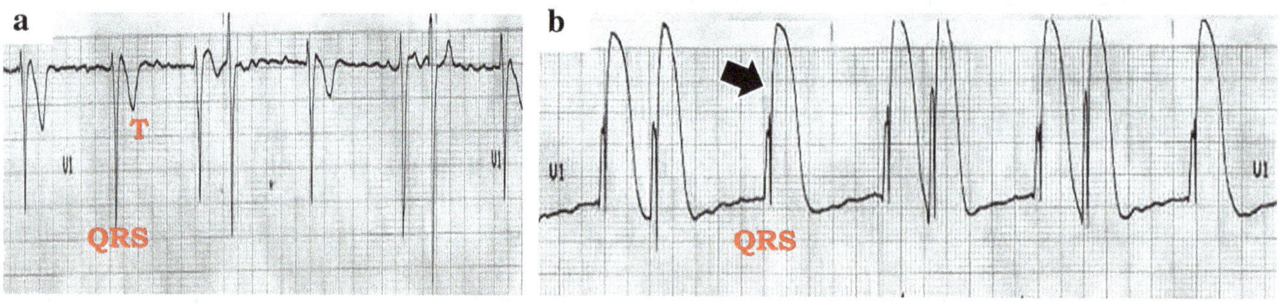

Fig. 4 Intracavitary ECG (lead V1) showing the cardiac electrical activity when the EC is free-floating into the RV (**a**) and when this is contacting the endocardium of the RV (**b**), as demonstrated by a subepicardial injury pattern (arrow)

lead position is into the RV, with the demonstration of a clear IVC and pulmonary artery [4].

After a subepicardial injury is demonstrated on intracavitary ECG and the lead is connected to the generator which is now turned on, ventricular capture is normally achieved at low stimulation thresholds. Surface ECG will ordinarily show the pacemaker spikes accompanied by broad QRS complexes of left bundle branch block (LBBB) morphology. Sensing will also be optimal at low thresholds. A "benign" captured right bundle branch pattern (RBBB), although rare, can also be recorded in some patients [14]. While RBBB is observed in left-sided catheters (perforations) as well as in coronary sinus (CS) insertion, TTE confirmation of the EC positioned into the RV is reassuring [15, 16].

Through the observation of the lead advancement by TTE, serious complications can be detected, such as septal perforations (interauricular and interventricular), RV free wall perforation and pericardial effusion, and eventually cardiac tamponade [16]. Misplacement into the pulmonary artery and IVC can also be readily detected by TTE [4, 8], allowing the redirection of the EC to an optimal position. The insertion in the coronary sinus (CS) [17] is another rare possibility, especially occurring when the CS is dilated or when a left-sided insertion (left IJV or subclavian vein) is attempted, and a persistent left superior vena cava is present. CS can be well-visualized in a foreshortened apical four-chamber view (Fig. 5) and, as previously mentioned, the captured QRS complexes will have a RBBB pattern. A lateral chest X-ray may aid in confirming a lead positioned in the CS. Of note, a CS lead placement allows for a more physiologic ventricular depolarization, with lesser degrees of inter- and intraventricular asynchrony in comparison with a RV position. Thus, there are lower risks of cardiac failure after TVP. In the absence of other complications or TVP malfunctioning, a CS lead can be safely kept in place [17]. The same principle of more physiologic ventricular depolarization applies also to RV leads that are not located in the ventricular apex, with lesser degrees of asynchrony in leads placed in the interventricular septum in comparison with apical leads. Unless the TVP is malfunctioning, these ECs do not usually require repositioning.

Once the capture and sensing of the device is adequate as demonstrated on the surface ECG, lung ultrasound is performed to rule in or out a pneumothorax (the presence or absence of lung sliding, along other signs of pneumothorax).

The complete technique is summarized in Fig. 6.

First step: Ultrasound-guided insertion of the introducer sheath (internal jugular vein or subclavian vein); arrow: needle into the internal jugular vein.	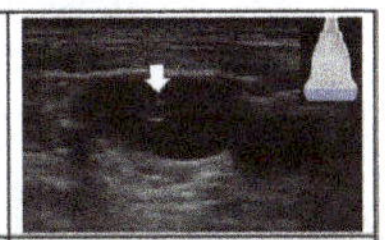
Second step: Transthoracic echocardiography is performed to observe the temporary pacing catheter electrode (EC) as it is advanced from the superior vena cava up to the right ventricle (RV); arrow: pacing lead into the RV.	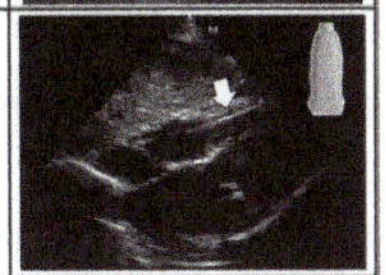
Third step: Intracavitary electrocardiography (ECG) is used to assess whether the EC is free-floating or in contact with the endocardium of the RV (subepicardial injury pattern, arrow).	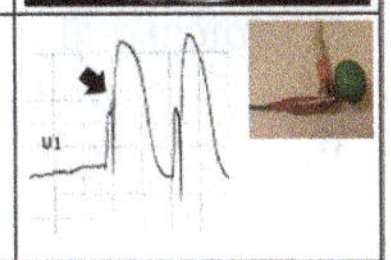
Fourth step: Surface ECG should demonstrate adequate capture and sensing, with QRS complexes showing a pattern of left bundle branch block; arrow: pacer spikes.	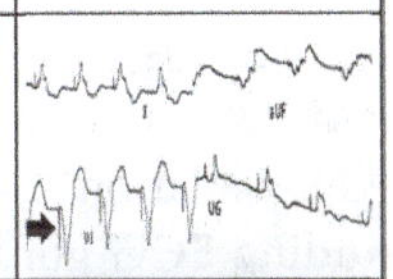
Five step: Lung ultrasound is performed for assessing lung sliding and rule in or out a pneumothorax.	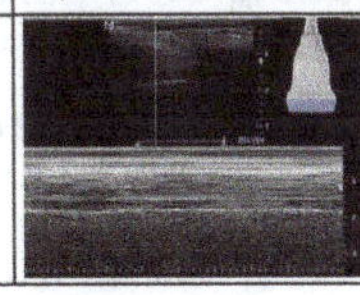

Fig. 6 Summary of the combined technique: ultrasound and intracavitary ECG technique for temporary transvenous pacing

Analysis of ultrasound plus intracavitary ECG-guidance to insert the EC

The combined use of US and intracavitary ECG to insert the EC appears as a potentially useful method for a secure lead placement in emergency settings. There are several benefits associated with this combined technique that need to be recognized. In the first place, the

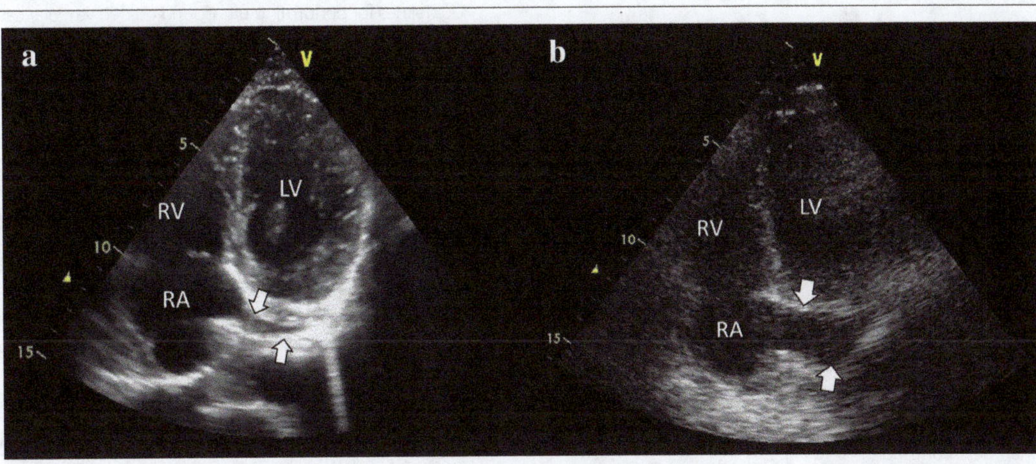

Fig. 5 Coronary sinus view, obtained from a foreshortened apical 4-chamber view. **a** Normal coronary sinus (arrow). **b** Dilated coronary sinus (arrows)

insertion of the introducer sheath under US guidance, which is associated with an improvement in first pass success and fewer complications in comparison with the landmark technique. Second, TTE may allow practitioners to quickly pass the EC to the RV, under direct visualization, thus allowing for the detection of complications or misplacements and the reposition of the EC in real time. Third, for intracavitary ECG, a rapid assessment of RV subepicardial injury pattern is achieved when the EC is in the RV, avoiding failed pacing captures and sensing. Finally, lung US is useful to rule in or out a pneumothorax in seconds, at the patient's bedside.

Limitations of ultrasound and intracavitary ECG are the same as the ones established for each method when used in isolation.

Adding ECG-guidance to TTE in this way is easy, does not seem to add unusual complexity or extra time spent on the procedure and may actually improve the times to active pacing, avoiding complications.

Limitations

This short communication is based on author's years of experience performing this procedure in this way, achieving excellent results. However, prospective studies are needed to validate this simultaneous technique in large populations.

Conclusions

While ultrasound is a feasible guidance to insert and monitor the EC placement at the patient's bedside, the addition of intracavitary ECG allows for a better determination of RV wall lead-contacting, enhancing a correct pacemaker capture and sensing, without adding unusual complexity or spending extra time in the procedure. Emergency and critical care physicians must be aware of the benefits of using this combined method when transvenous pacing is needed.

Additional files

Additional file 1: Video S1. Subcostal 4-chamber view showing in real time the entering of the temporary pacing electrode catheter (EC) into the RV, the intracavitary ECG when the EC is free-floating and when is contacting the endocardium, and the moment when the capture is achieved after connecting the electrodes of the EC to the generator device switched on.

Additional file 2: Video S2. Subcostal 4-chamber and apical 4-chamber view showing the pacing lead in the apex of the right ventricle, corresponding to Fig. 1.

Additional file 3: Video S3. Subcostal inferior vena cava (IVC) view demonstrating the pacing lead entering and getting out the IVC in direction of the right heart chambers, corresponding to Fig. 2.

Authors' contributions

The author wrote the manuscript, performed the ultrasound and ECG examinations, edited the multimedia material. The author read and approved the final manuscript.

Acknowledgements

The authors would like to thank Mrs. Julieta Vigna for the language guidance.

This work has not been presented at any conferences.

References

1. Competency-based training in intensive care medicine in Europe (CoBaTrICE programme): performs cardiac pacing (transvenous or transthoracic). http://www.cobatrice.org/Data/ModuleGestionDeContenu/PagesGenerees/en/03-Syllabus/0E-procedures/0E15-pacing//113.asp. Accessed 02 Mar 2015
2. Ahn J, Kharasch M, Aronwald R, Menon S, Du H, Calabrese N, Gitelis M, Aitchson P, Wang E (2013) Assessing the accreditation council for graduate medical education requirement for temporary cardiac pacing procedural competency through simulation. Simul Healthc 8(2):78–83
3. López Ayerbe J, Villuendas Sabaté R, García García C et al (2004) Temporary pacemakers: current use and complications. Rev Esp Cardiol 57(11):1045–1052
4. Blanco P, Nomura J (2014) An atypical misplacement of a temporary pacing catheter diagnosed and resolved by ultrasound. Am J Emerg Med 32(10):1296.e1–1296.e3
5. McCann P (2007) A review of temporary cardiac pacing wires. Indian Pacing Electrophysiol 7(1):40–49
6. Evans GL, Glasser SP (1971) Intracavitary electrocardiography as a guide to pacemaker positioning. JAMA 216(3):483–485
7. Harrigan RA, Chan TC, Moonblatt S, Vilke GM, Ufberg JW (2007) Temporary transvenous pacemaker placement in the emergency department. J Emerg Med 32(1):105–111
8. Aguilera PA, Durham BA, Riley DA (2000) Emergency transvenous cardiac pacing placement using ultrasound guidance. Ann Emerg Med 36(3):224–227
9. Pinneri F, Frea S, Najd K, Panella S, Franco E, Conti V, Corgnati G (2013) Echocardiography-guided versus fluoroscopy-guided temporary pacing in the emergency setting: an observational study. J Cardiovasc Med (Hagerstown) 14(3):242–246
10. Ferri LA, Farina A, Lenatti L, Ruffa F, Tiberti G, Piatti L, Savonitto S (2016) Emergent transvenous cardiac pacing using ultrasound guidance: a prospective study versus the standard fluoroscopy-guided procedure. Eur Heart J Acute Cardiovasc Care 5(2):125–129
11. Sullivan BL, Bartels K, Hamilton N (2016) Insertion and management of temporary pacemakers. Semin Cardiothorac Vasc Anesth 20(1):52–62
12. Councils on Intraoperative Echocardiography and Vascular Ultrasound of the American Society of Echocardiography, Troianos CA, Hartman GS, Glas KE, Skubas NJ, Eberhardt RT, Walker JD, Reeves ST (2011) Guidelines for performing ultrasound guided vascular cannulation: recommendations of the American Society of Echocardiography and the Society of Cardiovascular Anesthesiologists. J Am Soc Echocardiogr 24(12):1291–1318
13. Krishnan U, Karthikeyan VJ, Trinh J, Theologou T, Velavan P (2014) First report of the use of transesophageal echocardiography to position a temporary pacing wire. J Cardiothorac Vasc Anesth 28(1):110–111
14. Hemminger EJ, Criley JM (2006) Right ventricular enlargement mimicking electrocardiographic left ventricular pacing. J Electrocardiol 39(2):180–182
15. Yang YN, Yin WH, Young MS (2003) Safe right bundle branch block pattern during permanent right ventricular pacing. J Electrocardiol 36(1):67–71
16. Velibey Y, Yaylak B, Guvenc TS, Cinier G, Kalenderoglu K, Guzelburc O, Yildirimturk O (2018) Inadvertent left ventricle endocardial or uncomplicated right ventricular pacing: how to differentiate in the emergency department. J Emerg Med 54:e91–e95
17. Osman F, Ratib K, Krishnamoorthy S, Nadir A, Creamer J, Morley-Davies A (2008) Temporary pacing wire in the coronary sinus: a novel treatment of acute heart failure? Europace 10(7):877–879

Diagnostic value of whole-body-focused ultrasonography in high-acuity patients in the emergency department: a prospective single-center cross-sectional study

M. Riishede[1,2,3*], C. B. Laursen[2,4], L. S. Teglbjærg[3], E. Rancinger[1], P. B. Pedersen[2,3], S. M. Luef[4], J. H. Clausen[5], O. Graumann[2,6], A. T. Lassen[2,7] and G. Baatrup[1,2]

Abstract

Background: A fast and diagnostic accurate tool to assess the unselected category of high-acuity patients, in whom the underlying pathology is not always obvious, is needed in the emergency departments (ED). We aim to describe the feasibility, validity and diagnostic yield of a routine whole-body-focused ultrasonography (wbf-us) in an unselected group of high-acuity ED patients.

Methods: In a prospective observational study, a convenience sample of ED patients (≥ 18 years) with a high-acuity score or systolic blood pressure < 100 mmHg received a routine wbf-us of the heart, lungs, abdomen and deep veins by two non-expert sonographers. Final diagnosis was established by experienced auditors. Investigators were blinded to the patients' medical history and emergency physicians and auditors were blinded to the investigators assessments. Diagnostic accuracy was assessed by comparing the investigators' ultrasonography findings to a structured double-blinded clinical audit of patient files.

Results: We included 171 patients, initiated a whole-body-focused ultrasonography examination (wbf-us) in 160 and completed it in 128 patients with an average time of a full examination of 28 min. We found pathology in 65/171 (38%) of the patients whose most frequent symptoms upon arrival were cardiopulmonary. Among the patients who received wbf-us, we found the majority of pathology by wbf-us of the lungs ($n=50$, 31%), the heart ($n=26$, 16%), few in the abdomen ($n=5$, 3%) and none in the deep veins. The overall sensitivity was 50–100%, specificity 84–94%, positive predictive value 11–44% and negative predictive value 94–100%.

Conclusion: Focused cardiopulmonary ultrasonography might be considered for routine use in high-acuity ED patients with cardiopulmonary symptoms whereas focused ultrasonography of the abdomen and deep veins performed by non-expert sonographers only seems indicated in selected patients.

Trial registration Danish Data Protection Agency (ID 13/12076). Committee on Biomedical Research Ethics for the Region of Southern Denmark (ID S-20130047).

*Correspondence: Minna.Riishede@rsyd.dk
[1] The Research Section, Department of Surgery (A), Odense University Hospital, Baagoes Allé 15, 5700 Svendborg, Denmark
Full list of author information is available at the end of the article

Introduction

Rapid and accurate identification of the cause for severe illness in unselected high-acuity patients is often a challenge to the emergency physician (EP) [1, 2].

Focused ultrasonography (f-us) is a noninvasive bedside tool, generally free of pain and ionizing radiation, fairly easy to learn and associated with a reduction in the use of more cumbersome imaging [3–5]. The use of f-us in high-acuity patients has increased over the last decade [6].

Various studies have addressed symptoms using a range of single-organ f-us to whole-body f-us (wbf-us) in selected patients and shown that f-us can be both fast and accurate in identification of selected pathologies [7–9].

Moreover, studies have shown that f-us in selected patients can increase the diagnostic accuracy by increasing the sensitivity to up to 97% when adding f-us alongside standard clinical examination compared to a sensitivity as low as 50% by standard clinical examination alone indicating that f-us holds the potential to reduce the time to correct diagnosis and correct initial treatment [10].

Alongside these studies, evidence-based guidelines that describe indications, technical performance and interpretation of f-us as well as recommendations and guidelines of the implementation of f-us in ED or intensive care units have been published [11–13].

However, to our knowledge, the use of a wbf-us in an unselected group of high-acuity patients remains uninvestigated. Therefore, the aim of our study was to assess the feasibility (measured by duration and amount of evaluable wbf-us) and the validity and diagnostic yield (measured by sensitivity, specificity, negative and positive predictive values) of a wbf-us in an unselected group of high-acuity ED patients to clarify if the method of examination could be a helpful tool for the physician in the daily clinic. The wbf-us was performed by two physicians who are non-expert sonographers reflecting the daily clinical setting in most EDs.

Methods

A descriptive prospective, cross-sectional study was performed in the ED at Odense University Hospital, Svendborg, Denmark, which has approximately 29,000 visits per year of which around 4100 are triaged as high-acuity patients upon arrival.

Acute admissions in Denmark are to public hospitals via emergency call or referred to by the general practitioner. Selected patients bypass the ED and are transported directly to an expert department (e.g. with signs of acute myocardial infarction, pregnancy or trauma to head, thorax or column).

Initial diagnostic tests ordered for patients admitted to the ED are in general based on symptoms and signs and include blood sample analyses, ECG, microbiological analyses and imaging (e.g. X-ray, CT, MR). Ultrasonography examinations are mainly performed by summoned specialists and are not an integrated part of the initial examination of ED patients [14].

The inclusion took place from December 2013 to March 2016. Included patients constituted a convenience sample; consequently, inclusion only took place immediately after the patients' arrival to the ED. The investigators were blinded to the patients' medical history and only aware of the patients' direct cause of admittance upon inclusion. Patients were included after informed consent by the investigators if they were: (1) acutely admitted to the ED, (2) ≥ 18 years, (3) upon primary assessment they presented with a high-acuity score or systolic blood pressure < 100 mmHg. A high-acuity score was defined as the two highest levels of acuity in our ED triage system based on the patients' initial clinical scores (e.g. saturation, respiratory rate, heart rate) (Additional file 1: Appendix S1). Exclusion criteria were patients with mental disability or patients unable to sign informed consent.

The included patients constituted a mixture of both surgical and medical etiology with symptoms and signs of various diseases (e.g. respiratory problems, cerebral thrombosis or hip fracture). The investigators performed the wbf-us blinded to the EP and only in his absence. The wbf-us was performed with a Philips CX 50 ultrasound machine (Philips, USA) and consisted of wbf-us of the lungs (Flus), the heart (Fcu), the abdomen (Faus) and the deep veins of the legs (Lcu). The wbf-us was always performed in the same sequence commenced by Flus then Fcu, Faus and Lcu and only aborted or paused on demand of the patient (e.g. due to pain or nausea) or in case of urgent treatment or supplemental analysis (e.g. scans, blood samples). The wbf-us was not completed if not resumed within 1 h and the investigation time was defined as the time spent on the actual ultrasound examination. The time used at wbf-us examination time was measured from the first to the last gaze with the ultrasonography probe. Interruptions were not included.

Wbf-us diagnoses were assessed according to predefined diagnostic criteria (Additional file 2: Appendix S2) and performed according to the following predefined f-us protocols.

Focused lung ultrasonography (Flus): performed with a L12-5 linear array transducer (Philips) (12–5 MHz) or a C5-1 curved array transducer (Philips) (5–1 MHz) using a modification of the principles described by Lichtenstein, Volpicelli and colleagues as described by Laursen et al. [15–17]. We looked for pneumothorax, interstitial syndrome and pleural effusion.

Focused cardiac ultrasonography (Fcu): performed with a S5-1 sector transducer (Philips) (5–1 MHz) using the focus assessed transthoracic echocardiography (Fate) protocol [18]. We looked for reduced ejection fraction (EF) and pericardial effusion.

Focused abdominal ultrasonography (Faus): performed with a C5-1 broadband curved array transducer (Philips) (5–1 MHz) using the three abdominal windows from the RUSH protocol and including a transverse and oblique window of the abdominal aorta [7]. We looked for free abdominal fluid and abdominal aorta aneurism.

Limited compression ultrasonography (Lcu): performed with a L12-5 linear array transducer (Philips) (12–5 MHz) or C5-1 curved array transducer (Philips) (5–1 MHz) according to the American College of Emergency Medicine's imaging criteria compendium [19]. We looked for signs of a deep-vein thrombosis (DVT).

The investigators (ER and MR) had varying experience in wbf-us. Prior to inclusion MR performed: focused lung ultrasonography (Flus) > 80, Focused assessment with transthoracic echocardiography (Fate) > 50, focused assessment with sonography in trauma (Faus) > 40, limited compression ultrasonography (Lcu) > 50. Of these, 25 of each scanning area were supervised and evaluated during a period of f-us certification according to the national guidelines [13]. ER had no prior f-us skills and received an e-learn course of the wbf-us protocol including an oral presentation and hands on training followed by 5–10 supervised examinations until she was capable of performing the wbf-us protocol with an image quality sufficient for diagnostic evaluation (Additional file 2: Appendix S2).

A video clip from each window of the wbf-us examination (e.g. one respiratory cycle from each Flus window, 6 s of the heart from each Fcu projection) was saved to an external hard disc for later expert evaluations. With the exception of wbf-us findings of acute life-threatening conditions all wbf-us results were kept blinded from patients and EPs.

All wbf-us clips were finally assessed by expert physicians with European Federation of Societies for Ultrasound in Medicine and Biology (EFSUMB) for ultrasonography level 2–3 from specialties of respiratory medicine (Flus), cardiology (Fcu) and radiology (Faus, Lcu). The expert sonographers evaluated the investigators' wbf-us examinations and assessed the final diagnoses blinded to the investigators' interpretations and the EPs clinical evaluations.

All results from the wbf-us were compared to gold standard, which was defined as the final diagnoses assessed by blinded clinical audit of the medical record.

The blinded audit was performed according to predefined diagnostic criteria by two auditors who, independently of each other and blinded to all wbf-us clips and the interpretations of these, set the final diagnoses. In case of any discrepancy, a third auditor made the final decision (Additional file 3: Appendix S3).

Analyses

Data were reported as proportions with a 95% confidence interval (CI) based at binominal distribution. Diagnostic performances were established using sensitivity, specificity, positive and negative predictive values (PPV, NPV), their 95% CI and Fleiss kappa coefficients (K) using the results from the blinded medical record audit as gold standard.

Descriptive statistics, describing medical history, medication and vital parameters upon admission were performed. Data analysis was conducted using Stata version 14.0 (Stata Corporation LP®, Texas, USA).

The main analyses were performed by the 'intention to treat' principle. Missing data in the basic characteristics were handled by simple imputation: we kept patients with no or incomplete wbf-us in the study. Any cases of image quality inadequate for evaluation were handled as follows: (a) handled as non-pathologic in the analysis of total wbf-us diagnoses, (b) left out in the analysis of diagnostic accuracy and inter-observer agreement.

Ethics

Patients were included after informed consent. Any wbf-us that revealed signs of a predefined acute life-threatening condition was immediately non-blinded to the EP in charge (e.g. pericardial effusion, ejection fraction ≤ 45%, pulmonary edema, massive pleural effusion, pneumothorax, pulmonary emboli or deep-vein thrombosis (DVT). Subsequently, it was up to the clinician to assess whether further action should be taken. The study was undertaken in accordance with the Helsinki Declaration and approved by the Committee on Biomedical Research Ethics for the Region of Southern Denmark (ID S-20130047) and the Danish Data Protection Agency (ID 13/12076).

Results

We included 171 patients (Fig. 1). Median age was 69 years (range 18–97) and 94 (55%) were women (Table 1).

With the wbf-us we found one or more pathologies in 65/171 (38%) patients allocated to the departments as follows: Medical Department 58/147 (39%); Surgical Departments (abdominal and orthopedic) 4/17 (24%) and from other departments 3/7 (43%).

Based on the wbf-us, we found most pathology by the protocols of Flus 50/160 patients (31%), Fcu 26/160 patients (16%) and few cases by Faus 5/148 patients (3%) and none by Lcu 0/128 patients (0%) (Table 2).

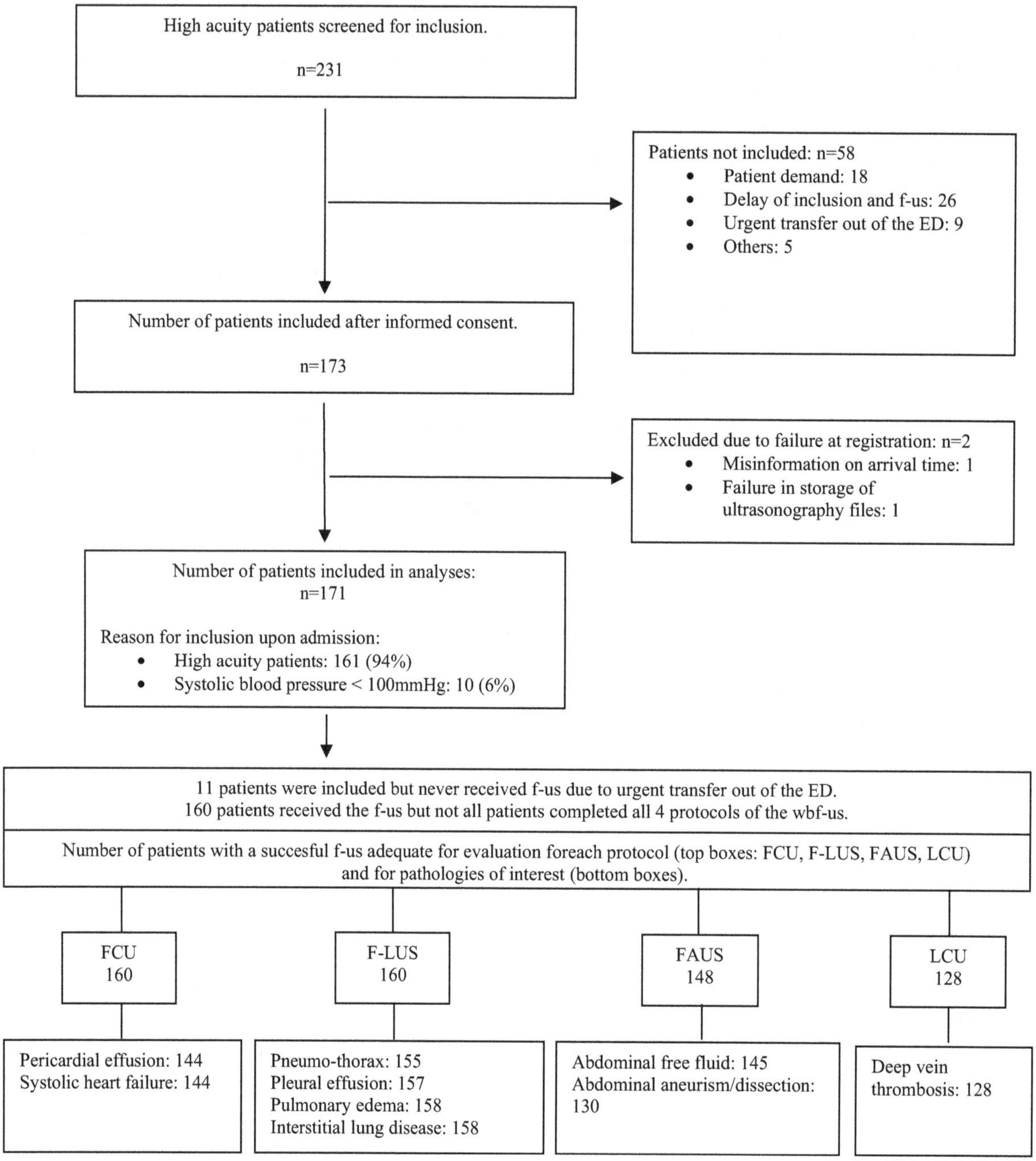

* The Surgical Department includes the abdominal and orthopedic surgical departments.

Abbreviations: n (number of patients), ED (emergency department), f-us (focused ultrasonography), wbf-us (whole body focused ultrasonography), FCU (Focused cardiac ultrasonography), F-LUS (focused lung ultrasonography), FAUS (focused abdominal ultrasonography), LCU (limited compression ultrasonography).

Fig. 1 Flow chart of inclusion of adult high acuity patients admitted to the Emergency Department

The most frequent specific pathological findings were pleural effusion $n=39$, interstitial syndrome/pulmonary edema $n=25$ and systolic heart failure $n=19$. For prevalence of pathological wbf-us findings, see Table 2.

A wbf-us adequate to answer questions from all 4 scanning protocols could be performed in 128 (75%) patients with a median examination time of 28 min (IQR 24–32). The wbf-us was never initiated in 11 (6%)

Table 1 Baseline characteristics of adult high acuity patients included upon admission to the emergency department

Characteristics ($n=171$)	Value
Age (years), median (range)	69 (18–97)
Gender (*n* (%))	
Female	94 (55)
Male	77 (45)
Vital parameters upon admission	
Heart rate (beats/min) ($n=170$), median (IQR)	87 (72–100)
Systolic BP (mmHg) ($n=170$), median (IQR)	135 (119–153)
Diastolic BP (mmHg) ($n=170$), median (IQR)	75 (65–87)
Respiration rate (breaths/min) ($n=164$), median (IQR)	18 (16–21)
Saturation (%)	
Patients with oxygen supply ($n=34$), median (IQR)	95 (93–98)
Saturation (%)	
Patients without oxygen supply ($n=152$), median (IQR)	97 (93–99)
Temperature (°C) ($n=170$), median (IQR)	37.0 (36.0–37.7)
Glascow Coma Score ($n=170$), median (IQR)	15 (15–15)
Blood glucose ($n=144$), median (IQR)	6.7 (6–8.6)
Former medical history among the 171 included patients, *n* (%)	
Coronary artery disease	11 (6)
Heart failure	29 (17)
Arterial hypertension	44 (25)
Diabetes mellitus	24 (14)
Chronic obstructive pulmonary disease	33 (19)
Asthma	15 (9)
Thromboembolic disease	14 (8)
Other Pulmonary disease	8 (5)
Psychiatric disorder	30 (18)
Stroke	6 (4)
Chronic kidney disease	7 (4)
Reason for inclusion upon admission among the 171 included patients, *n* (%)	
High acuity patients	161 (94)
Systolic blood pressure < 100 mmHg	10 (6)
Affiliated department upon admission among the 171 included patients, *n* (%)	
Medical	147 (86)
Surgical[a]	17 (10)
Others	7 (4)

Number of patients with an ultrasonography examination sufficient for diagnostic evaluation for each protocol (*N*) and for the individual pathology (*n*). Cases of no ultrasonography clips are left out

Fcu focused cardiac ultrasonography, *Flus* focused lung ultrasonography, *Faus* focused abdominal ultrasonography, *Lcu* limited compression ultrasonography

[a] Surgical includes the general and orthopedic surgical departments

patients and not completed in 43 (25%) primarily due to acute clinical procedures (e.g. imaging and blood samples).

The investigators' ultrasonography findings were confirmed by expert evaluations with an internal total agreement of 89–100%.

Final diagnostic gold standard was established by chart review by two independent researchers and had an overall inter-observer agreement of 97.6% (Kappa 0.74).

Based on the gold standard evaluation of the 171 included patients, we found pleural effusion in 22 (13%), interstitial syndrome 3 (2%), pulmonary edema in 6 (4%) and systolic heart failure in 4 (2%). For the complete list of final diagnoses, see Table 3 and Additional file 4.

Finally, we performed a 'per protocol' contingency table analysis of the correlation between the pathology found by wbf-us and gold standard diagnoses and found that according to the most frequent diagnostic findings

Table 2 Distribution of pathology found by whole body focused ultrasonography in adult high acuity ED patients

Diagnoses	Investigators' prevalence of pathology in each subgroup, *n* (%)
Lungs (Flus): $N=160$	
Pathological findings in the 50 patients with positive findings	
Pneumothorax, (of 155 investigated)	0 (0%)
Pleural effusion, (of 157 investigated)	39 (25%)
Pulmonary edema, (of 158 investigated)	25 (16%)
Interstitial lung disease, (of 158 investigated)	25 (16%)
Cardiac (Fcu): $N=160$	
Pathological findings in the 26 patients with positive findings	
Pericardial effusion, (of 144 investigated)	10 (7%)
Systolic heart failure (EF < 45%), $n=144$	19 (13%)
Abdomen (Faus): $N=148$	
Pathological findings in the 5 patients with positive findings	
Free fluid abdomen, (of 145 investigated)	4 (3%)
Abdominal aorta aneurism/dissection[a], (of 130 investigated)	1 (1%)
Veins (Lcu): $N=128$	
Pathological findings in 0 patients	
Deep vein thrombosis, (of 128 investigated)	0 (0%)

ED Emergency Department

[a] Signs of aorta aneurism or dissection are defined as a deviation from the normal diameter (women < 2.9 cm, men < 3.2 cm) of the abdominal aorta

the wbf-us revealed 100% of patients with interstitial lung disease (3/3) and pericardial effusion (2/2), 89% of patients with pleural effusion (17/19) and 50% of the patients with pulmonary edema (3/6) and systolic heart failure (2/4) (Table 4 and Additional file 5a, b).

This resulted in an overall sensitivity of 50–100%, specificity of 84–94%, PPV of 11–44% and a NPV of 94–100%. Diagnostic accuracy values and their 95% CI are provided in Table 5.

Discussion

We initiated wbf-us in 160 high-acuity ED patients in an unselected group of 171 patients and found pathology in a little more than 1/3 patients. The most frequent pathological ultrasonography findings were of cardiopulmonary origin and were mainly found in patients admitted with respiratory or circulatory symptoms.

Similar to other studies of f-us of the heart and lungs in dyspneic ED patients, we found cardiopulmonary diagnoses as heart failure, pneumonia and pleural effusion among the most common pathologies [10, 20, 21]. In parallel, our findings are consistent with the low number of free abdominal fluid, abdominal aorta aneurisms/dissection and DVT found by gold standard as well as the uneven distribution of patients to the medical (147) and surgical (17) departments.

The f-us examination time included f-us examination, filing of f-us clips and patient handling in relation to the f-us examination, and interruptions from other persons or procedures were not included. Comparable to similar studies of selected f-us of the heart, lungs ± the abdomen and the deep veins, we had an average time for a complete wbf-us of 28 min (IQR 28–32) [9, 20, 22, 23]. This made the examination susceptible to numerous interruptions due to the urgency of treatment.

Our study hereby shows that a routine wbf-us approach might not be pertinent in all high-acuity ED patients. It supports the idea of a more rational approach where Flus and Fcu are routinely applied in patients with signs or symptoms of disease in the chest and where Faus and Lcu might be relevant in selected patients.

Diagnostic accuracy of the f-us examinations

The investigators found several pathologies that were not found by gold standard. The most common diagnoses were: (a) pericardial effusion in 8 patients, with a majority of final diagnoses of infection with extrapulmonary focus and pneumonia; (b) systolic heart failure in 17 patients with the majority of final diagnoses of cardiopulmonary origin; and (c) pleural effusion, pulmonary edema and interstitial lung disease in 22 patients with the majority of final diagnoses of cardiopulmonary origin.

The inter-observer agreement on 89–100% on the wbf-us images emphasizes that the investigators' images are of acceptable quality.

Table 3 Gold standard defined as final diagnoses established by blinded audit of the medical records

Diagnoses (found in all 171 patients)	Number of final diagnosis, *n* (%)
Cerebral diseases	
Cerebral stroke	12 (7)
Cerebral hemorrhagia	2 (1)
Pulmonary diseases	
COPD	17 (11)
Suspected COPD with exacerbation	5 (3)
Asthma	4 (2)
Interstitial lung disease[a]	3 (2)
Pneumonia	24 (14)
Pulmonary oedema[a]	6 (4)
Pleural effusion[a]	22 (13)
Parapneumonic effusion	6 (4)
Empyema	0 (0)
Pulmonary embolism	3 (2)
Pneumothorax[a]	0 (0)
Heart diseases	
Systolic heart failure[a]	4 (2)
Nonsystolic heart failure	2 (1)
Myocardial infarction (acute or recent evolved)	4 (2)
Pericardial effusion[a]	2 (1)
Valvular heart disease	12 (7)
Infective endocarditis	0 (0)
Cardiac arrythmia	26 (15)
Chest pain (myocardial infarction ruled out)	9 (5)
Abdominal diseases	
Ileus	0 (0)
Appendicitis	2 (1)
Free abdominal fluid[a]	1 (1)
Pancreatitis/kidney stone	8 (5)
Dissection/aneurism of the abdominal aorta[a]	0 (0)
Orthopedic diseases	
Fracture	8 (5)
Luxation	5 (3)
Orthopedic injuries	6 (4)
Other diseases or symptoms	
DVT[a]	0 (0)
Anemia	14 (8)
Malignancy	7 (4)
Poisoning	4 (2)
Lipotymi/dizziness/discomfort	10 (6)
Infection with extrapulmonary focus	31 (18)
No diagnostic criteria met	28 (16)

Final diagnoses are established on all included patients, $n = 171$

Ultrasound examination clips deemed not evaluable by novice sonographers or experts are treated as normal in this analysis

COPD chronic obstructive pulmonary disease, *DVT* deep vein thrombosis

[a] Diagnoses for which we looked for in the whole body focused ultrasonography examination

Several studies of cardiopulmonary f-us has demonstrated that f-us is superior to the often used gold standard (chest radiography) when it comes to the detection of certain pathologies of acute cardiopulmonary disease [20, 24]. This increases the amount of false-positive f-us findings and leads to a drop in PPV which hereby becomes falsely low. A study of ED patients with respiratory symptoms demonstrated that f-us of the heart, lungs and deep veins in the legs increased the prescription of advanced diagnostic tests earlier in the hospital stay, which confirmed the suspected f-us diagnoses and identified missed life-threatening diseases. When compared to the control group during the entire stay at hospital, there was no significant difference in amount of prescribed advanced diagnostic tests [17]. Similar to these studies we find many false-positive results as we also find an overall diagnostic accuracy comparable with similar studies (Table 4) [8, 10, 17, 25, 26].

The investigators overlooked the pathology according to final diagnosis as follows: (a) systolic heart failure in two patients (one was due to strict diagnostic criteria, the other might be due to lack of skills among the investigators since the expert sonographer diagnosed the systolic heart failure when reviewing the f-us clips); (b) pleural effusion in two patients (expert evaluation found no pathology in one patient and deemed the f-us clips unevaluable in the other patient); and (c) pulmonary edema in three patients where the expert sonographer found no pulmonary edema either.

Similar to the previously mentioned studies we find that the wbf-us is a reliable tool to find pathology in highly acute ED patients as well as the wbf-us can find pathology that would otherwise be missed at clinical assessment [10, 17]. The f-us thereby holds the potential to reduce the time to correct diagnosis, proper treatment and the amount of X-rays we expose our patients to.

Strengths and limitations

Recommendations and guidelines have been made to increase f-us competencies and uniformity of assessment [13, 27], however, several studies of individual f-us procedures show that even with a short introduction novices can assess patients with a diagnostic accuracy similar to that of experts [4, 25]. The wbf-us was performed in an unselected group of high-acuity patients in a clinically realistic ED setting which provided us the possibility to investigate if certain patient categories are redundant or missed in the search of who to perform the wbf-us on and which f-us modalities to use. To reduce the subjective bias often seen in blinded auditing, the final diagnoses were performed by three auditors. The third auditor only set a diagnosis in case of disagreement between the

Table 4 Per protocol: correlation and diagnostic accuracy between investigators pathological ultrasonography findings and gold standard pathology

Interstitial lung disease			
Investigator	**Gold standard**		**Total**
	1	**0**	
1	3	22	25
0	0	133	133
Total	3	155	158
Pericardial effusion			
Investigator	**Gold standard**		**Total**
	1	**0**	
1	2	8	10
0	0	134	134
Total	2	142	144
Pleural effusion			
Investigator	**Gold standard**		**Total**
	1	**0**	
1	17	22	39
0	2	116	118
Total	19	138	157
Pulmonary edema			
Investigator	**Gold standard**		**Total**
	1	**0**	
1	3	22	25
0	3	130	133
Total	6	152	158
Systolic heart failure			
Investigator	**Gold standard**		**Total**
	1	**0**	
1	2	17	19
0	2	123	125
Total	4	140	144

PPV positive predictive value, *NPV* negative predictive value, *CI* 95% confidence interval

two first auditors whose agreement was 97.6% (Kappa 0.74).

The study also has limitations: being a single-center study performed by only two investigators, this study might not be generalizable to all other EDs. The basic characteristics in our study population mimic those found in similar studies in high-acuity ED patients [27]. However, the distribution of patients between the departments was uneven which mimics the patient category in tertiary hospital EDs, but it mainly gives us a picture of the wbf-us in medical ED patients.

Selection bias is present; the inclusion only took place when the investigators were present (daytime), some eligible patients were included but received no f-us due to urgent need of treatment in expert departments, others bypassed the ED due to administrative decisions and finally some patients were too ill to cooperate to f-us or to give informed consent. We believe that the selection bias could not be avoided.

The wbf-us protocol was designed to look for the most critical but reversible conditions that can be visualized by ultrasonography and that are most often found in

Table 5 Diagnostic accuracy of investigators pathology found with focused ultrasonography compared to gold standard

Diagnoses	Gold standard positive/f-us positive	Sensitivity % (95% CI)	Specificity % (95% CI)	PPV % (95% CI)	NPV % (95% CI)
Heart (Fcu): $N=160$					
Pericardial effusion, $n=144$	2/10	100 (16–100)	94 (89–8)	26 (3–56)	100 (97–100)
Systolic heart failure (EF < 45%), $n=144$	4/19	50 (7–93)	88 (81–93)	11 (1–33)	98 (94–100)
Lungs (Flus): $N=160$					
Pneumothorax[a], $n=155$	0/0				
Pleural effusion, $n=157$	19/39	89 (67–99)	84 (77–90)	44 (28–60)	98 (94–100)
Pulmonary edema, $n=158$	6/25	50 (12–88)	86 (79–91)	12 (3–31)	98 (94–100)
Interstitial lung disease, $n=158$	3/25	100 (29–100)	86 (79–91)	12 (3–31)	100 (97–100)
Abdomen (Faus): $N=148$					
Abdominal aorta aneurism/dissection[b], $n=130$	0/1				
Free fluid abdomen[c], $n=145$	1/4	100 (CI 3–100)	98 (CI 94–100)	25 (CI 1–81)	100 (CI 97–100)
Veins (Lcu): $N=128$					
Deep-vein thrombosis, $n=128$[a]	0/0				

Gold standard: final diagnoses of blinded medical record audit

Statistical analyses are made using the statistical concept 'per protocol': cases of no ultrasonography clips are left out

Number of patients with an ultrasonography examination sufficient for diagnostic evaluation for each protocol (*N*) and for each pathology (*n*)

F-us focused ultrasonography, *Fcu* focused cardiac ultrasonography, *Flus* focused lung ultrasonography, *Faus* focused abdominal ultrasonography, *Lcu* limited compression ultrasonography

[a] Due to a low number of events the sensitivity and specificity could not be calculated

[b] Signs of aorta aneurism or dissection are defined as a deviation from the normal diameter (women < 2.9 cm, men < 3.2 cm) of the abdominal aorta

[c] Free fluid abdomen' is assessed from the 3 views of the abdominal f-us. If any region of the abdominal f-us showed any sign of free fluid the FAUS was regarded as pathological

high-acuity ED patients. The wbf-us protocol was also designed to be simple and fast so that it could be used by ED physicians who not all are expert sonographers. We, therefore, excluded a lot of pathologies from the wbf-us protocol that could have been relevant in some patients such as patients with abdominal pain (e.g. cholecystitis, ectopic pregnancy, pneumoperitoneum).

Despite these actions, the wbf-us examination was time consuming. In addition, the research context of the study increased the amount of data registration which increased the amount of interruptions due to other clinical procedures which again increased the number of non-completed f-us examinations (Fig. 1). Consequently, the feasibility of the wbf-us in the clinical setting is influenced by the duration of the scanning procedure.

Furthermore, the wbf-us diagnoses were based on predefined criteria but the investigators were not blinded to the patients' clinical presentation and could have been influenced by the patients' clinical appearance to increase or decrease the probability of distinctive pathological patterns.

However, final diagnoses could only be obtained if diagnosed or confirmed during the actual stay at hospital. Therefore, the high number of false-positive findings and the related low PPV is partly explained by the fact that patients admitted with other pathological conditions than those diagnosed at previous admissions (e.g. heart failure) had these well-known pathologies confirmed by the wbf-us. But if patients were asymptomatic and the EP did not take action on the unblinded f-us findings or found them relevant enough to be listed in the medical record, then these pathologies were not reconfirmed during the actual stay and, therefore, not included as a final diagnosis. Furthermore, some final diagnoses could have occurred during the hospital stay (e.g. pleural effusion or pulmonary edema) and not have been present at the patients arrival the ED where the wbf-us was performed. This could partly explain the unexpected poor diagnostic accuracy (low sensitivity and PPV) in these findings. Unfortunately, our study was not designed to take these factors into account.

Moreover, we performed a routine wbf-us in all included patients regardless their symptoms and found unexpected pathology (e.g. pleural effusion in a patient with hip fracture). The dilemma is that we do not know the clinical relevance of these unexpected ultrasonography findings in asymptomatic patients and our study is not designed to investigate this.

Conclusion

F-us in the hands of non-expert sonographers seems to be a useful diagnostic bedside tool in adult high-acuity medical ED patients. However, Flus and Fcu seem indicated in patients with cardiopulmonary symptoms whereas Faus and Lcu seem indicated in selected patients. F-us holds the potential to reduce the time to correct diagnosis and to find pathology that is missed at initial diagnostic assessment.

Additional files

Additional file 1: Appendix S1. Definition of high acuity patients included in this study.

Additional file 2: Appendix S2. Sonographic definitions and diagnostic criteria of the focused ultrasonography examination.

Additional file 3: Appendix S3. Blinded audit and audit diagnostic criteria of final diagnoses.

Additional file 4. Number of pathological ultrasonography findings compared to gold standard diagnoses in the adult high acuity patients admitted to the emergency department.

Additional file 5. a Per protocol correlation and diagnostic accuracy between investigators pathological ultrasonography findings and gold standard pathology found in adult high acuity patients admitted to the emergency department. Contingency tables and calculations are made according to the statistical concept 'per protocol', hence only including the patients who received a focused ultrasonography examination. **b** Per intention to treat correlation and diagnostic accuracy between investigators pathological ultrasonography and gold standard pathology found in adult high acuity patients admitted to the emergency department. Contingency tables and calculations are made according to the statistical concept 'intention to treat' including the entire study population. N = 171.

Abbreviations

CI: confidence interval; COPD: chronic obstructive pulmonary disease; DVT: deep-vein thrombosis; ED: Emergency Department; EP: Emergency Physician; Faus: focused abdominal ultrasonography; Fcu: focused cardiac ultrasonography; Flus: focused lung ultrasonography; IQR: inter quartile range; K: kappa coefficients; Lcu: limited compression ultrasonography; N: number of patients; NPV: negative predictive value; PPV: positive predictive value.

Acknowledgements

We are deeply indebted to the participating patients and the entire staff at the Emergency Department at Odense University Hospital, Svendborg, Denmark for their support and participation in this project.

Authors' contributions

Eligibility for authorship is gained according to the Vancouver guidelines. MR: contributed to the conception and design of the study, conducted the inclusion and acquisition of data, analysis and interpretation of data, drafting the submitted article and approved the final version for publication. CBL: contributed to the conception and design of the study, data analysis and interpretation of data, drafting the submitted article and approved the final version for publication. LST: contributed to the conception and design of the study, drafting the submitted article and approved the final version for publication. ES: contributed to the acquisition of data and approved the final version of the article for publication. P. B. Pedersen: contributed to the acquisition of data and approved the final version of the article for publication. SML: contributed to the acquisition of data and approved the final version of the article for publication. JHC: contributed to the acquisition of data and approved the final version of the article for publication. OG: contributed to the acquisition of data and approved the final version of the article for publication. ATL: contributed to the data analysis and interpretation of data, drafting the submitted article and approved the final version for publication. GB: contributed to the conception and design of the study, the interpretation of data, drafting the submitted article. All authors read and approved the final manuscript.

Author details

[1] The Research Section, Department of Surgery (A), Odense University Hospital, Baagoes Allé 15, 5700 Svendborg, Denmark. [2] Department of Clinical Research, University of Southern Denmark, SDU, Odense, Denmark. [3] Department of Internal Medicine & Emergency Medicine (M/FAM), Odense University Hospital, Svendborg, Denmark. [4] Department of Respiratory Medicine, Odense University Hospital, Odense, Denmark. [5] Department of Cardiology, Hospital of Southern Jutland, Aabenraa, Denmark. [6] Department of Radiology, Odense University Hospital, Odense, Denmark. [7] Department of Emergency Medicine, Odense University Hospital, Odense, Denmark.

References

1. Croucher B (2014) The challenge of diagnosing dyspnea. AACN Adv Crit Care 25(3):284–290
2. Lien CT, Gillespie ND, Struthers AD et al (2002) Heart failure in frail elderly patients: diagnostic difficulties, co-morbidities, polypharmacy and treatment dilemmas. Eur J Heart Fail 4(1):91–98
3. Laursen CB, Sloth E, Lassen AT et al (2015) Does point-of-care ultrasonography cause discomfort in patients admitted with respiratory symptoms? Scand J Trauma Resusc Emerg Med 23:46
4. Frederiksen CA, Juhl-Olsen P, Andersen NH et al (2013) Assessment of cardiac pathology by point-of-care ultrasonography performed by a novice examiner is comparable to the gold standard. Scand J Trauma Resusc Emerg Med 21:87
5. Peris A, Tutino L, Zagli G et al (2010) The use of point-of-care bedside lung ultrasound significantly reduces the number of radiographs and computed tomography scans in critically ill patients. Anesth Analg 111(3):687–692
6. Lichtenstein D, van Hooland S, Elbers P et al (2014) Ten good reasons to practice ultrasound in critical care. Anaesthesiol Intensive Ther 46(5):323–335
7. Perera P, Mailhot T, Riley D et al (2010) The RUSH exam: rapid ultrasound in SHock in the evaluation of the critically ill. Emerg Med Clin North Am 28(1):29–56, vii
8. Lichtenstein DA, Meziere GA (2008) Relevance of lung ultrasound in the diagnosis of acute respiratory failure: the BLUE protocol. Chest 134(1):117–125
9. Russell FM, Ehrman RR, Cosby K et al (2015) Diagnosing acute heart failure in patients with undifferentiated dyspnea: a lung and cardiac ultrasound (LuCUS) protocol. Acad Emerg Med 22(2):182–191
10. Laursen CB, Sloth E, Lassen AT et al (2014) Point-of-care ultrasonography in patients admitted with respiratory symptoms: a single-blind, randomised controlled trial. Lancet Respir Med 2(8):638–646
11. Volpicelli G, Elbarbary M, Blaivas M et al (2012) International evidence-based recommendations for point-of-care lung ultrasound. Intensive Care Med 38(4):577–591
12. Via G, Hussain A, Wells M et al (2014) International evidence-based recommendations for focused cardiac ultrasound. J Am Soc Echocardiogr 27(7):683.e1–683.e33
13. Laursen CB, Nielsen K, Riishede M et al (2014) A framework for implementation, education, research and clinical use of ultrasound in emergency departments by the Danish Society for Emergency Medicine. Scand J Trauma Resusc Emerg Med 22:25
14. Nielsen K, Lauridsen JR, Laursen CB et al (2015) Physicians using ultrasound in Danish emergency departments are mostly summoned specialists. Scand J Trauma Resusc Emerg Med 23:51
15. Lichtenstein D (2007) General ultrasound in the critically ill. Springer-Verlag, Berlin Heidelberg

16. Volpicelli G, Mussa A, Garofalo G et al (2006) Bedside lung ultrasound in the assessment of alveolar-interstitial syndrome. Am J Emerg Med 24(6):689–696
17. Laursen CB, Sloth E, Lambrechtsen J et al (2013) Focused sonography of the heart, lungs, and deep veins identifies missed life-threatening conditions in admitted patients with acute respiratory symptoms. Chest 144(6):1868–1875
18. Jensen MB, Sloth E, Larsen KM et al (2004) Transthoracic echocardiography for cardiopulmonary monitoring in intensive care. Eur J Anaesthesiol 21(9):700–707
19. American College of Emergency Physicians (2006) Emergency ultrasound imaging criteria compendium. Ann Emerg Med 48(4):487–510
20. Zanobetti M, Scorpiniti M, Gigli C et al (2017) Point-of-care ultrasonography for evaluation of acute dyspnea in the ED. Chest 151(6):1295–1301
21. Guttikonda SNR, Vadapalli K (2018) Approach to undifferentiated dyspnea in emergency department: aids in rapid clinical decision-making. Int J Emerg Med. 11(1):21
22. Crowhurst TD, Dunn RJ (2013) Sensitivity and specificity of three-point compression ultrasonography performed by emergency physicians for proximal lower extremity deep venous thrombosis. Emerg Med Australas 25(6):588–596
23. Ghane MR, Gharib MH, Ebrahimi A et al (2015) Accuracy of rapid ultrasound in shock (RUSH) exam for diagnosis of shock in critically ill patients. Trauma Mon 20(1):e20095
24. Xirouchaki N, Magkanas E, Vaporidi K et al (2011) Lung ultrasound in critically ill patients: comparison with bedside chest radiography. Intensive Care Med 37(9):1488–1493
25. Chiem AT, Chan CH, Ander DS et al (2015) Comparison of expert and novice sonographers' performance in focused lung ultrasonography in dyspnea (FLUID) to diagnose patients with acute heart failure syndrome. Acad Emerg Med 22(5):564–573
26. Ghafouri HB, Zare M, Bazrafshan A et al (2016) Diagnostic accuracy of emergency-performed focused assessment with sonography for trauma (FAST) in blunt abdominal trauma. Electron Physician 8(9):2950–2953
27. American College of Emergency Physicians (2009) Emergency ultrasound guidelines. Ann Emerg Med. 53(4):550–570

14

Interscalene brachial plexus nerve block in the emergency department: an effective and practice-changing workshop

Tyler Beals[1*], Kay Odashima[2], Lawrence E. Haines[2], Antonios Likourezos[2], Jefferson Drapkin[2] and Eitan Dickman[2]

Abstract

Background: The interscalene brachial plexus nerve block (ISNB) is a potentially useful method of regional analgesia for humerus fracture and shoulder dislocation reduction in the Emergency Department (ED). We examined the effectiveness of an ISNB workshop given to emergency medicine (EM) residents. We also explored complication rates and effectiveness of ISNBs performed in the ED.

Methods: One-hour evidence-based ISNB workshops were conducted with EM residents. Participants were given pre-, post-, and 3-month post-workshop knowledge and technical assessments. Results were analyzed using descriptive statistics. A pre- and post-workshop chart review examined ISNB utilization, complications, post-ISNB opiate administration, and post-ISNB procedural sedation.

Results: 41 residents enrolled in the workshop. Pre-workshop pass rate: knowledge assessment 22%. Immediate post-workshop pass rates: knowledge assessment 100%, image acquisition 93%, needle placement 100%. Three months post-workshop pass rates: knowledge assessment 73%, image acquisition 76%, needle placement 100%. Areas of poorest knowledge retention were anatomical landmarks, block distribution, and early signs of LAST. In the chart review, 2 ISNBs were performed in the pre-workshop period, and 12 in the post-workshop period. No serious complications were recorded. 78.5% of attempted ISNBs were successful, without need for procedural sedation. Of the 11 successfully performed ISNBs, 91% received no opiates after the procedure.

Conclusions: Our study suggests that EM residents can learn the ISNB, perform it safely in the emergency department, and that the ISNB may be an alternative to procedural sedation and opiate use for shoulder dislocation. Residents are adept at ISNB technical skills but demonstrate some deficits in knowledge retention.

Keywords: Emergency medicine, Point of care ultrasound, Regional anesthesia, Interscalene brachial plexus nerve block, Shoulder dislocation, Pain management, Medical education

Background

Ultrasound-guided regional anesthesia (UGRA) has been used in peri-operative settings by anesthesiologists for decades and is now becoming increasingly common in Emergency Departments (EDs) [4]. Particularly in the setting of the current opioid crisis, there is growing interest in opioid-sparing analgesic techniques [3, 7, 21, 23]. A recent AAEM position paper on the management of acute pain in the ED calls for "pain-syndrome targeted" strategies including regional anesthesia [13].

The interscalene brachial plexus nerve block (ISNB) is well established in anesthesia and orthopedic literature to provide effective analgesia for shoulder surgery and humerus fractures [1, 12, 18]. A small body of literature supports the usefulness of brachial plexus nerve blocks for ED-relevant indications including humerus fracture, shoulder reduction, and deltoid abscess drainage [5, 17,

*Correspondence: tbeals@bidmc.harvard.edu
[1] Beth Israel Deaconess Medical Center, 1 Deaconess Rd, Rosenberg 2, Boston, MA 02215, USA
Full list of author information is available at the end of the article

20, 22]. In addition to analgesia, regional anesthesia can decrease length of stay (LOS) through avoidance of procedural sedation [5, 17, 20, 22].

Bedside ultrasound training is the standard in American emergency medicine (EM) residencies, and EPs are facile in its various applications. The 2013 Council of Emergency Medicine Residency Directors-Academy of Emergency Ultrasound (CORD-AEUS) consensus document recommends UGRA, and specifically the ISNB, as advanced skills to be taught in emergency medicine residency [9].

However, there is currently a paucity of literature describing effective educational techniques for EM residents in UGRA. Until recently, UGRA education was largely limited to descriptions in the anesthesia literature, and even there, universal agreement on the most effective methods does not exist [16]. Akthar et al. demonstrated femoral nerve block competency in EM residents after a brief workshop [2]. This workshop was 1-h long and included didactic and simulator training. Bretholz et al. showed increased self-reported confidence in pediatric EM residents' performance of ulnar and femoral nerve blocks after a half-day workshop but did not assess competency [6]. Other literature suggests that use of simulators and dedicated workshops are effective methods of teaching UGRA [10, 11, 15, 19]. Regarding the ISNB specifically, EPs have been found to be capable of identifying the relevant anatomy and needle path after a brief educational course [8].

The goal of this study is to assess the feasibility of implementing a 1-h workshop teaching the ISNB to EM residents. A secondary aim is a retrospective examination of the clinical utilization, safety, and efficacy of ISNBs performed in the ED before and after the workshop.

Materials and methods

This study was approved by Maimonides Medical Center Institutional Review Board. All participants in the workshop provided written informed consent to participate in this study. The training sessions took place at a large urban tertiary academic medical center with an active emergency ultrasound program, including fellowship training. The workshop design was adapted from a previous study of the ultrasound-guided femoral nerve block [2] as well as other evidence-based educational methods described in the literature. Educational goals of the workshop, as described in the sections below, were based upon UGRA educational guidelines set forth by the American Society of Regional Anesthesia and Pain Medicine and the European Society of Regional Anaesthesia and Pain Therapy Joint Committee [14]. The 1-h workshop was taught by an emergency ultrasound fellowship trained physician and a senior EM resident. Multiple workshop dates were held over the course of 6 months with groups of 2–4 residents in their 1st, 2nd, or 3rd year of training. Residents involved had prior training in core emergency ultrasound applications and US-guided needle placement for vascular access as part of their residency training.

The workshop consisted of four sections:

1. General knowledge and safety: This section consisted of a brief lecture covering the indications for an ISNB, its distribution of analgesia, appropriate dose and type of anesthetic, aseptic technique, visualization of the needle and anesthetic spread, avoidance of complications, and management of local anesthetic systemic toxicity. A video demonstration of the procedure was shown.
2. Image recognition: Residents were shown a series of ultrasound images of the interscalene brachial plexus and its surrounding anatomy. They were taught relevant sonographic landmarks and appropriate needle trajectories for performing a successful block.
3. Image acquisition: Residents identified sonographic landmarks and located the interscalene brachial plexus on themselves and each other.
4. Motor skill: Finally, they practiced in-plane needle placement on an ISNB simulation model.

Pre-, immediate post-, and 3 months post-workshop assessments were conducted to examine the effectiveness of the workshop and skill retention. The assessment consisted of three parts:

1. Paper assessment: This was a 10-item multiple choice exam covering general knowledge of UGRA and the ISNB in particular (Fig. 1). A score of 80% was considered passing.
2. Image acquisition assessment: Using healthy volunteers, residents identified the sternocleidomastoid, anterior scalene, middle scalene, brachial plexus roots, carotid artery, injection site, and planned needle path (Fig. 2). Correct identification of all of this was required for passage.
3. Needle placement assessment: Using an interscalene nerve block trainer with simulated neck anatomy, residents were graded on their ability to guide a needle using in-plane technique into proper position under ultrasound guidance. Scoring was based upon the validated Modified Cheung Checklist (Fig. 3) [24, 25]. Passage was defined as successful placement of the needle at the target site and the presence of fewer than 5 "quality compromising behaviors."

1. Which of the following is an indication for an interscalene brachial plexus nerve block (ISNB)? Check all that apply.

2. Which of the following is a contraindication for an ISNB? Check all that apply.

3. What is the most common complication of the ISNB?

4. What nerves are reliably anesthetized by the ISNB?

5. Approximately what are the maximum therapeutic doses of lidocaine without epinephrine and bupivacaine without epinephrine, respectively?

6. The most important concept for avoidance of complications from ultrasound guided nerve blocks is:

7. What organ system is the first to display signs of lidocaine and bupivacaine toxicity?

8. Lidocaine and bupivacaine toxicity can cause severe refractory cardiac dysrhythmias. In addition to standard ACLS, these patients may benefit from intravenous fat emulsion (Intralipid) therapy. The correct IV fat emulsion regimen consists of:

9. Immediately after performing an ISNB for your patient, she maintains intact sensation over the entire affected extremity. Your next step is:

10. Needle path for the ISNB passes:

Fig. 1 Paper assessment. Multiple choice answers not shown

Assessments were made by the principal investigator (an ultrasound fellowship trained EP), and a senior EM resident who had undergone training in the ISNB with ultrasound faculty. Assessments were initially performed solely by the PI until an adequate kappa value was calculated for agreement between assessors at which point assessments were variably made by the resident or PI.

The paper, image acquisition, and needle placement assessments were given at the immediate post- and 3 months post-workshop times. Only the paper assessment was given pre-workshop because the practical assessments would hold little value in participants with no prior experience with the ISNB.

For our secondary aim, we performed a retrospective chart review of ED patients receiving the ISNB during 8 months following first workshop compared to the same calendar dates in the year prior. The ED's electronic medical record was searched for discharge diagnoses of humerus fracture and shoulder dislocation from July 2015 to April 2106 for the "pre-workshop" period and July 2016 to April 2017 for the "post-workshop" period. ICD9 codes were 812 and 831 and ICD10 codes were S42 and S43, respectively (the switch from ICD9 to ICD10 occurred in October 2015). Charts with matching diagnoses were examined for documentation of ISNB administration. Data extraction was performed by a research assistant and included the indication for ISNB, whether procedural sedation was needed after ISNB, and if opiate analgesics were used after ISNB placement.

Results

Forty-one residents (PGY 1–3) participated in the workshop. Only 3 (7%) reported having previously performed an ISNB. Kappa calculated for inter-rater reliability of the practical assessments showed 100% agreement. Immediately post-workshop, 100% of the participants passed the knowledge and needle placement assessments, and 93% passed the image acquisition assessment. Three months post-workshop, 73% of the residents passed the knowledge assessment, 76% passed the image acquisition assessment, and 100% passed the needle placement assessment (Table 1). Questions' number 1, 4, 5, and 7 were missed by at least 20% of participants in the 3-month post-workshop assessment. These dealt with block indications, anatomy, anesthetic dosages, and recognition of local anesthetic systemic toxicity, respectively. There were no intraneural or intravascular injections during the needle placement assessments.

During the needle placement assessments, there were no intraneural or intravascular injections, and all participants ultimately placed the needle tip at the intended target. In the immediate post-workshop assessment, no resident lost more than 2 points. The most-missed points were for failure to use Doppler and failure to aspirate

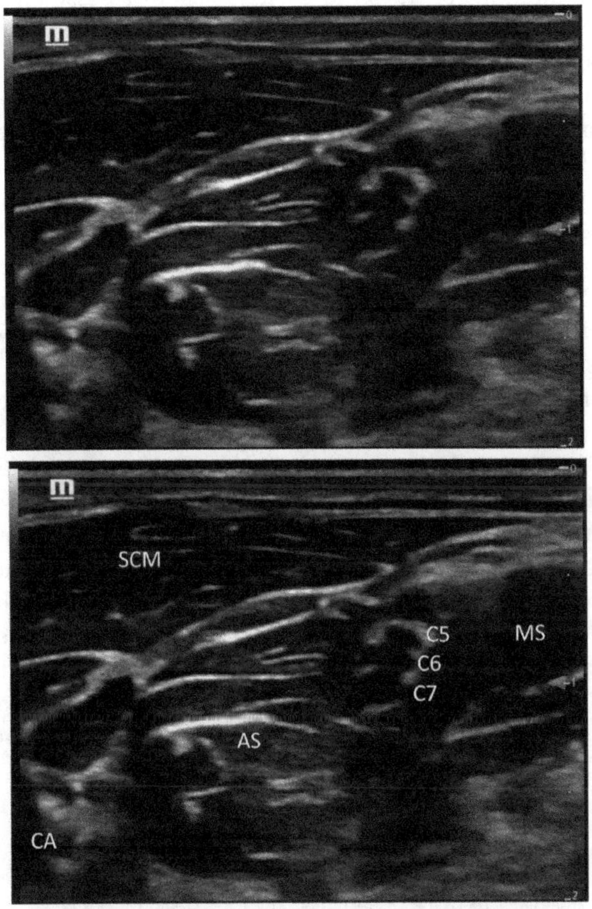

Fig. 2 Image acquisition. To pass this assessment, residents needed to acquire an ultrasound image on a healthy volunteer and identify the sternocleidomastoid (SCM), anterior scalene (AS), middle scalene (MS), interscalene groove (C5–7), and carotid artery (CA). They also had to indicate the needle path and site of injection

prior to injecting (27% and 17% of participants, respectively). Three months post-workshop, 2 participants lost 3 points and the remainder lost 2 or fewer. The most-missed points were for failure to use Doppler and failure to always maintain needle tip visualization during needle advancement (34% and 24% of participants, respectively).

In our chart review, there were 2 ISNBs performed in the pre-workshop period and 12 ISNBs performed in the post-workshop period. One was for a proximal humerus fracture and the rest for shoulder dislocation reduction. Pre-workshop, one ISNB was performed by the PI of this study and the other by an EM faculty member. Post-workshop, 6 blocks were performed by residents who attended the workshop, 3 were performed by the PI, and 3 were performed by other EM faculty. Blocks performed by residents were supervised by EM faculty who are not study authors. Lidocaine or bupivacaine was used based on provider preference. There were no immediate complications documented; however, patients were not followed beyond discharge for peripheral nerve injury or other delayed complications. Three patients (21%) required procedural sedation after ISNB, suggesting failed blocks. Two patients (14%) required opiate analgesia after ISNB placement. Ten patients (71%) required neither procedural sedation nor opiate analgesia following ISNB (Table 2).

Discussion

Our study suggests that emergency residents can learn the ISNB, demonstrate competency in practical assessments after a single workshop, and that the ISNB may be an alternative to procedural sedation and opiate use for shoulder dislocation. While residents are particularly

1. Does not optimize patient position (prone and turned away from proceduralist)
2. Does not position ultrasound machine on opposite side of patient (US machine should be less than 45 degrees off line-of-sight from needle insertion)
3. Choses incorrect transducer (linear)
4. Makes significant error in depth, gain, or focal zone
5. Does not use Doppler to rule out vascular structures
6. Uses unstable grip (part of hand/finger should be anchored to patient)
7. Does not know which side of screen corresponds to which side of probe
8. Does not maintain image of interscalene target throughout procedure
9. Does not maintain needle tip visualization during needle advancement, or does not immediately stop needle advancement if visualization is lost
10. Does not efficiently regain needle tip visualization if lost (should take <10 seconds)
11. Fails to recognize that the needle tip is intraneural or intravascular
12. Does not ask for syringe aspiration prior to injection

Fig. 3 Needle placement scoring metric. Passage of this assessment required identification of the needle tip in the interscalene groove along with the presence of 4 or fewer of the following behaviors (adapted from Wong et al. [25])

Table 1 Workshop passage rates

	Pre-workshop	Post-workshop	3 months post-workshop
Paper assessment	9/41 (22%)	41/41 (100%)	30/41 (73%)
Image acquisition	[a]	38/41 (93%)	31/41 (76%)
Needle placement	[a]	41/41 (100%)	41/41 (100%)

[a] Image acquisition and needle placement assessments were not performed pre-workshop due to participants' lack of exposure to the ISNB at baseline. Passage rate would be anticipated to approach 0%

Table 2 Chart review performed over 8 months starting at date of first workshop

	Pre-workshop	Post-workshop
Number of ISNBs	2	12
Complications recorded	0	0
Patients requiring procedural sedation after ISNB	0	3
Patients requiring opiate analgesia after ISNB	0	2

Comparison was same calendar dates in prior academic year. One post-workshop ISNB was for humerus fracture. All others were performed for shoulder reduction

adept at ultrasound-guided needle placement, they demonstrated poorest retention of knowledge regarding anatomical landmarks, anesthesia distribution, and early signs of LAST. We recommend that this be used to direct future ISNB instruction and in creation of a bedside reference document that can be reviewed just prior to the procedure.

Regarding our workshop design, we feel that the small group setting (2–4 participants) was an important factor in its success. This allowed for close observation of participants' performance of procedural skills and quick correction of improper techniques. In addition, much of the instructional energy during workshops was put into foundational knowledge and skills needed for all UGRA applications. While it may seem very labor-intensive for instructors to conduct 15 1-h workshops, the skills learned here greatly simplify future instruction of other nerve blocks. Finally, the overall structure of the workshop—general didactics with image recognition, followed by hands-on image acquisition, and ending with hands-on long-axis needle guidance—is one that we feel can be emulated elsewhere. For others using this workshop design, consideration can be given to pre-workshop study material, as this may enhance knowledge retention. Additional workshops and practice sessions with simulators over the course of residency would also strengthen procedural skills and guard against skill atrophy.

Limitations of the study include lack of assessment of ISNB placement on live patients. While previous studies have suggested that the ability to perform UGRA on a simulator predicts actual performance, it cannot replace real-world experience. Limitations of the chart review include its retrospective nature, single site design, small sample size, and lack of control group. Conclusions about causality cannot be made regarding participation in the workshop and ISNB performance in clinical practice. While no definitive conclusions can be drawn regarding opiate-sparing effects of the ISNB, we do believe that our results are consistent with previous prospective literature demonstrating brachial plexus anesthesia as an alternative to procedural sedation for shoulder reduction. In addition, conclusions regarding the safety of these blocks are limited by lack of patient follow-up beyond discharge. However, the most concerning immediate complications including local anesthetic systemic toxicity, pneumothorax, and respiratory distress from diaphragmatic paralysis were not observed. Finally, this study was performed early on in our group's collective experience with the ISNB in the ED. We feel that with time and accumulation of experience, ISNB performance and patient outcomes will continue to improve.

Abbreviations

ISNB: interscalene brachial plexus nerve block; ED: emergency department; EM: emergency medicine; UGRA: ultrasound-guided regional anesthesia.

Acknowledgements

Special thanks to Ralph Monfort for his help with assessments.

Declarations

This study was conducted with approval of the Maimonides Medical Center Institutional Review Board and in accordance with the principles of the Declaration of Helsinki.

Authors' contributions

TB, KO, LH, and ED conceived this project. TB and KO designed and conducted the workshop. JD performed the chart review. AL performed statistical analysis. TB drafted the manuscript, and KO, LH, and ED contributed substantially to its revision. TB takes responsibility for the paper as a whole. All authors read and approved the final manuscript.

Author details

[1] Beth Israel Deaconess Medical Center, 1 Deaconess Rd, Rosenberg 2, Boston, MA 02215, USA. [2] Maimonides Medical Center, Brooklyn, NY, USA.

References

1. Abdallah FW, Halpern SH, Aoyama K, Brull R (2015) Will the real benefits of single-shot interscalene block please stand up? A systematic review and meta-analysis. Anesth Analg 120:1114–1129. https://doi.org/10.1213/ANE.0000000000000688
2. Akhtar S, Hwang U, Dickman E, Nelson BP, Morrison RS, Todd KH (2013) A brief educational intervention is effective in teaching the femoral nerve block procedure to first-year emergency medicine residents. J Emerg Med 45:726–730. https://doi.org/10.1016/j.jemermed.2013.04.051
3. Barnett ML, Olenski AR, Jena AB (2017) Opioid-prescribing patterns of emergency physicians and risk of long-term use. N Engl J Med 376:663–673. https://doi.org/10.1056/NEJMsa1610524

4. Bhoi S, Chandra A, Galwankar S (2010) Ultrasound-guided nerve blocks in the emergency department. J Emerg Trauma Shock 3:82–88. https://doi.org/10.4103/0974-2700.58655
5. Blaivas M, Adhikari S, Lander L (2011) A prospective comparison of procedural sedation and ultrasound-guided interscalene nerve block for shoulder reduction in the emergency department. Acad Emerg Med 18:922–927. https://doi.org/10.1111/j.1553-2712.2011.01140.x
6. Bretholz A, Doan Q, Cheng A, Lauder G (2012) A presurvey and postsurvey of a web- and simulation-based course of ultrasound-guided nerve blocks for pediatric emergency medicine. Pediatr Emerg Care 28:506–509. https://doi.org/10.1097/PEC.0b013e3182586f42
7. Carter D, Sendziuk P, Eliott JA, Braunack-Mayer A (2016) Why is pain still under-treated in the emergency department? Two new hypotheses. Bioethics 30:195–202. https://doi.org/10.1111/bioe.12170
8. Ching B, Anaebere T, Herring AA (2014) Emergency physician performance using ultrasound to identify anatomy relevant to interscalene brachial plexus nerve blocks. Annals Emerg Med 64:S122–S123. https://doi.org/10.1016/j.annemergmed.2014.07.375
9. Lewiss RE et al (2013) CORD-AEUS: consensus document for the emergency ultrasound milestone project. Acad Emerg Med 20:740–745. https://doi.org/10.1111/acem.12164
10. Mariano ER et al (2015) Evaluation of a standardized program for training practicing anesthesiologists in ultrasound-guided regional anesthesia skills. J Ultrasound Med 34:1883–1893. https://doi.org/10.7863/ultra.14.12035
11. Martinelli SM, Monroe H, Coombs R, Miller N, Borstov A, Salo-Coombs V (2012) Assessing the impact of a regional anesthesia workshop on anesthesiology residents' perceived comfort in performing peripheral nerve blocks. J Educ Perioper Med 14:E061
12. Mian A, Chaudhry I, Huang R, Rizk E, Tubbs RS, Loukas M (2014) Brachial plexus anesthesia: a review of the relevant anatomy, complications, and anatomical variations. Clin Anatomy 27:210–221. https://doi.org/10.1002/ca.22254
13. Motov S et al (2018) The treatment of acute pain in the emergency department: a white paper position statement prepared for the american academy of emergency medicine. J Emerg Med 54:731–736. https://doi.org/10.1016/j.jemermed.2018.01.020
14. Narouze SN et al (2012) The American Society of Regional Anesthesia and Pain Medicine, the European Society of Regional Anaesthesia and Pain Therapy, and the Asian Australasian Federation of Pain Societies Joint Committee recommendations for education and training in ultrasound-guided interventional pain procedures. Reg Anesth Pain Med 37:657–664. https://doi.org/10.1097/aap.0b013e318269c189
15. Niazi AU, Haldipur N, Prasad AG, Chan VW (2012) Ultrasound-guided regional anesthesia performance in the early learning period: effect of simulation training. Reg Anesth Pain Med 37:51–54. https://doi.org/10.1097/AAP.0b013e31823dc340
16. Nix CM, Margarido CB, Awad IT, Avila A, Cheung JJ, Dubrowski A, McCartney CJ (2013) A scoping review of the evidence for teaching ultrasound-guided regional anesthesia. Reg Anesth Pain Med 38:471–480. https://doi.org/10.1097/AAP.0b013e3182a4ed7a
17. Raeyat Doost E, Heiran MM, Movahedi M, Mirafzal A (2017) Ultrasound-guided interscalene nerve block vs procedural sedation by propofol and fentanyl for anterior shoulder dislocations. Am J Emerg Med 35:1435–1439. https://doi.org/10.1016/j.ajem.2017.04.032
18. Roberts JR, Custalow CB, Thomsen TW (2019) Roberts and Hedges' clinical procedures in emergency medicine and acute care, vol 7. Elsevier, New York
19. Sites BD, Spence BC, Gallagher JD, Wiley CW, Bertrand ML, Blike GT (2007) Characterizing novice behavior associated with learning ultrasound-guided peripheral regional anesthesia. Reg Anesth Pain Med 32:107–115. https://doi.org/10.1016/j.rapm.2006.11.006
20. Stone MB, Wang R, Price DD (2008) Ultrasound-guided supraclavicular brachial plexus nerve block vs procedural sedation for the treatment of upper extremity emergencies. Am J Emerg Med 26:706–710. https://doi.org/10.1016/j.ajem.2007.09.011
21. Tadros A, Layman SM, Davis SM, Davidov DM, Cimino S (2015) Emergency visits for prescription opioid poisonings. J Emerg Med 49:871–877. https://doi.org/10.1016/j.jemermed.2015.06.035
22. Tezel O et al (2014) A comparison of suprascapular nerve block and procedural sedation analgesia in shoulder dislocation reduction. Am J Emerg Med 32:549–552. https://doi.org/10.1016/j.ajem.2014.02.014
23. Todd KH et al (2007) Pain in the emergency department: results of the pain and emergency medicine initiative (PEMI) multicenter study. J Pain 8:460–466. https://doi.org/10.1016/j.jpain.2006.12.005
24. Watson MJ et al (2014) Psychometric evaluation of a direct observation of procedural skills assessment tool for ultrasound-guided regional anaesthesia. Anaesthesia 69:604–612. https://doi.org/10.1111/anae.12625
25. Wong DM et al (2014) Evaluation of a task-specific checklist and global rating scale for ultrasound-guided regional anesthesia. Reg Anesth Pain Med 39:399–408. https://doi.org/10.1097/AAP.0000000000000126

15

Renal resistive index: a new reversible tool for the early diagnosis and evaluation of organ perfusion in critically ill patients

Antonio Anile[1], Silvia Ferrario[2*], Lorena Campanello[3], Maria Antonietta Orban[3] and Giacomo Castiglione[1]

Abstract

Background: We reported a case of early detection of peripheral hypoperfusion trough the evaluation of a new index in intensive care: Renal Doppler Resistive Index (RRI).

Case presentation: We admitted a 76-year-old man who underwent ileostomy and hernioplasty because of an intestinal occlusion due to obstructive strangulated right inguinal hernia. The post-operative period was characterised by hemodynamic instability and he needed an invasive hemodynamic monitoring, administration of vasopressors and continuous renal replacement therapy (CRRT). Then, hemodynamic stability was obtained and vasopressors interrupted. RRI was lower than 0.7. In the eleventh post-operative day, despite stable macrocirculatory parameters, we found increased values of RRI. An abdomen ultrasound first and then a CT scan revealed the presence of bleeding from the previous ileostomy. Hence, the patient immediately underwent another surgical operation.

Conclusions: RRI modification appears to be more precocious than any other hemodynamic, microcirculatory and metabolic parameter routinely used. RRI has been widely used to assess renal function in critically ill patients; now, we presume that RRI could represent a common and useful tool to manage target therapy in critical condition.

Keywords: Renal Doppler Resistive Index (RRI), Organ perfusion, Fluid challenge

Background

The macrohemodynamics targets, such as blood mean arterial pressure (MAP), cardiac output (CO), peripheral resistance, etc., have been used to drive goal-directed therapy in case of circulatory shock. However, it has been reported that conditions of microcirculatory disfunction could persist and evolve initially in hypoperfusion and then in cryptic shock [1] in spite of improvement or stability of macrocirculatory parameters. In cases of circulatory shock, monitoring microcirculatory parameters could be the most important endopoint to optimize the treatment, since microcirculatory disfunction could persist despite the improvement of macrocirculatory parameters [2]. Routine microcirculatory monitoring parameters, such as venous oxygen saturation (SvO2) and venous central oxygen saturation (SvcO2), remain fundamental but have several limits to consider [3]. SvO2 measurement implicates a pulmonary artery catheter. Collecting a sample of blood from superior caval vein allows to obtain a value of SvcO2 that reflects the O2 saturation of the superior vascular tree, that is slightly different as compared to O2 saturation of inferior vascular tree (as the abdominal vascular district) [1, 4]. Indeed, usually oxygen consumption (VO2) is independent of oxygen delivery (DO2) until tissues can satisfy metabolic requirement increasing oxygen extraction when DO2 decreases. This mechanism has an intrinsic limit: beyond critic DO2, the compensatory increasing of O2 extraction run out and VO2 become dependent from DO2.

Bloos et al. demonstrated that in patients with protract cardiac arrest, in case of microcirculatory artero-venous shunt or cellular apoptosis due to severe tissue damage, SvO2 and SvcO2 could show normal or increased values in spite of dangerous tissue hypoxia [3]. Consequently,

*Correspondence: silvia.ferrario88@hotmail.it
[2] Section of Nephrology, Department of Clinical and Experimental Medicine, Policlinico Universitario, University of Catania, Catania, Italy
Full list of author information is available at the end of the article

tissue hypoxia develops and increased serum lactate and lactic acidosis may be observed [5–7].

Doppler-based renal resistive index measurement is a rapid and non-invasive tool that may be useful to detect tissue hypoperfusion and oxygenation, and to measure resistance to arterial blood flow in renal vessels in intensive care unit (ICU) patients [8, 9]. Sampling renal interlobar or arcuate arteries with pulsed wave Doppler ultrasound allows to obtain a "low resistance" profile typical of the downstream territories with high resting perfusion. Doppler waveform recorded in those territories shows a steep systolic rise that is the "early systolic peak", followed by a decreasing component representing the diastolic flow.

RRI can be calculated as (peak systolic velocity − end diastolic velocity)/peak systolic velocity [10].

Evidence of a direct correlation between RRI and cardiovascular damages is more and more frequently reported; therefore, RRI has been proposed as a new tool in ICU patients monitoring [11, 12].

In normal conditions, renal artery blood flow occurs during both systolic and diastolic phase. On the contrary, in several pathologic conditions (such as shock, systemic inflammation, obstruction, etc.), renal arterial blood flow decreases and becomes even reverted during the diastolic phase consequently provoking an increase of RRI [8–12].

Nevertheless, RRI is the result of complex, and often not fully understood, interactions between arterial characteristics and systemic hemodynamic factors; in fact, many systemic parameters correlate with these ultrasonographic (US) measures. RRI does not always selectively indicate organ damage, but under particular conditions, it reflects systemic vascular disease. Increased values are associated with extrarenal factors such as age, vascular disease, pulse pressure, systemic vascular compliance, heart rate and cardiac function and with renal factor as end-stage renal disease and renal capillary wedge pressure. Thus, the hemodynamic factors involved have to be considered to understand RRI clinical meaning. Ageing provokes a progressive rigidity of the aorta with a great increase in the arterial pulse pressure. Pulse pressure is connected with cardiac function and systemic arterial compliance affecting the value of peak systolic velocity. The vascular compliance of large arteries determines the blood pressure pulsatility; consequently, in the condition of reduced systemic compliance, RRI results are strongly modified. The cardiac function, with its components such as heart rate and left ventricular outflow, can also strongly affect RRI.

Moreover, RRI is considered as a marker of progression of renal damage and an indicator of irreversible damage in chronic kidney failure.

Renal capillary wedge pressure develops from the combination of renal interstitial and venous pressure; therefore, conditions of systemic venous congestion could increase renal capillary wedge pressure with a subsequent elevation of RRI indexes [13].

Due to these confounding factors, as it has been previously suggested, it might be important to compare RRI with Splenic Doppler Resistive Index (SRI) [14]. Corradi et al. showed that the evaluation of SRI allows the early detection of occult hemorrhagic shock and persistent occult hypoperfusion after polytrauma in adult patients [15].

Since SRI variations after fluid administration could be an effective tool to monitor systemic hemodynamic, also SRI may represent a useful method in the detection of organ perfusion [16].

Case report

A 76-year-old man was admitted to our hospital for abdominal pain and biliary vomiting. He had a past medical history of Alzheimer disease, chronic obstructive pulmonary disease and myelodysplastic syndrome recently treated with blood transfusion. He was diagnosed for intestinal occlusion due to obstructive right inguinal hernia and he was submitted to a surgical resection of an ischemic intestinal loop, ileostomy and hernioplasty. Due to hemodynamic instability, he was transferred to our ICU.

The post-operative period upon admission was characterised by hypotension non-responsive to fluid challenge and vasoplegia that required the administration of dopamine at the dosage of 6 mcg/kg/min to obtain hemodynamic stability. To achieve a better hemodynamic evaluation, an arterial catheter was inserted into femoral artery and a central venous catheter was inserted into internal jugular vein to monitor hemodynamic status using transpulmonary thermodilution (EV1000 system: Edwards Lifesciences, Irvine, CA). Cardiac index (CI) and mean arterial pressure were maintained > 4 l/min/m^2 and 65–75 mmHg, respectively.

We recorded values of systemic vascular resistance index (SVRI) between 1000 and 1500 dyn s/cm^5 m^2. Administration of vasopressors was managed by hemodynamic monitoring with EV1000 (norepinephrine until 0.4 mcg/kg/min). During the first 24 h, a reduction of urine output was noted; hence, a fluid load was performed in association with high doses of diuretics. No response was obtained and we started calcium-citrate continuous venous–venous haemodialysis (calcium-citrate CVVHD Multifiltrate Fresenius System) with blood flow 100 ml/min, ultrafiltration 100 ml/h and dialysate flow 2000 ml/h. In the fourth postoperative day, we observed a recovery of renal function and we could suspend CVVHD.

We monitored haemoglobin (Hb) level and we had to administrate blood transfusion to keep values of Hb > of 7.5 mg/dl. We also measured RRI in the first post-operative day and then every 48 h and we found values lower than 0.7 in each situation. Serum lactate constantly remained lower than 1.5 mEq/l. During the following days, the hemodynamic parameters recorded by EV1000 allowed to reduce vasopressors dosage until interruption of dopamine and decrease of norepinephrine to 0.08 mcg/kg/min. In the eleventh post-operative day, we performed another renal Doppler ultrasound to evaluate organ perfusion because of a condition of slightly tense abdomen and the need to increase norepinephrine dose.

Table 1 Macrocirculatory parameters from pre- (T0) and post-surgical (T1) intervention of re-ileostomy

	T0	T1
Lac	1	1.3
SvcO2	57	75
SVV %	4	13
SVRI	1018	1003
CI	4.6	5.3

LAC lactate (mmol/L), *SvcO2* venous central oxygen saturation (%), *SVV%* stroke volume variation (%), *SVRI* systemic vascular resistance index (dyn s/cm^5 m^2), *CI* cardiac index (L/min/m^2)

Despite stable macrocirculatory parameters recorded by EV1000, acceptable arterial blood gas analyses, normal level of SvcO2 (Table 1), we found increased values of RRI (0.86) (Fig. 1). Hence, we performed an abdomen Focused assessment with sonography for trauma (FAST) that allowed us to detect free intraabdominal fluid, and then we requested a CT scan that revealed the presence of bleeding from the previous ileostomy. We also measured the intra-abdominal pressure (IAP) that was 19 mmHg. Immediately afterwards, laboratory tests detected anaemia that required blood transfusion. The patient immediately underwent another surgical operation of blood evacuation (above 1000 ml), resection of the ileal loop responsible for the bleeding and new ileostomy was performed. After the operation, we measured IAP lesser of 11 mmHg. The hemodynamic monitoring with EV1000, arterial and venous blood gas analysis (Table 1) overlapped with the ones performed before the surgical operation. Despite the evidence of active bleeding from the previous ileostomy, detected with CT scan, the macroemodinamic parameters routinely used were still in normal range and weren't able to reveal hypoperfusion and haemodynamic instability. RRI instead showed an improvement of diastolic (perfusional) phase decreasing to normal values (0.58) (Fig. 1) and demonstrating the enhancement of organ perfusion.

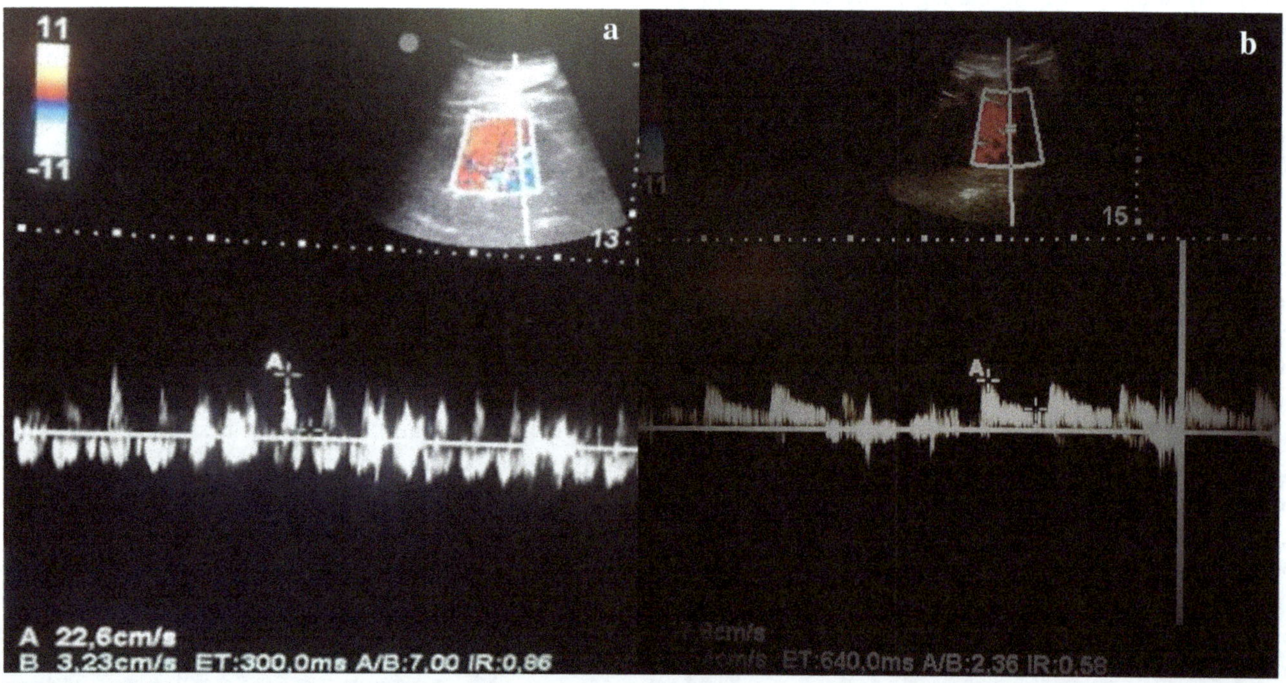

Fig. 1 Renal Resistive Index. Pre- (**a**) and post- (**b**) surgical intervention of re-ileostomy

Discussion

It must be considered that the evaluation of RRI and SRI has limitations. First, all members of the medical équipe have to be able to evaluate these two ultrasonographic measures to establish a protocol of hemodynamic monitoring. Secondly, measuring RRI and SRI in not cooperative patients is not so easy. Thirdly, as mentioned above, RRI is influenced by many systemic extra-renal and renal factors that could conceal modifications caused by changes in organ perfusion.

Nevertheless, what we observed in our case suggests that RRI is an early and sensitive index of insufficient oxygen delivery and tissue hypoperfusion, probably reflecting vascular regulation even in initial phases of hypoxia. In addition, after the restoration of a sufficient microcirculatory blood flow and organ perfusion, the decrease in normal values shows the early reversibility of this index. The notion that shock or haemodynamic instability is a condition that does not imply necessarily a state of hypotension has been largely confirmed [17, 18]. Corradi et al reported that in haemodynamically stable multiple trauma patients, increased values of RRI could reliably predict a state of hidden or early haemorrhagic shock. Furthermore, in their study, serum lactate and Hb detected during the event were in normal ranges, showing that RRI is completely independent of MAP, CO and Hb [17, 18]. Moreover it is reported that BP and CO could not be considered unconditionally as markers of a shock developing [17]. Maynard et al. showed that peripheral hypoperfusion and "core organs" (splanchnic and mesenteric) hypoperfusion was an effective predictor of outcome other than regional perfusion [4]. Acting as functional supply reservoir, "core organs" protect themselves from hypotension until the insufficient DO2 determines cellular apoptosis and organ failure [2] becoming a multi-organ dysfunction syndrome (MODS) etiopathogenetic factor [1], as it has been demonstrated in animal and human models. A likely explanation could be found in the high sensitivity of kidney to ischemic damage owing to its complex microvascular structure along with its high metabolic needs [10]. Deruddre et al. showed that measurement of RRI could represent a new tool to identify the optimal individual MAP to sustain renal blood flow and could help managing norepinephrine titration during septic shock treatment [19]. More interesting is the early modification of RRI compared to SvcO2 which could be explained with a delay in SvcO2 increment hidden by a temporary increase of O2 extraction (up to a given limit) [3] that cannot be otherwise detectable or predictable by any other parameter.

In the early phase of shock in our patient, the routine hemodynamic parameters that conventionally indicate a state of hypoperfusion appeared to be unchanged; whereas RRI was significantly sensitive to hypoperfusion caused by IAP increment, that commonly determines renal injury and heart failure [20, 21].

To be also noted is the early reversibility of RRI, while the other haemodynamic monitored parameters (CO, SVV, MAP, blood gas analysis, SvcO2, Lactate and urine output) did not show perioperative modifications. To our knowledge, the only demonstration of a quantitative reversibility of intrarenal perfusion response was reported in animal models [22]. A meta-analysis recently published with the purpose to investigate the role of RRI as diagnostic tool showed that RRI may be considered as a predictor of persistent acute kidney injury (AKI) and its reversibility in critically ill patients [23].

If our observations were supported by large clinical trials, RRI could be considered as an early and reversible marker of organ perfusion that could be employed along with the other haemodynamic parameters routinely used.

Abbreviations

RRI: Renal Doppler Resistive Index; CRRT: continuous renal replacement therapy; MAP: mean arterial pressure; CO: cardiac output; SvO2: venous oxygen saturation; SvcO2: venous central oxygen saturation; VO2: oxygen consumption; DO2: oxygen delivery; ICU: intensive care unit; CI: cardiac index; SVRI: systemic vascular resistance index; calcium-citrate CVVHD: calcium-citrate continuous venous–venous haemodialysis; Hb: haemoglobin; FAST: focused assessment with sonography for trauma; IAP: intra-abdominal pressure; AKI: acute kidney injury; SRI: Splenic Doppler Resistive Index.

Acknowledgements

Not applicable.

Authors' contributions

All authors contributed to the manuscript equally. All authors read and approved the final manuscript.

Author details

[1] Intensive Care Unit, Ospedale Vittorio Emanuele, AOU Policlinico–Vittorio Emanuele, Catania, Italy. [2] Section of Nephrology, Department of Clinical and Experimental Medicine, Policlinico Universitario, University of Catania, Catania, Italy. [3] School of Anaesthesia and Intensive Care, University Hospital "G. Rodolico", University of Catania, Catania, Italy.

References

1. Pusckarich MA, Trzeciak S, Shapiro NI, Heffner AC, Kline JA, Jones AE, Emergency Medicine Shock Research Network (EMSHOCKNET) (2011) Outcomes of patients underground early sepsis resuscitation for cryptic shock compared with overt shock. Resuscitation 82:1289–1293
2. Aya HD, Carsetti A, Bazurro S, Bastoni D, Malbrain ML, Cecconi M (2015) From cardiac output to blood flow auto-regulation in shock. Anesthesiol Intensive Ther. https://doi.org/10.5603/AIT.a2015.0077
3. Bloos F, Rheinart K (2005) Ossimetria venosa. Intensive Care Med 31:911–913
4. Maynard N, Bihari D, Beale R, Smithies M, Baldock G, Mason R, McColl I (1993) Assesment of splanchnic oxygenation by gastric tonometry in patient with acute circolatoryfaylure. JAMA 10:1203–1210
5. Rivers EP, Rady MY, Martin GB, Fenn NM, Smithline HA, Alexander ME, Nowak RM (1992) Venous hyperoxia after cardiac arrest. Characterization of a defect in systemic oxygen utilization. Chest 102:1787–1793

6. Vincent JL, Backer De (2004) Oxygen transport the oxygen delivery controversy. Intensive Care Med 30:1990–1996
7. Cohen R, Woods HF (1976) Clinical and biochemical aspects of lactic acidosis. Br Med J 2:762
8. La Dorze M, Bouglé A, Deruddre S, Duranteau J (2012) Renal Doppler ultrasound: a new tool to asses renal perfusion in critically ill patients. Shock 37:360–365
9. Rozemeiler S, Haitsma Mulier JLG, Röttgering JG, Elbers PWG, Spoelstra-de Man AME, Tuinman PR, de Waard MC, Oudemans-van Straaten HM (2018) Renal resistive index: response to shock and its determinants in critically ill patients. Shock. https://doi.org/10.1097/SHK1246
10. Di Nicolò P, Granata A (2018) Renal intraparenchymal resistive index: the ultrasonographic answer to many clinical questions. J Nephrol. https://doi.org/10.1007/s40620-018-00567-x
11. Meco M, Giustiniano E (2012) Renal resistivity index as a guide for treatment of severe postoperative renal failure in cardiac surgery: a case report. J Anesth Clin Res. https://doi.org/10.4172/2155-6148.1000260
12. Corradi F, Brusasco C, Paparo F, Manca T, Santori G, Benassi F, Molardi A, Gallingani A, Ramelli A, Gherli T, Vezzani A (2015) Renal Doppler resistive index as a marker of oxygen supply and demand mismatch in postoperative cardiac surgery patients. Biomed Res Int. https://doi.org/10.1155/2015/763940
13. Di Nicolò P, Granata A (2017) Renal resistive index: not only kidney. Clin Exp Nephrol 21:359–366
14. Grün OS, Herath E, Weihrauch A, Flügge F, Rogacev KS, Fliser D, Heine GH (2012) Does the measurement of the difference of resistive indexes in spleen and kidney allow a selective assessment of chronic kidney injury? Radiology 264(3):894–902
15. Corradi F, Brusasco C, Garlaschi A, Santori G, Vezzani A, Moscatelli P, Pelosi P (2012) Splenic Doppler resistive index for early detection of occult hemorrhagic shock after polytrauma in adult patients. Shock 38:466–473
16. Brusasco C, Tavazzi G, Robba C, Santori G, Vezzani A, Manca T, Corradi F (2018) Splenic Doppler resistive index variation mirrors cardiac responsiveness and systemic hemodynamics upon fluid challenge resuscitation in postoperative mechanically ventilated patients. Biomed Res Int. https://doi.org/10.1155/2018/1978968
17. Antonelli M, Levy M, Andrews PJ, Chastre J, Hudson LD, Manthous C, Meduri GU, Moreno RP, Putensen C, Stewart T, Torres A (2007) Hemodynamic monitoring in shock and implication for management. Intensive Care Med 33:575–590
18. Corradi F, Brusasco C, Vezzani A, Palermo S, Altomonte F, Moscatelli P, Pelosi P (2011) Hemorrhagic shock in polytrauma patients: early detection with renal Doppler resistive index measurements. Radiology 1:112–118
19. Deruddre S, Cheisson G, Mazoit JX, Vicaut E, Benhamou D, Duranteau J (2007) Renal arterial resistance in septic shock: effects of increasing mean arterial pressure with norepinephrine on the renal resistive index assessed with Doppler ultrasonography. Intensive Care Med 33:1557–1562
20. Whitehouse T, Stotz M, Taylor V, Stidwill R, Singer M (2006) Tissue oxygen and hemodynamics in renal medulla, cortex, and corticomedullary junction during hemorrhage-reperfusion. Am J Physiol Renal Physiol 291:647–653
21. Ninet S, Schnell D, Dewitte A, Zeni F, Meziani F, Darmon M (2015) Doppler-based renal resistive index for prediction of renal dysfunction reversibility: a systematic review and meta-analysis. J Crit Care 30:629–635
22. Mullens W, Abrahams Z, Skouri HN, Francis GS, Taylor DO, Starling RC, Paganini E, Tang WH (2008) Elevated intra-abdominal pressure in acute decompensated heart failure: a potential contributor to worsening renal function? J Am Coll Cardiol 51:300–306
23. Kirkpatrick AW, Colistro R, Laupland KB, Fox DL, Konkin DE, Kock V, Mayo JR, Nicolaou S (2007) Renal arterial resistive index response to intraabdominal hypertension in a porcine model. Crit Care Med 35:207–213

16

Unanticipated critical findings on echocardiography in septic patients

Sarah J. Beesley[1,2,6*], Ezekiel Egan[3], Michael J. Lanspa[1,2,4], Emily L. Wilson[1], Elliotte L. Hirshberg[1,2,4,5], Colin K. Grissom[1,2,4], Rebecca Burk[1,4] and Samuel M. Brown[1,2,4]

Abstract

Background: Echocardiography is increasingly performed among septic patients as a routine part of evaluation and management in the intensive care unit (ICU). The rate of unanticipated critical findings (e.g., severe left or right ventricular dysfunction or pericardial tamponade) on such echocardiograms is unknown. We evaluated a retrospective cohort of septic ICU patients in whom transthoracic echocardiography was performed as a routine part of sepsis management. In addition to identifying critical findings, we defined whether each critical finding was anticipated, and whether the clinical team responded to the critical finding. The primary outcome was rate of unanticipated critical findings, which we hypothesized would occur in fewer than 5% of patients. We also performed an exploratory analysis of the association between unanticipated critical finding and mortality, controlling for severity of illness.

Results: We studied 393 patients. Unanticipated critical findings were identified in 5% (95% CI 3–7%) of patients ($n = 20$). Among the 20 patients with unanticipated critical findings, a response to the unanticipated critical finding was identified in 12 (60%) patients. An unanticipated critical finding was not significantly associated with 28-day mortality when controlling for admission APACHE II ($p = 0.27$).

Conclusions: Unanticipated critical findings on echocardiograms in septic ICU patients are uncommon. The potential therapeutic relevance of echocardiography to sepsis is more likely related to hemodynamic management than to traditional cardiac diagnoses. Research studies that employ blinded echocardiograms in septic patients may anticipate unblinding for critical findings approximately 1 in every 20 echocardiograms.

Keywords: Echocardiography, Intensive care, Sepsis, Septic shock

Background

Echocardiography is increasingly performed among patients with sepsis as a routine part of management [1–3]. Opinion and/or consensus statements in favor of broader application of focused critical care echocardiography and instructional guides [4–8] manifest increasing momentum in favor of the broad use of these focused echocardiograms. Critical care echocardiography now supports a board certification process [9–11].

Appropriateness criteria suggest that transthoracic echocardiogram (TTE) is appropriate in the case of shock or situations where TTE is likely to change management, and a variety of studies suggest that TTE identifies findings that change management [12–18]. Admittedly, these studies have either been in populations with high likelihood of relevant findings (e.g., perioperative management of cardiac surgery patients) or have been analyzed under the assumption that echocardiography should direct management and then reporting that echocardiography changes management [19]. Currently, the application of echocardiography in septic patients is often related to hemodynamic management, especially fluid administration [20–22].

*Correspondence: Sarah.beesley@imail.org
[6] Shock Trauma Intensive Care Unit, 5121 South Cottonwood Street, Murray, UT 84107, USA
Full list of author information is available at the end of the article

However, for healthcare systems evaluating the implications of screening echocardiograms and for clinical researchers wondering how often a research echocardiogram may identify an unanticipated critical finding (such as severe left or right ventricular dysfunction or pericardial tamponade, which may necessitate new study procedures and/or unblinding), it is important to know how often an echocardiogram obtained for sepsis identifies an unexpected critical finding. In a prior study of an unselected ICU population ($N=467$), a high proportion (36%) of unanticipated cardiac abnormalities were identified on echocardiogram [23]. This study included many findings not normally considered critical and was not specific to sepsis patients.

We thus sought to clarify how often unanticipated critical findings are identified in the echocardiograms of septic patients admitted to the ICU. We performed an analysis of patients in our registry of septic patients in whom TTE had been performed as a routine part of the management of sepsis. We hypothesized that unanticipated critical findings on echocardiogram would be present in less than 5% of echocardiograms.

Methods

Patients

Participants included patients (age at least 18 years) with severe sepsis or septic shock (Sepsis-2 definition [24], which applied at the time of cohort assembly) admitted to study ICUs between October 2012 and November 2015. Patients had clinically suspected infection defined by study coordinator chart review, two or more systemic inflammatory response syndrome criteria and had either shock (systolic blood pressure (SBP) < 90 mmHg despite IVF challenge of ≥ 20 mL/kg or infusion of vasopressors) or severe sepsis (lactate > 4 mmol/L) [24, 25]. We included only patients who had an echocardiogram obtained within 24 h of admission; in the study ICU, this is approximately 50% of patients with sepsis and 75% of patients with septic shock (unpublished data). Exclusion criteria included known pregnancy, primary diagnosis of acute coronary syndrome or major cardiac dysrhythmia, or known alternative diagnosis for shock (trauma, anaphylaxis, hemorrhage) on coordinator review, confirmed by an investigator.

Critical findings on echocardiogram

We reviewed all echocardiogram reports to identify critical findings. Echocardiograms were performed by trained, credentialed sonographers and over-read by either board-certified cardiologists or Level II critical care echocardiographers who were testamurs of the National Board of Echocardiography ASCeXAM. We employed the American Society of Echocardiography definitions of critical findings: (1) cardiac tamponade or new large pericardial effusion, (2) new left ventricular ejection fraction (LVEF) < 30%, (3) new severe right ventricular systolic dysfunction [26], (4) evidence of aortic dissection, (5) new cardiac masses or thrombi, or (6) new, severe valvular dysfunction [27]. We also included (7) left ventricular outflow obstruction or hypertrophic cardiomyopathy with velocities > 4 m/s, or (8) moderate or greater right to left shunt [28], as those may be immediately relevant in a critical care environment.

We defined whether the critical finding was anticipated or not based on the following algorithm: (1) was the finding present on a prior echocardiogram? (if so ⟶ anticipated); or (2) was the finding referenced in clinical documentation as being of diagnostic concern before the echocardiogram had been performed (if so ⟶ anticipated). See process outline in Fig. 1. Of note, when a vegetation was identified on TTE, this was not considered an unanticipated critical finding if endocarditis was considered prior to obtaining the TTE; we considered positive blood cultures with a typical organism before the echocardiogram was ordered as suggesting that endocarditis was under diagnostic consideration.

We also evaluated the response to the identification of an unanticipated critical finding. If the finding was unanticipated, the clinical response was noted in the following categories: no response, monitoring response, or intervention. No response means that we could find no evidence in the electronic medical record (EMR) that the treating team incorporated the critical finding into their monitoring or management. Monitoring response means that the EMR indicated either increased or additional monitoring explicitly tied to the critical finding. This included both non-invasive monitoring (e.g., repeat echocardiogram or other imaging), and invasive monitoring (e.g., left or right heart catheterization). Intervention was considered present if there was a change in treatment associated with the critical finding and included both non-invasive intervention (e.g., antibiotics, afterload reduction, diuresis) and invasive intervention (e.g., percutaneous coronary intervention, transcatheter aortic valve replacement, surgery).

A critical finding was designated as a false-positive finding if subsequent testing refuted the apparent findings from the initial echocardiogram report.

Analysis plan

We estimated a priori that the proportion of unanticipated critical findings would be < 5%. We estimated the precision of our estimate to be within 2.3% for a proportion of 5% with a sample size of 390 and a 95% confidence level. This was calculated using PASS 12.0.3 [29].

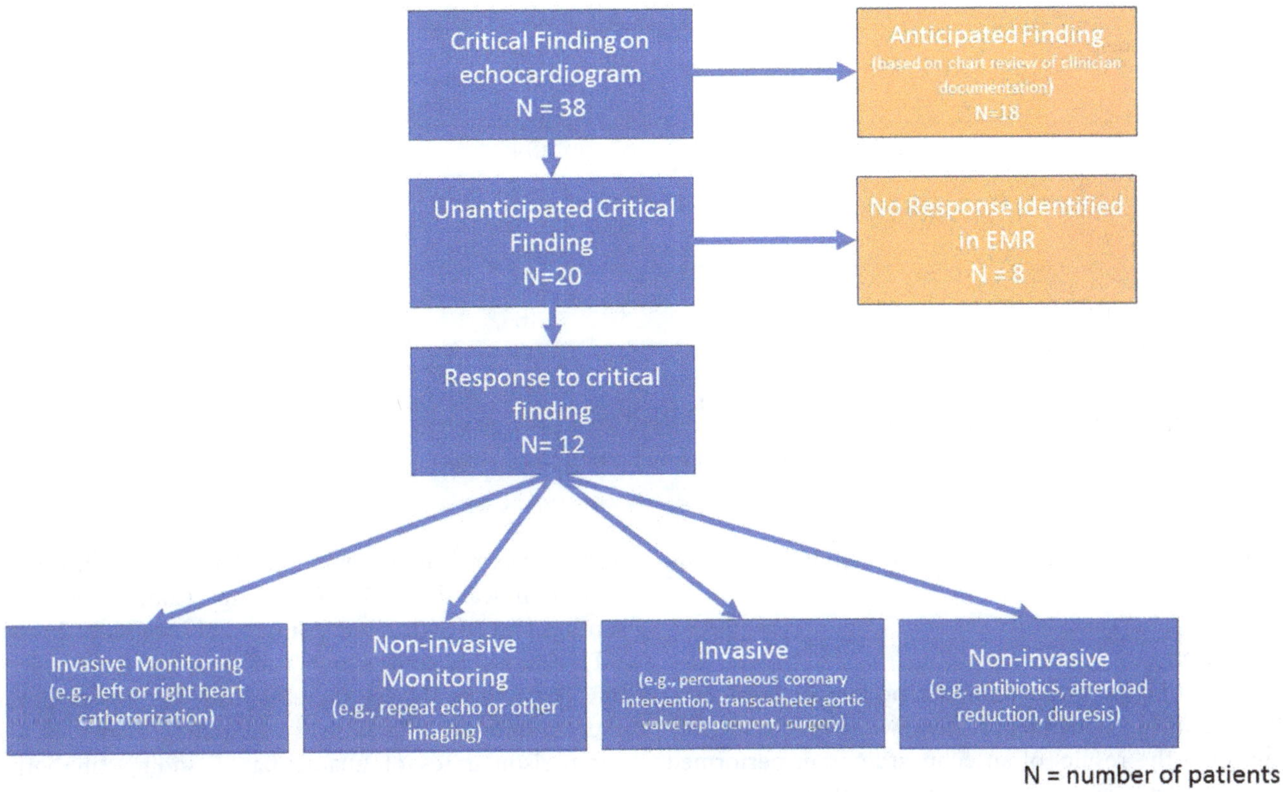

Fig. 1 Study flowchart

The prespecified primary analysis was to estimate the proportion of unanticipated critical findings identified on TTE. As a secondary exploratory analysis, we evaluated the association between critical findings and 28-day mortality, adjusted for severity of illness, using multivariate logistic regression. All analyses were conducted using the R Statistical Package, version 3.5.1 [30].

The study was approved with waiver of informed consent by the Intermountain Institutional Review Board (Intermountain IRB #1009957).

Results

This cohort of septic patients included 393 patients. There were 222 (56%) patients in shock (systolic blood pressure < 90 mmHg) at the time of the echocardiogram; 151 of these were on vasopressors. Mean APACHE II score for the cohort was 26 (SD = 10). Overall 28-day mortality was 24% (n = 93).

Unanticipated critical findings were identified in 5% (95% CI 3–7%) of patients (n = 20). In total, 40 critical findings were identified on TTE in 38 (10%) patients (two patients had two critical findings). Of these 40 findings, 21 (53%) were unanticipated (see Table 1). Twelve of the 19 anticipated critical findings had been identified on prior echo, and the remaining 7 anticipated critical findings were previously suspected by the treating team based on EMR documentation.

Out of the 20 patients with unanticipated critical findings, a response to the unanticipated critical finding was identified in 12 (60%) patients. The response was non-invasive monitoring in 11 patients (primarily repeat echocardiograms) and non-invasive intervention in 6 patients (primarily blood pressure or fluid management). Some patients had multiple responses to the unanticipated critical findings, i.e., both a change in monitoring and a non-invasive intervention. No patients with unanticipated critical findings underwent either invasive monitoring or invasive interventions for that finding. Four unanticipated critical findings (one aortic dissection and three intracardiac masses) were found to be false-positives on repeat imaging with either CT angiogram or echocardiogram. In the 8 patients whose critical finding elicited no response, 50% died within 48 h of ICU admission; among the 12 patients whose critical findings elicited a response, 1 (8%) died within 48 h of ICU admission.

An unanticipated critical finding was not significantly associated with 28-day mortality when adjusted for admission APACHE II (p = 0.27). A critical finding (whether anticipated or unanticipated) on echocardiogram was also not significantly associated with 28-day

Table 1 Critical findings

Type of critical finding	Critical finding ($N=40$)	Unanticipated critical finding ($N=21$)
Tamponade	0 (0%)	0 (0%)
New depressed LV EF < 30%	9 (22%)	7 (33%)
New severe right ventricular systolic dysfunction	5 (12%)	2 (9%)
Aortic dissection	1 (2%)	1 (5%)
Cardiac mass, thrombus or vegetation	13 (32%)	7 (33%)
LVOT obstruction or HCM, > 4 m/s	3 (7%)	2 (9%)
Right to left shunt, moderate or severe	1 (2%)	1 (5%)
Severe valvular dysfunction	8 (20%)	1 (5%)

Data presented as *N* (%); *N* represents number of critical findings (there are two patients with two critical findings)

LVEF left ventricular ejection fraction, *LVOT* left ventricular outflow track, *HCM* hypertrophic cardiomyopathy

mortality when adjusted for admission APACHE II score ($p=0.85$).

Discussion

As echocardiograms are frequently performed both clinically and within research protocols, we sought to identify how often the results of an echocardiogram performed among septic ICU patients were unexpected and critical. In our large single-center cohort that makes extensive use of echocardiography in the early management of septic patients, unanticipated critical findings were identified in 5% of septic patients. This confirmed our prespecified hypothesis before this study that approximately 1 in 20 echocardiograms in septic patients identified an unanticipated critical finding. Mortality in this study is comparable to other studies on similar populations [31, 32].

Our findings provide useful estimates for researchers performing blinded echocardiograms in septic patients of the probability that unblinding may be required. Our findings also suggest to clinicians how often unexpected results may be anticipated on echocardiograms performed as part of the management of sepsis. We also believe that our findings suggest that the key target for building evidence for efficacy of critical care echocardiography in septic patients will emphasize hemodynamic guidance, which is likely to be much more important than unanticipated diagnoses.

Our findings contribute to preexisting literature on critical care echocardiography. In a study of pediatric ICU patients, echocardiography introduced a new diagnosis unrelated to the echo indication in 13%; an echo ordered as stat was more likely to change management and diagnosis than a routinely ordered echo [33]. In another study of critically ill patients, TTE changed diagnosis in 19% of cases and management in 34% of cases with "adequate clinical data". TTE changed diagnosis in 56% of cases and management in 58% of cases with "inadequate clinical data" [34]. For comparison, patients presenting to ED with chest pain and shortness of breath, TTE changed diagnosis in 25% of cases and management in 37% of cases. It also increased the diagnosing physician's confidence in diagnosis and management [35]. For comparison, rates of unanticipated findings in outpatients undergoing echocardiography for dyspnea or chest pain were found to be 22% in one study of 368 outpatient TTEs [36]. These comparable studies reflect a variety of settings and methods, but with the similar conclusion that, occasionally, unanticipated findings that change management may be identified by echocardiogram.

Our study findings may not be fully generalizable because they represent patients treated at one academic referral center and was performed on a retrospective cohort. Many emergency room physicians at this center have an interest in point of care ultrasound and patients are also often frequently ultrasounded at the bedside while in the emergency room. This could have potentially led to an underestimation of unanticipated critical findings compared to other sites if findings were identified prior to ICU transfer and documented in the medical chart. We also note the contextuality of our findings: the rate of unanticipated findings on echo may correlate with the breadth of clinicians' differential diagnoses. At this academic referral center, ICU patients are generally cared for by a team of clinicians prior to ICU transfer, as well as an ICU resident, fellow and attending once in the ICU; having several different clinicians involved in creating and documenting a differential diagnosis may make this less of an issue, although we did not formally address this question. In addition, while a TTE is generally obtained in septic patients admitted to the study ICU, if sicker patients at higher risk of an unanticipated critical finding preferentially underwent echocardiography, our estimate of the prevalence of such findings may be inaccurately high. We did not perform a bubble study on all patients, so the rate of right to left shunt in this population might have been underestimated. We acknowledge that our study is not adequately powered to determine whether unanticipated critical findings—or responses to them—are associated with mortality; much larger cohorts would be required for such an analysis.

Conclusion

Unanticipated critical findings on routine echocardiograms in septic ICU patients are uncommon. The potential relevance of echocardiography to sepsis management is more likely related to hemodynamic management than to traditional cardiologic diagnoses. Secondarily, research studies that employ blinded echocardiograms in septic patients may anticipate unblinding of approximately 1 in every 20 echocardiograms based on the unanticipated critical findings.

Abbreviations

APACHE: Acute Physiology and Chronic Health Evaluation; CT: Computed tomography; CI: Confidence interval; EMR: Electronic medical record; IRB: Institutional Review Board; ICU: Intensive care unit; IVF: Intravenous fluid; LVEF: Left ventricular ejection fraction; SD: Standard deviation; SBP: Systolic blood pressure; TTE: Transthoracic echocardiogram.

Acknowledgements

Not applicable.

Authors' contributions

SJB, EE, SMB, EH, ML, and CG designed the study. EE, SJB, ML, and SMB analyzed and interpreted the data. SJB, ML, and SMB drafted the report, and all other authors revised it. All authors read and approved the final manuscript.

Author details

[1] Pulmonary Division, Intermountain Medical Center, Salt Lake City, UT, USA. [2] Pulmonary Division, University of Utah School of Medicine, Salt Lake City, UT, USA. [3] University of Utah School of Medicine, Salt Lake City, UT, USA. [4] Critical Care Echocardiography Service, Intermountain Medical Center, Salt Lake City, UT, USA. [5] Department of Pediatrics, University of Utah School of Medicine, Salt Lake City, UT, USA. [6] Shock Trauma Intensive Care Unit, 5121 South Cottonwood Street, Murray, UT 84107, USA.

References

1. Griffee MJ, Merkel MJ, Wei KS (2010) The role of echocardiography in hemodynamic assessment of septic shock. Crit Care Clin 26(2):365–382. https://doi.org/10.1016/j.ccc.2010.01.001 **(Table of contents)**
2. McLean AS (2016) Echocardiography in shock management. Crit Care 20:275. https://doi.org/10.1186/s13054-016-1401-7
3. Schmidt GA (2009) ICU ultrasound. The coming boom. Chest 135(6):1407–1408. https://doi.org/10.1378/chest.09-0502
4. Beaulieu Y (2007) Bedside echocardiography in the assessment of the critically ill. Crit Care Med 35(5 Suppl):S235–S249
5. Beaulieu Y, Marik PE (2005) Bedside ultrasonography in the ICU: part 2. Chest 128(3):1766–1781. https://doi.org/10.1378/chest.128.3.1766
6. Beaulieu Y, Marik PE (2005) Bedside ultrasonography in the ICU: part 1. Chest 128(2):881–895
7. Donovan KD, Colreavy F (1999) Echocardiography in intensive care: the basics. Part I. Crit Care Resusc 1(3):291–295
8. Donovan KD, Colreavy F (1999) Echocardiography in intensive care: the basics. Part II. Crit Care Resusc 1(3):296–310
9. Mayo PH, Beaulieu Y, Doelken P, Feller-Kopman D, Harrod C, Kaplan A, Oropello J, Vieillard-Baron A, Axler O, Lichtenstein D, Maury E, Slama M, Vignon P (2009) American College of Chest Physicians/La Societe de Reanimation de Langue Francaise statement on competence in critical care ultrasonography. Chest 135(4):1050–1060. https://doi.org/10.1378/chest.08-2305
10. Skaarup SH, Laursen CB, Bjerrum AS, Hilberg O (2017) Objective and structured assessment of lung ultrasound competence. A multispecialty Delphi consensus and construct validity study. Ann Am Thorac Soc 14(4):555–560. https://doi.org/10.1513/annalsats.201611-894oc
11. Vieillard-Baron A, Mayo PH, Vignon P, Cholley BP, Slama M, Pinsky M, McLean A, Choi G, Beaulieu Y, Arntfield R, Koenig S (2014) International consensus statement on training standards for advanced critical care echocardiography. Intensive Care Med 40(5):654–666. https://doi.org/10.1007/s00134-014-3228-5
12. Chenzbraun A, Pinto FJ, Schnittger I (1994) Transesophageal echocardiography in the intensive care unit: impact on diagnosis and decision-making. Clin Cardiol 17(8):438–444
13. Colreavy FB, Donovan K, Lee KY, Weekes J (2002) Transesophageal echocardiography in critically ill patients. Crit Care Med 30(5):989–996
14. Heidenreich PA, Stainback RF, Redberg RF, Schiller NB, Cohen NH, Foster E (1995) Transesophageal echocardiography predicts mortality in critically ill patients with unexplained hypotension. J Am Coll Cardiol 26(1):152–158
15. Benjamin E, Griffin K, Leibowitz AB, Manasia A, Oropello JM, Geffroy V, DelGiudice R, Hufanda J, Rosen S, Goldman M (1998) Goal directed transesophageal echocardiography performed by intensivists to assess left ventricular function: comparison with pulmonary artery catheterization. J Cardiothorac Vasc Anesth 12(1):10–15
16. Bruch C, Comber M, Schmermund A, Eggebrecht H, Bartel T, Erbel R (2003) Diagnostic usefulness and impact on management of transesophageal echocardiography in surgical intensive care units. Am J Cardiol 91(4):510–513
17. Vignon P, Mentec H, Terre S, Gastinne H, Gueret P, Lemaire F (1994) Diagnostic accuracy and therapeutic impact of transthoracic and transesophageal echocardiography in mechanically ventilated patients in the ICU. Chest 106(6):1829–1834
18. American College of Cardiology Foundation Appropriate Use Criteria Task F, American Society of E, American Heart A, American Society of Nuclear C, Heart Failure Society of A, Heart Rhythm S, Society for Cardiovascular A, Interventions, Society of Critical Care M, Society of Cardiovascular Computed T, Society for Cardiovascular Magnetic R, American College of Chest P, Douglas PS, Garcia MJ, Haines DE, Lai WW, Manning WJ, Patel AR, Picard MH, Polk DM, Ragosta M, Parker Ward R, Weiner RB (2011) ACCF/ASE/AHA/ASNC/HFSA/HRS/SCAI/SCCM/SCCT/SCMR 2011 appropriate use criteria for echocardiography. A report of the American College of Cardiology Foundation Appropriate Use Criteria Task Force, American Society of Echocardiography, American Heart Association, American Society of Nuclear Cardiology, Heart Failure Society of America, Heart Rhythm Society, Society for Cardiovascular Angiography and Interventions, Society of Critical Care Medicine, Society of Cardiovascular Computed Tomography, Society for Cardiovascular Magnetic Resonance American College of Chest Physicians. J Am Soc Echocardiogr 24(3):229–267. https://doi.org/10.1016/j.echo.2010.12.008
19. Manasia AR, Nagaraj HM, Kodali RB, Croft LB, Oropello JM, Kohli-Seth R, Leibowitz AB, DelGiudice R, Hufanda JF, Benjamin E, Goldman ME (2005) Feasibility and potential clinical utility of goal-directed transthoracic echocardiography performed by noncardiologist intensivists using a small hand-carried device (SonoHeart) in critically ill patients. J Cardiothorac Vasc Anesth 19(2):155–159
20. Beigel R, Cercek B, Arsanjani R, Siegel RJ (2014) Echocardiography in the use of noninvasive hemodynamic monitoring. J Crit Care 29(1):184.e181–184.e188. https://doi.org/10.1016/j.jcrc.2013.09.003
21. Price S, Nicol E, Gibson DG, Evans TW (2006) Echocardiography in the critically ill: current and potential roles. Intensive Care Med 32(1):48–59. https://doi.org/10.1007/s00134-005-2834-7

22. Boyd JH, Sirounis D, Maizel J, Slama M (2016) Echocardiography as a guide for fluid management. Crit Care 20(1):274. https://doi.org/10.1186/s13054-016-1407-1
23. Bossone E, DiGiovine B, Watts S, Marcovitz PA, Carey L, Watts C, Armstrong WF (2002) Range and prevalence of cardiac abnormalities in patients hospitalized in a medical ICU. Chest 122(4):1370–1376
24. Levy MM, Fink MP, Marshall JC, Abraham E, Angus D, Cook D, Cohen J, Opal SM, Vincent JL, Ramsay G (2003) 2001 SCCM/ESICM/ACCP/ATS/SIS international sepsis definitions conference. Crit Care Med 31(4):1250–1256. https://doi.org/10.1097/01.CCM.0000050454.01978.3B
25. Singer M, Deutschman CS, Seymour CW, Shankar-Hari M, Annane D, Bauer M, Bellomo R, Bernard GR, Chiche JD, Coopersmith CM, Hotchkiss RS, Levy MM, Marshall JC, Martin GS, Opal SM, Rubenfeld GD, van der Poll T, Vincent JL, Angus DC (2016) The third international consensus definitions for sepsis and septic shock (Sepsis-3). JAMA 315(8):801–810. https://doi.org/10.1001/jama.2016.0287
26. McConnell MV, Solomon SD, Rayan ME, Come PC, Goldhaber SZ, Lee RT (1996) Regional right ventricular dysfunction detected by echocardiography in acute pulmonary embolism. Am J Cardiol 78(4):469–473
27. Picard MH, Adams D, Bierig SM, Dent JM, Douglas PS, Gillam LD, Keller AM, Malenka DJ, Masoudi FA, McCulloch M, Pellikka PA, Peters PJ, Stainback RF, Strachan GM, Zoghbi WA (2011) American Society of Echocardiography recommendations for quality echocardiography laboratory operations. J Am Soc Echocardiogr 24(1):1–10. https://doi.org/10.1016/j.echo.2010.11.006
28. Chauvet JL, El-Dash S, Delastre O, Bouffandeau B, Jusserand D, Michot JB, Bauer F, Maizel J, Slama M (2015) Early dynamic left intraventricular obstruction is associated with hypovolemia and high mortality in septic shock patients. Crit Care. https://doi.org/10.1186/s13054-015-0980-z
29. Hintze J (2013) PASS 12. NCSS, LLC, Kaysville
30. R Development Core Team (2014) R: A language and environment for statistical computing. R Foundation for Statistical Computing, Vienna, Austria
31. Capuzzo M, Volta C, Tassinati T, Moreno R, Valentin A, Guidet B, Iapichino G, Martin C, Perneger T, Combescure C, Poncet A, Rhodes A, Working Group on Health Economics of the European Society of Intensive Care M (2014) Hospital mortality of adults admitted to Intensive Care Units in hospitals with and without Intermediate Care Units: a multicentre European cohort study. Crit Care 18(5):551. https://doi.org/10.1186/s13054-014-0551-8
32. Liu V, Escobar GJ, Greene JD, Soule J, Whippy A, Angus DC, Iwashyna TJ (2014) Hospital deaths in patients with sepsis from 2 independent cohorts. JAMA 312(1):90–92. https://doi.org/10.1001/jama.2014.5804
33. Kutty S, Attebery JE, Yeager EM, Natarajan S, Li L, Peng Q, Truemper E, Hammel JM, Danford DA (2014) Transthoracic echocardiography in pediatric intensive care: impact on medical and surgical management. Pediatr Crit Care Med 15(4):329–335. https://doi.org/10.1097/PCC.0000000000000099
34. Stanko LK, Jacobsohn E, Tam JW, De Wet CJ, Avidan M (2005) Transthoracic echocardiography: impact on diagnosis and management in tertiary care intensive care units. Anaesth Intensive Care 33(4):492–496. https://doi.org/10.1177/0310057x0503300411
35. Levitt MA, Jan BA (2002) The effect of real time 2-D-echocardiography on medical decision-making in the emergency department. J Emerg Med 22(3):229–233
36. Kirkpatrick JN, Ky B, Rahmouni HW, Chirinos JA, Farmer SA, Fields AV, Ogbara J, Eberman KM, Ferrari VA, Silvestry FE, Keane MG, Opotowsky AR, Sutton MS, Wiegers SE (2009) Application of appropriateness criteria in outpatient transthoracic echocardiography. J Am Soc Echocardiogr 22(1):53–59. https://doi.org/10.1016/j.echo.2008.10.020

17

Basic critical care echocardiography training of intensivists allows reproducible and reliable measurements of cardiac output

Christian Villavicencio[1*], Julen Leache[1], Judith Marin[2], Iban Oliva[1], Alejandro Rodriguez[1], María Bodí[1] and Nilam J. Soni[3,4,5]

Abstract

Background: Although pulmonary artery catheters (PACs) have been the reference standard for calculating cardiac output, echocardiographic estimation of cardiac output (CO) by cardiologists has shown high accuracy compared to PAC measurements. A few studies have assessed the accuracy of echocardiographic estimation of CO in critically ill patients by intensivists with basic training. The aim of this study was to evaluate the accuracy of CO measurements by intensivists with basic training using pulsed-wave Doppler ultrasound vs. PACs in critically ill patients.

Methods: Critically ill patients who required hemodynamic monitoring with a PAC were eligible for the study. Three different intensivists with basic critical care echocardiography training obtained three measurements of CO on each patient. The maximum of three separate left-ventricular outflow tract diameter measurements and the mean of three LVOT velocity time integral measurements were used. The inter-observer reliability and correlation of CO measured by PACs vs. critical care echocardiography were assessed.

Results: A total of 20 patients were included. Data were analyzed comparing the measurements of CO by PAC vs. echocardiography. The inter-observer reliability for measuring CO by echocardiography was good based on a coefficient of intraclass correlation of 0.6 (95% CI 0.48–0.86, $p < 0.001$). Bias and limits of agreement between the two techniques were acceptable (0.64 ± 1.18 L/min, 95% limits of agreement of − 1.73 to 3.01 L/min). In patients with CO < 6.5 L/min, the agreement between CO measured by PAC vs. echocardiography improved (0.13 ± 0.89 L/min; 95% limits of agreement of − 1.64 to 2.22 L/min). The mean percentage of error between the two methods was 17%.

Conclusions: Critical care echocardiography performed at the bedside by intensivists with basic critical care echocardiography training is an accurate and reproducible technique to measure cardiac output in critically ill patients.

Keywords: Pulmonary artery catheter, Critical care echocardiography, Cardiac output, Pulsed-wave Doppler

Background

Cardiac output (CO) is the reference standard measurement for assessing target organ perfusion and oxygen delivery in shock. Assessing CO in critically ill patients allows physicians to determine hemodynamic status, identify the most appropriate therapeutic strategy, and monitor the effects of therapy.

Insertion of a pulmonary artery catheter (PAC) has been historically required to calculate CO by thermodilution [1]. However, routine use of PACs in patients with shock is no longer recommended, except in those patients presenting refractory shock, cardiogenic shock, or right-ventricular dysfunction [2]. In recent years, there has been increasing interest to develop non-invasive or minimally invasive technologies to measure CO. Among them, critical care echocardiography (CCE) has emerged as a promising technique that is commonly available, less expensive, and non-invasive (transthoracic

*Correspondence: christiananda@hotmail.com
[1] Critical Care Department, Joan XXIII-University Hospital, Mallafre Guasch 4, 43007 Tarragona, Spain
Full list of author information is available at the end of the article

echocardiography), or minimally invasive (transesophageal echocardiography) [3, 4].

In stable patients, estimation of CO by CCE has been shown to be accurate when compared to the standard thermodilution technique using a PAC [5–7]. A few studies have compared the accuracy of these techniques in critically ill patients [8], likely due to limited ability to acquire high-quality images in critically ill patients [9]. Despite this, technological advancements are making it easier to obtain high-quality images, and as recommendations on appropriate use of CCE in intensive-care units (ICUs) have emerged [10–13], CCE has become standard practice in many ICUs to evaluate cardiac function.

The primary objective of this study was to compare CO measured by intensivists with basic CCE skills using pulsed-wave Doppler (PWD) vs. PAC in critically ill patients. The secondary objective was to evaluate the inter-observer reliability of PWD-CO measured amongst intensivists with basic CCE skills, as well as identify factors associated with difficult acquisition of PWD-CO measurements with CCE.

Methods

Study population

We performed an observational study in a 30-bed medical ICU at Joan XXIII University Hospital in Spain. Approval was obtained from the Joan XXIII University hospital Ethics Committee (IRB # 88/2013), and the study was considered to present minimal risk to subjects. Informed consent was obtained from each subject or their next of kin.

Critically ill patients who required hemodynamic monitoring and were admitted to the ICU were eligible for enrollment from May 2013 to May 2015. Additional eligibility criteria included age >18, monitoring with a PAC, and interpretable images acquired by CCE. Exclusion criteria included a medical history of congenital heart disease, severe tricuspid regurgitation, severe aortic regurgitation, aortic stenosis, pregnancy, and atrial fibrillation. CO measurements were acquired independent of the subject's medical and nursing care, and investigators did not change medical management based on findings of this study.

Training

Before study enrolment, three intensivists were trained to measure CO with a portable ultrasound machine by attending a CCE course that included 10 h of didactics and 4 h of hands-on instruction on acquisition of high-quality parasternal long-axis and apical 5-chamber views. Training also included 10 h of didactics and 6 h of hands-on instruction for advanced cardiac training to learn how to use cardiac software to measure left-ventricular outflow tract diameter (LVOTd) and the left-ventricular outflow tract velocity time integral (VTI).

Study protocol and data measurements

Subjects were enrolled during the first 24 h of being invasively monitored with a PAC. Decision to insert a PAC was at the discretion of the treating physician. The following demographic, clinical, and physiologic data were collected: age, sex, weight, height, heart rate (HR), central venous pressure (CVP), mean arterial blood pressure (MAP), Acute Physiology and Chronic Health Evaluation II score (APACHE II) [14], the Sequential Organ-Failure Assessment (SOFA) score [15], use of mechanical ventilation (MV), positive end-expiratory pressure (PEEP), use of renal replacement therapy, need for vasoactive drugs, and interpretability of the ultrasound images.

All echocardiographic measurements were done with an Esaote MyLab 30 GOLD cardiovascular ultrasound system (Esaote, Geneva, Italy) equipped with a 3.5 MHz phased-array transducer. Measurements were obtained independently by three blinded intensivists that included a set of hemodynamic parameters with LVOTd, VTI, and HR. All ultrasound images obtained by the three intensivists were stored in digital format and analyzed independently by two blinded investigators to assess the interpretability of the images using a standardized rating scale [16].

Once a subject was enrolled, the three intensivists performed sequential measurements of PWD-CO. The PAC-CO was obtained after each echocardiographic measurement. The PWD-CO was calculated using the maximum value of three LVOTd measurements and the average of three VTI values [17]. The PWD-CO was calculated as follows:

$$\text{PWD-CO} = \text{Stroke volume (SV)} \times \text{HR},$$

$$\text{where SV} = \left[(3.1416) \times (\text{LVOTd}/2)^2\right] \times \text{VTI}.$$

The LVOTd was measured from a parasternal long-axis view (Fig. 1). The distance from the inner edge to inner edge of the LVOT was measured in a line parallel to the aortic annulus from the base of the right aortic valve coronary cusp to the base of the non-coronary cusp. The VTI was measured by obtaining an apical 5-chamber view and then placing a pulsed-wave Doppler cursor in the LVOT below the aortic valve annulus (Fig. 2). We measured the VTI, at the same time, in the respiratory cycle, ideally at the end of expiration.

The Doppler signal was traced using cardiac software to calculate the VTI, and an average of three measurements

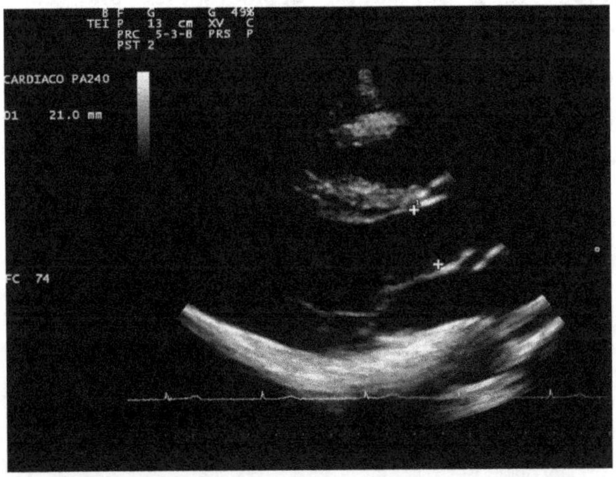

Fig. 1 Measurement of the LVOTd from a parasternal long-axis view

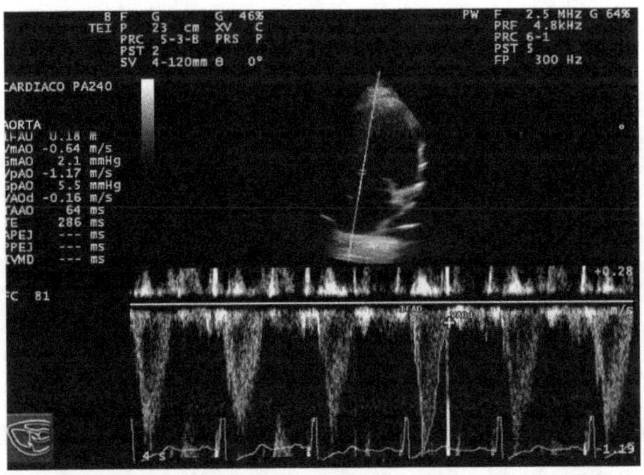

Fig. 2 Measurement of the LVOT VTI from an apical 5-chamber view

was used. The HR was calculated using the ultrasound cardiac software and not by physical examination or telemetry.

The PAC-CO was performed using a 7-French balloon-tipped standard four-lumen PAC model 131HF7 (Edwards Lifesciences Corp, Irvine, CA, USA) connected to a cardiac output monitor LCD medical display-model MOLVL 150-05 (General Electrics, Milwaukee, Wisconsin). PAC-CO measurements were obtained by injecting 10 mL of cold 0.9% saline throughout the respiratory cycle. The CO was measured three times and the results were averaged [18].

All the PWD-CO and PAC-CO measurements were obtained within a maximum of 1 h. The intensivists obtaining the thermodilution results (PAC-CO) were blinded to the PWD-CO measurements and vice versa.

Statistical analysis

First, a descriptive analysis was performed. Normal distribution of the study variables was confirmed using the Kolmogorov–Smirnov test. Discrete variables were expressed as counts and percentages, and continuous variables were expressed as means with standard deviations (SD) or as medians with interquartile ranges (25th–75th percentile). Differences between groups were assessed using a Chi-squared test or Fisher's exact test, and Student's t test or Mann–Whitney U test, as appropriate. A $p<0.05$ was considered statistically significant.

The measurement of PAC-CO was considered to be the gold standard measurement for comparison. PWD-CO measurements were compared to the PAC-CO measurements for each individual time-point. Comparisons between these measurements were performed by the linear technique described by Bland and Altman [19]. We defined a clinically acceptable level of agreement between the two techniques when the percentage of error was less than 30% as described by Critchley and Critchley [20]. This cut-off is based on an assumption that a new device destined to monitor CO should have a similar level of precision as the gold standard technique, which in this case is the PAC-CO [21].

The mean differences between the two techniques (bias), the standard deviation (SD) and precision and percentage of error (PE), together with the 95% limits of agreement (LOA) were determined for both techniques. PE for agreement between the two techniques was calculated using the following equation:

$$\text{PE PAC-PWD} = \sqrt{\left[(\text{precision PAC})^2 + (\text{precision PWD})^2\right]}.$$

The coefficient of variation (CV) and coefficient of error (CE) were also calculated for both techniques and between them.

The intra- and inter-observer variability was measured by the coefficient of intraclass correlation (CIC) and organized according to the Fleiss kappa scale (Fleiss index). A CIC greater > 0.6 was consider acceptable. Data were analyzed using the SPSS Statistics for windows version 15.0 (IBM corp. Armonk, NY, USA).

Results

Patients

A total of 42 critically ill patients were assessed for enrolment in this study. Among them, 14 patients (33.3%) were excluded due to inability to acquire a high-quality image from the parasternal long-axis view to measure LVOTd or apical 5-chamber view to measure VTI. An additional eight patients (19%) were excluded due to atrial fibrillation ($n=5$), aortic valve disease ($n=2$), or technical difficulties in obtaining the PAC-CO measurement ($n=1$).

Data were analyzed from 20 subjects [mean age 67 (±14) years), 70% males]. Baseline characteristics of the study population are shown in Table 1. Briefly, the most common diagnosis for ICU admission was septic shock (45%). The majority of patients were receiving mechanical ventilation (90%) and vasopressor medications (80%).

Compared to included patients, the excluded patients had a faster heart rate and required higher norepinephrine doses. Variables associated with inability to acquire high-quality echocardiographic views were an abdominal wall dressing ($p=0.043$) and high tidal volumes ($p=0.008$) (Table 2).

Data measurements

PWD-CO was acquired successfully in 20 patients. To acquire the desired measurements with PWD-CO and PAC-CO, a mean of 54 (±23) min elapsed to perform a complete examination, from setting up the ultrasound machine for the PWD-CO measurement to acquiring the PAC-CO measurement. For measurement of the PWD-CO alone, a mean of 12 (±4) min elapsed. The mean LVOTd was 1.92 cm (±0.13 cm) and the mean VTI was 20.85 cm (±3.72 cm). The average PWD-CO was 5.22 L/min (±1.17 L/min), which was less than the average PAC-CO of 6.26 L/min (±1.96 L/min).

Pearson correlation index demonstrated a reasonable correlation between PWD-CO and PAC-CO measurements ($r=0.78$, $p<0.0001$) (Fig. 3). To compare CO by both techniques, a Bland–Altman analysis was performed and showed a bias of 1.03 L/min (±1.27 L/min) with 95% limits of agreement ranging from −1.50 to 3.56 L/min (Fig. 4). Less difference was seen between both techniques in patients with reduced cardiac output. In those patients with CO < 6.5 L/min, a bias of 0.46 L/min (±0.88 L/min) with 95% limits of agreement of −1.29 to 2.22 L/min was found.

The bias, precision, level of agreement, percentage of error, coefficient of variation, and coefficient of error are listed in Table 3. The mean PE between PWD-CO and PAC-CO was 17%. In one patient, the mean PE was higher than 30%. In this case, cardiac rate was normal with a high stroke volume and we could not explain the reason for this outlier.

Finally, we found an excellent intra-observer and a good inter-observer agreement between the LVOTd and VTI measurements using the Fleiss kappa scale. Detailed results are shown in Table 4.

Table 1 Study population demographics and clinical characteristics

Characteristics	Number of patients (%)
Demographics	
Age, years[a]	67 (±14)
Sex-male, *n* (%)	14 (70)
Time ICU admission—CO study, days[a]	6 (±6)
Primary diagnosis, *n* (%)	
Septic shock	9 (45)
Respiratory failure	2 (10)
Surgical	2 (10)
Trauma	1 (5)
Other	6 (30)
Secondary diagnoses, *n* (%)	
DM	8 (40)
Hepatic cirrhosis	2 (10)
COPD	2 (10)
Solid cancer	6 (30)
CRF	2 (10)
Vital signs	
Heart rate, bpm[a]	88 (±12)
MAP, mmHg[a]	75 (±9)
BMI, kg/m^2[a]	27 (±3)
Vasopressors and inotropes	
Noradrenaline, *n* (%)	16 (80)
Noradrenaline, mcg/kg/min[a]	0.34 (±0.24)
Dobutamine, *n* (%)	2 (10)
Dobutamine, mcg/kg/min[a]	5.56 (±1.71)
Hemodynamics	
CVP, mmHg[a]	13 (±4)
PAP, mmHg[a]	31 (±6)
PCWP, mmHg[a]	15 (±5)
Ventilation	
Mechanical ventilation, *n* (%)	18 (90)
FiO_2, %[a]	40 (±10)
PEEP, cmH_2O[a]	7.78 (±3.12)
Tidal volume, mL[a]	543 (±70)
PaO_2, mmHg[a]	83 (±15)
PaO_2/FiO_2[a]	216 (±90)
Severity of illness	
SOFA[a]	8 (±3)
APACHE II[a]	22 (±9)
Mortality, *n* (%)	5 (25)

BMI: body mass index; DM: diabetes mellitus; COPD: chronic obstructive pulmonary disease; CRF: chronic renal failure; SOFA: sequential organ-failure assessment; APACHE II: acute physiology and chronic health evaluation; MAP: mean arterial pressure; CVP: central venous pressure; PAP: systolic pulmonary arterial pressure; PCWP: pulmonary capillary wedge pressure; PEEP: positive end-expiratory pressure; VAC: vacuum-assisted closure; FiO_2: fraction of inspired oxygen; PaO_2: partial arterial pressure of oxygen

[a] Mean ± standard deviation

Table 2 Factors associated with inability to acquire echocardiographic views

	Possible to acquire			Not possible to acquire			*p*
	n (%)	Mean	SD	*n* (%)	Mean	SD	
Age	34	66	13	8	68	19	0.721
BMI	33	28	5	7	29	9	0.631
Mechanical ventilation	27 (77)			8 (23)			0.563
Tidal volume (mL)	26	542	63	7	616	53	0.008
PEEP	26	7	3	8	6	1	0.116
Thoracic drain	7 (87)			1 (12)			0.503
Abdominal dressing	2 (40)			3 (60)			0.043

BMI: body mass index; mL: milliliters; PEEP: positive end-expiratory pressure; SD: standard deviation

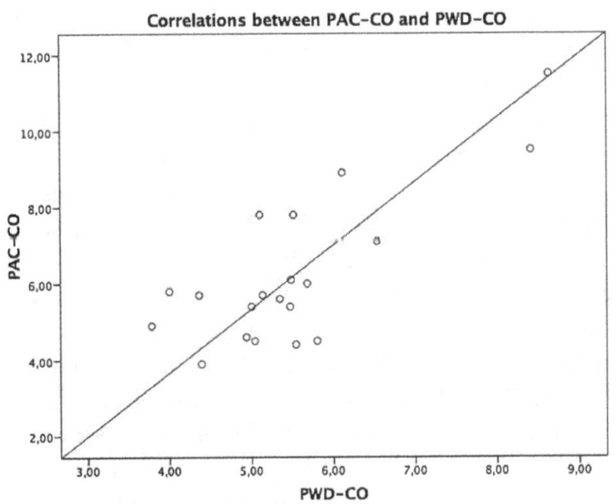

Fig. 3 Correlation of PAC-CO and PWD-CO ($r=0.78$, $p<0.0001$)

Discussion

In this study, we found an acceptable agreement of CO measured by CCE vs. PAC with thermodilution, and the inter- and intra-observer reliability was high. These findings suggest that CO can be accurately measured in critically ill patients by intensivists with the basic CCE training. However, it is important to recognize that high-quality transthoracic images to calculate CO could only be obtained in about half of eligible patients.

Although studies since the 1980s have shown that PWD measurements can accurately determine CO [4–9], a few studies have compared PWD-CO vs. PAC-CO in non-selected, critically ill patients. A recently systematic review of cardiac output measurements by echocardiography vs. thermodilution [22] concluded that the two techniques are not interchangeable. Twenty-four studies of critically ill and non-critically ill patients were included and both transesophageal and transthoracic echocardiography were used in these studies. None of the studies assessed inter- and intra-observer variability. Important limitations of the studies in this systematic review were small sample sizes, heterogeneity, and inadequate statistical analyses.

To our knowledge, one study that compared the use of PWD-CO vs. PAC-CO in critically ill patients found high accuracy and precision between the two techniques [23]. Although the design of this study is comparable to our study, the PWC-CO measurements were obtained by intensivists with extensive experience in CCE.

Similar to previously published studies, our bias analysis showed a systematic underestimation of CO by PDW compared to thermodilution by PAC [24]. This discrepancy was more notable in patients with high cardiac outputs (Fig. 4), probably related to the influence of high flow velocities and turbulent flow over the PWD signal, variability of the VTI angle [25], physiologic fluctuations in stroke volume, and size of the aortic valve orifice [26].

Strengths and limitations

Our study demonstrated that intensivists with basic CCE training can assess cardiac output in an unselected population of critically ill patients with an acceptable level of agreement between the PWD-CO and PAC-CO measurements. Although isolated CO values should be interpreted with caution, our findings indicate that PWD-CO measurements were accurate over a wide range of cardiac outputs, showing an even stronger correlation in patients with a cardiac output < 6.5 L/min, which can have important implications for the management of vasopressors and fluid therapy.

Additionally, our study is one of the few studies that assessed the inter- and intra-observer variability, and reported the challenges of acquiring high-quality transthoracic images by intensivists with basic CCE training. The intra-observer agreement was excellent and inter-observer agreement was good for ultrasound measurements of LVOT diameter, VTI, and CO. The coefficients of intraclass correlation were acceptable and similar to

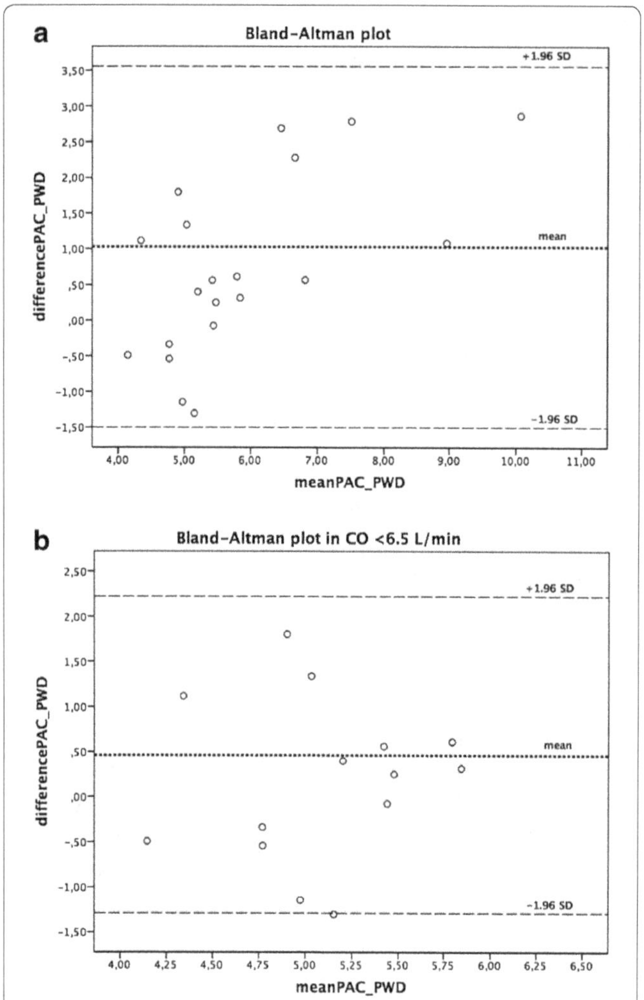

Fig. 4 Bland–Altman plots. **a** Difference in PAC-CO and PWD-CO in all patients, and **b** difference in PAC-CO and PWD-CO in patients with CO < 6.5 L/min

values described in the literature [27], suggesting that serial measurements, even if performed by different observers with basic training, can be sufficiently reproducible in clinical practice. We also found a significant association between abdominal wall dressings and poor-quality images.

Our study has several limitations. First, the total number of subjects from whom data was analyzed was small ($n=20$). Approximately half of the patients were excluded due to difficulty in acquiring high-quality images. This limitation of our study is similar to the other studies [28, 29] where high-quality images were not acquired due to use of mechanical ventilation and high levels of PEEP. Furthermore, use of PACs for hemodynamic monitoring has been progressively decreasing in our intensive care unit given the availability of non-invasive methods to measure CO. Thus, use of a PAC was left to the discretion of the attending physician when another less invasive methods of monitoring CO could not be utilized.

Another limitation of our study is the time required to acquire the CO measurements, which averaged close to an hour for a complete examination [mean 54 (±23) min]. Although this amount of time would be impractical in clinical practice, it is important to note that several measurements were obtained to follow our research study protocol. Most important, the mean time to acquire only the PWD-CO was 12 min, which is realistic to perform in clinical practice. The time and accuracy of these measurements could potentially be improved if acquired by experienced intensivists or cardiac sonographers.

Finally, limited experience of the intensivists in our study was likely an important factor that reduced the accuracy of the PWD-CO measurements. This limited experience is probably due in part to the fact that standards for CCE education currently vary by country, and there is no widely accepted consensus on the training of intensivists [30], despite the recommendations of professional societies to define competencies for basic and advanced training levels [10, 11].

Although an acceptable level of agreement was achieved between CO measured by CCE vs. PAC, the effect of individual or serial measurements of CO on clinical outcomes in critically ill patients is unknown. A

Table 3 Agreement between PWD-CO and PAC-CO

	CO (mean, SD)	Prec.	Bias	95% LOA	PE	CE	CV
PAC	6.26 (1.96)	6%	–	–	–	0.03	0.05
PAC (CO < 6.5 L/min)	5.18 (0.70)	6%	–	–	–	0.03	0.05
PWD	5.22 (1.17)	15%	–	–	–	0.08	0.13
PWD (CO < 6.5 L/min)	4.72 (0.59)	16%	–	–	–	0.08	0.14
PWD-CO vs. PAC-CO	–	–	1.03	− 1.50 to 3.56	17%	0.09	–
PWD-CO vs. PAC-CO[a]	–	–	0.46	− 1.29 to 2.22	12%	0.06	–

CO: cardiac output; Prec.: precision; LOA: limits of agreement; IC: interval confidence; PE: percentage of error; CV: coefficient of variation; CE: coefficient of error; PWD-CO: cardiac output measured by pulse wave Doppler; PAC-CO: cardiac output measured by pulmonary artery catheter

[a] Cohort of patients with CO < 6.5 L/min

Table 4 Intra- and inter-observer variability

	CIC	95% CI	*p* value	Fleiss index
Intra-observer				
LVOTd				
Observer 1	0.7	0.47–0.85	<0.001	Good
Observer 2	0.8	0.65–0.91	<0.001	Excellent
Observer 3	0.9	0.71–0.94	<0.001	Excellent
VTI				
Observer 1	0.9	0.85–0.97	<0.001	Excellent
Observer 2	0.9	0.79–0.95	<0.001	Excellent
Observer 3	0.9	0.73–0.94	<0.001	Excellent
Inter-observer				
CO	0.6	0.31–0.82	<0.001	Good

CIC: coefficient of intraclass correlation; CI: confidence interval; LVOTd: left-ventricular outflow tract diameter; VTI: velocity time integral; CO: cardiac output

recent study found a moderate level of agreement in the hemodynamic assessments performed using transpulmonary thermodilution (TPT) vs. CCE in ventilated patients with septic shock. However, there was no impact in mortality or lactate clearance [31]. Future studies should explore the impact of assessing CO by CCE on mortality and other important clinical outcomes.

Conclusion

In conclusion, our findings demonstrate that intensivists with basic critical care echocardiography training can accurately and reliably measure CO in critically ill patients compared to gold standard measurements using a pulmonary artery catheter. However, an important limitation is the inability to obtain high-quality transthoracic images to calculate CO in approximately half of eligible patients.

Additional file

Additional file 1. PWD-CO vs. PAC-CO Data.

Abbreviations

CO: cardiac output; PAC: pulmonary artery catheter; TTE: transthoracic echocardiography; TEE: transesophageal echocardiography; CCE: critical care echocardiography; ICUs: intensive-care units; PWD: pulsed-wave Doppler ultrasound; LVOTd: left-ventricular outflow tract diameter; VTI: left-ventricular outflow tract velocity time integral; HR: heart rate; CVP: central venous pressure; MAP: mean arterial blood pressure; APACHE II: Acute Physiology and Chronic Health Evaluation II score; SOFA: Sequential Organ-Failure Assessment score; MV: mechanical ventilation; PEEP: positive end-expiratory pressure; SV: stroke volume; SD: standard deviations; LOA: limits of agreement; PE: precision; CV: coefficient of variation; CE: coefficient of error; CIC: coefficient of intraclass correlation.

Authors' contributions

All authors contributed to study conception and design, data analysis, and drafting the manuscript. All authors read and approved the final manuscript.

Author details

[1] Critical Care Department, Joan XXIII-University Hospital, Mallafre Guasch 4, 43007 Tarragona, Spain. [2] Critical Care Department, Hospital del Mar-Research Group in Critical Illness (GREPAC), Institut Hospital del Mar d'investigacions Mèdiques (IMIM), Barcelona, Spain. [3] Division of Pulmonary & Critical Care Medicine, University of Texas Health San Antonio, San Antonio, TX, USA. [4] Division of General & Hospital Medicine, University of Texas Health San Antonio, San Antonio, TX, USA. [5] Section of Hospital Medicine, South Texas Veterans Health Care System, San Antonio, TX, USA.

References

1. Connors AF Jr, Speroff T, Dawson NV (1996) The effectiveness of right heart catheterization in the initial care of critically ill patients. JAMA 276(11):889–897
2. Cecconi M, De Backer D, Antonelli M, Beale R, Bakker J, Hofer C, Jaeschke R, Mebazaa A, Pinsky MR, Teboul JL, Vincent JL, Rhodes A (2014) Consensus on circulatory shock and hemodynamic monitoring. Task force of the European Society of Intensive Care Medicine. Intensive Care Med 40(12):1795–1815
3. Ihlen H, Amlie JP, Dale J (1984) Determination of cardiac output by Doppler echocardiography. Br Heart J 51(1):54–60
4. McLean AS, Needham A, Stewart D, Parkin R (1997) Estimation of cardiac output by noninvasive echocardiographic techniques in the critically ill subject. Anaesth Intensive Care 25(3):250–254
5. Axler O, Megarbane B, Lentschener C (2003) Comparison of cardiac output measured with echocardiographic volumes and aortic Doppler methods during mechanical ventilation. Intensive Care Med 29(1):208–217
6. Evangelista A, Garcia-Dorado D, Del Castillo H (1995) Cardiac index quantification by Doppler ultrasound in patients without left ventricular outflow tract abnormalities. J Am Coll Cardiol 25(3):710–716
7. Schuster AH, Nanda NC (1984) Doppler echocardiographic measurement of cardiac output: comparison with a non-golden standard. Am J Cardiol 53(1):257–259
8. Mayer SA, Sherman D, Fink ME (1995) Noninvasive monitoring of cardiac output by Doppler echocardiography in patients treated with volume expansion after subarachnoid hemorrhage. Crit Care Med 23(9):1470–1474
9. Vignon P, Mentec H, Terre S (1994) Diagnostic accuracy and therapeutic impact of transthoracic and transesophageal echocardiography in mechanically ventilated patients in the ICU. Chest 106(6):1829–1834
10. Mayo PH, Beaulieu Y, Doelken P (2009) American College of Chest Physicians/La Société de Réanimation de Langue Française statement on competence in critical care ultrasonography. Chest 135(4):1050–1060
11. Expert Round Table on Ultrasound in ICU (2011) International expert statement on standards for critical care ultrasonography. Intensive Care Med 37(7):1077–1083
12. Orde S, Slama M, Hilton A, Yastreboy K, McLean A (2017) Pearls and pitfalls in comprehensive critical care echocardiography. Crit Care 21(1):279
13. Price S, Via G, Sloth E, Guarracino F, Breitkreutz R, Catena E, Talmor D, World Interactive Network Focused On Critical UltraSound ECHO-ICU Group (2008) Echocardiography practice, training and accreditation in the intensive care: document for the World Interactive Network Focused on Critical Ultrasound (WINFOCUS). Cardiovasc Ultrasound 6:49
14. Knaus WA, Draper EA, Wagner DP, Zimmerman JE (1985) APACHE II: a severity of disease classification system. Crit Care Med 13(10):818–829
15. Vincent JL, de Mendonca A, Cantraine F (1998) Use of the SOFA score to assess the incidence of organ dysfunction/failure in intensive care units: results of a multicenter, prospective study. Crit Care Med 26(11):1793–1800
16. Dinh VA, Ko HS, Rao R, Bansal RC, Smith DD, Kim TE, Nguyen HB (2012) Measuring cardiac index with a focused cardiac ultrasound examination in the ED. Am J Emerg Med 30(9):1845–1851

17. Armstrong W, Ryan T (2000) Feigenbaum's echocardiography, 7th edn. Lippincott Williams & Wilkins, Philadelphia
18. Jansen JRC, Schreuder JJ, Bogaard JM, Van Rooyen W, Versprille A (1981) Thermodilution technique for measurement of cardiac output during artificial ventilation. J Appl Physiol Respir Environ Exerc Physiol 51(3):584–591
19. Bland JM, Altman DG (1986) Statistical methods for assessing agreement between two methods of clinical measurement. Lancet 1(8476):307–310
20. Critchley LA, Critchley JA (1999) A meta-analysis of studies using bias and precision statistics to compare cardiac output measurement techniques. J Clin Monit Comput 15(2):85–91
21. Taylor RW, Clavin JE, Matuschat GM (1997) Pulmonary artery catheter consensus conference: the first step. Crit Care Med 25(12):910–925
22. Wetterslev M, Møller-Sørensen H, Johansen RR, Perner A (2016) Systematic review of cardiac output measurements by echocardiography vs. thermodilution: the techniques are not interchangeable. Intensive Care Med 42(8):1223–1233
23. Mercado P, Maize J, Beyls C, Titeca-Beauport D, Joris M, Kontar L, Riviere A, Bonef O, Soupison T, Tribouilloy C, de Cagny B, Slama M (2017) Transthoracic echocardiography: an accurate and precise method for estimating cardiac output in the critically ill patient. Crit Care 21(1):136
24. Valtier B, Cholley BP, Belot JP (1998) Noninvasive monitoring of cardiac output in critically ill patients using transesophageal Doppler. Am J Respir Crit Care Med 158:77–83
25. Espersen K, Jensen EW, Rosenborg D (1995) Comparison of cardiac output measurement techniques: thermodilution, Doppler, CO_2-rebreathing and the direct Fick method. Acta Anaesthesiol Scand 39(2):245–251
26. Fisher DC, Sahn DJ, Friedman MJ, Larson D, Valdes-Cruz LM, Horowitz S, Goldberg SJ, Allen HD (1983) The mitral valve orifice method for non invasive two-dimensional echo Doppler determinations of cardiac output. Circulation 67(4):872–877
27. Prieto L, Lamarca R, Casado A (1998) Assessment of the reliability of clinical findings: the intraclass correlation coefficient. Med Clín 110(4):142–145
28. Boussuges A, Blanc P, Molenat F (2002) Evaluation of left ventricular filling pressure by transthoracic Doppler echocardiography in the intensive care unit. Crit Care Med 30(2):362–367
29. Nagueh SF, Kopelen HA, Zoghbi WA (1995) Feasibility and accuracy of Doppler echocardiographic estimation of pulmonary artery occlusive pressure in the intensive care unit. Am J Cardiol 75(17):1256–1262
30. Labbé V, Ederhy S, Pasquet B, Miguel-Montanes R, Rafat C, Hajage D, Gaudry S, Dreyfuss D, Cohen A, Fartoukh M, Ricard JD (2016) Can we improve transthoracic echocardiography training in non-cardiologist residents? Experience of two training programs in the intensive care unit. Ann Intensive Care 6(1):44
31. Vignon P, Begot E, Mari A, Silva S, Chimot L, Delour P, Vargas F, Filloux B, Vandroux D, Jabot J, François B, Pichon N, Clavel M, Levy B, Slama M, Riupoulene B (2018) Hemodynamic assessment of patients with septic shock using transpulmonary thermodilution and critical care echocardiography: a comparative study. Chest 153(1):55–64

18

Bedside lung ultrasonography by emergency department residents as an aid for identifying heart failure in patients with acute dyspnea after a 2-h training course

Mohamed Amine Msolli[1,3], Adel Sekma[1,3], Maryem Ben Marzouk[1,3], Wael Chaabane[2,3], Khaoula Bel Haj Ali[1,3*], Lotfi Boukadida[2,3], Nasri Bzeouich[1,3], Imen Gannoun[3], Imen Trabelssi[3], Kamel Laaouiti[1,3], Mohamed Habib Grissa[1,3], Kaouthar Beltaief[1,3], Zohra Dridi[4], Asma Belguith[5], Mehdi Methamem[6], Wahid Bouida[1,3], Riadh Boukef[2,3], Hamdi Boubaker[1,3] and Semir Nouira[1,3] on behalf of the GREAT Network

Abstract

Background: Ultrasonographic B-lines have recently emerged as a bedside imaging tool for the differential diagnosis of acute dyspnea in the Emergency Department (ED). However, despite its simplicity, LUS has not fully penetrated emergency department. This study aimed to assess the accuracy and reproducibility of ultrasonographic B-lines performed by emergency medicine (EM) residents for the diagnosis of congestive heart failure (CHF) in patients admitted to ED for acute dyspnea.

Patients and methods: This is a cross-sectional prospective study conducted between January 2016 and October 2017 including patients aged over 18 years admitted to ED for acute dyspnea. At admission, two consecutive bedside LUS study were performed by a pair of EM residents who received a 2-h course for recognition of sonographic B-lines to determine independently B-lines score and B-profile pattern. All participating sonographers were blinded to patients' clinical data. B-lines score ≥ 15 or a B-profile pattern was considered as suggestive of CHF. The final leading diagnosis was assessed by two expert sonographers, who were blinded to the residents' interpretations, based on clinical findings, chest X-ray, brain natriuretic peptide, cardiac and lung ultrasound testing. Accuracy and agreement of B-lines score and B-profile pattern were calculated.

Results: We included 700 patients with a mean age of 68 ± 12.6 years and a sex ratio (M/F) of 1.43. The diagnosis of CHF was recorded in 371 patients (53%). The diagnostic performance of B-lines score at a cut-off 15 and B-profile pattern was, respectively, 88% and 82.5% for sensitivity, 75% and 84% for specificity, 80% and 85% for positive predictive value, 84% and 81% for negative predictive value. The area under receiver operating characteristic curve was 0.86 [0.83–0.89] and 0.83 [0.80–0.86], respectively, for B-lines score and B-profile pattern. There was an excellent agreement between residents for the diagnosis of CHF using both scores (kappa = 0.81 and 0.85, respectively, for ordinal scale B-lines score and B-profile pattern).

Conclusion: Lung ultrasound B-lines assessment has a good accuracy and an excellent reproducibility in the diagnosis of CHF in the hand of EM residents following a short training program.

*Correspondence: belhajalikhaoula@yahoo.fr
[1] Emergency Department, Fattouma Bourguiba University Hospital, 5000 Monastir, Tunisia
Full list of author information is available at the end of the article

Keywords: Lung ultrasonography, B-lines, Congestive heart failure, Diagnosis, Accuracy, Reproducibility

Introduction

Acute dyspnea is a common clinical emergency and a leading cause of hospital admissions [1]. While the differential diagnosis is broad, congestive heart failure (CHF) is one of the most frequent causes that can be difficult to differentiate from other etiologies. Although immediate and accurate diagnosis is critical, available diagnostic modalities of CHF among dyspneic patients, lack either specificity or sensitivity [2–4]. Echocardiography was shown to be pivotal in the diagnostic workup of CHF, but such facility requires high skills and is not always available in many emergency departments [5, 6]. Recently, lung ultrasound (LUS) has emerged as a promising alternative tool that can be performed by novice sonographers [7–13]. This easy non-invasive bedside method provides rapid diagnostic information allowing an earlier and targeted treatment. Consequently, LUS is increasingly used in clinical practice particularly in acute care settings [10]. Nonetheless, before accepting the widespread use of LUS, there is still need to assess its accuracy and reproducibility in the hand of non-experts.

The purpose of our study is to evaluate the accuracy and reproducibility of B-lines testing assessed by emergency medicine (EM) residents after 2-h training in the diagnosis of CHF in patients admitted to the emergency department with acute dyspnea.

Patients and methods

Patients

This is prospective cross-sectional study conducted in the Emergency Department (ED) of three University Hospitals (Fattouma Bourguiba University Hospital, Sahloul University Hospital, and Farhat Hached University Hospital, Tunisia) from January 2016 to October 2017.

A convenience sampling approach, including all patients admitted to the ED for acute dyspnea as chief complaint, was used. Exclusion criteria were: age less than 18 years, impossibility to give consent to participate in the study, post-traumatic dyspnea, pregnant women, and need for endotracheal intubation or inotropic drugs patients who were deemed too unstable for sonography by the treating team were also excluded.

Methodology

All eligible patients underwent a complete physical examination. Blood pressure, heart rate, and pulse oximetry were measured and oxygen was delivered by face mask as needed. Research associates collected the following data: name, age, sex, previous medical history, ongoing treatment, and physical examination findings. The following additional tests were performed for all included patients: blood gas, hemoglobin, serum creatinine, BNP, electrocardiogram, chest X-ray, and echocardiogram. Lung ultrasonography was performed by EM residents using two ultrasound machines (Philips EnVisor C, Nederland; SonoSite M-Turbo, Sonosite Inc., Bothell, WA) and broadband curved array probes (3.5–5 MHz). The study period overlapped one and half academic year in three university hospitals, so a total of 40 residents were eligible to participate. ED residents were appointed to carry out this examination less than 4 h following patients' admission. None of the ED residents used LUS for the assessment of B-lines prior to the study. All participating residents were previously attended a 2-h training session with at least 10 clinical tests supervised by a certified emergency physicians who had accomplished a full mentoring program for "Ultra-Sound Life Support". The first 30 min of the training course included basic ultrasound physics, use of ultrasound equipment, probe positioning, and lung ultrasound interpretation (A-lines, B-lines, consolidation, lung sliding, lung pulse, and miscellaneous artifacts). In the second 30 min, real-time LUS was performed in healthy volunteers describing the technique and findings. The rest of the training was hands-on training on actual patients. Trainees had to identify the presence of lung sliding, A-lines, B-lines and consolidation.

For each patient, two LUS tests were performed by two independent residents who were not aware of patient's clinical data and did not participate in the patient's management. We recorded the ED residents' interpretation and images were recorded for each LUS study for later expert review. To not break the blind protocol, patients were asked to not provide information on their medical history to the operators during LUS. Patients were placed in a semi-recumbent or supine position depending on their respiratory tolerance. For each side of the chest, 4 zones have to be assessed (Fig. 1): 2 anterior and 2 lateral. The anterior chest wall was delineated from the sternum to the anterior axillary line and was subdivided into upper and lower halves (approximately from clavicle to the second–third intercostal spaces and from the third space to diaphragm). The lateral chest was delineated from the anterior to the posterior axillary line and was subdivided into upper and basal halves. The operator was

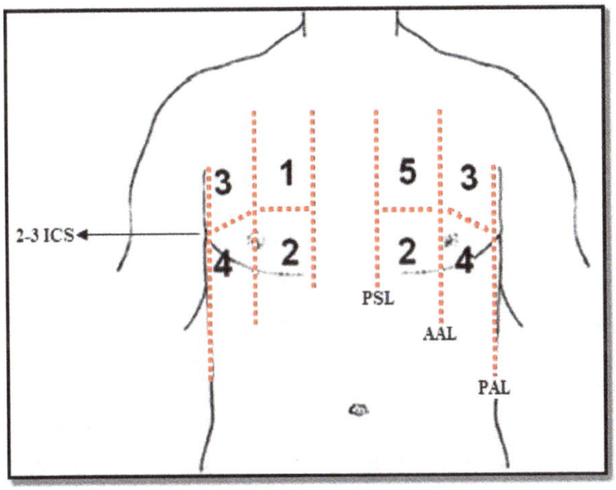

Fig. 1 The four chest ultrasound areas per side. Areas 1 and 2 denote the upper anterior and lower anterior chest areas, respectively. Areas 3 and 4 denote the upper lateral and basal lateral chest areas, respectively. *PSL* parasternal line, *AAL* anterior axillary line, *PAL* posterior axillary line, *ICS* intercostal space

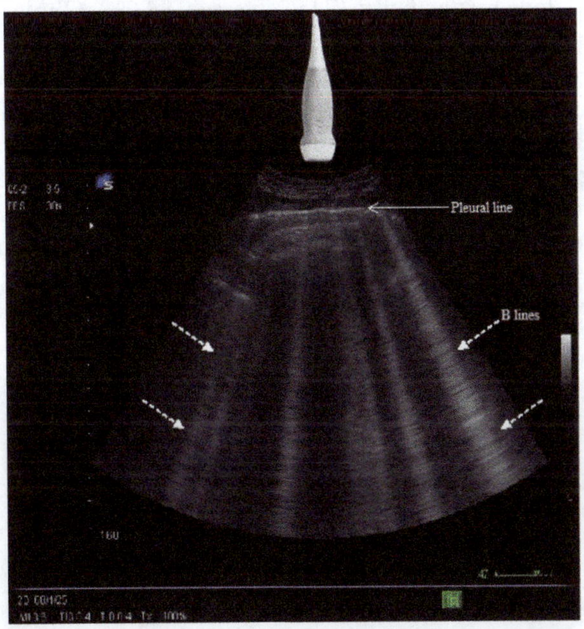

Fig. 2 B-lines represented by vertical hyperechoic images starting from the pleural line and extending to the whole ultrasound field (discontinuous arrows)

asked to calculate the B-lines score which is the sum of the B-lines found in both sides (8 zones) [14]; the intercostal space with the greatest number of B-lines within each zone was used for scoring. B-line was defined as a vertical bright echogenic bundle with a narrow basis, spreading from the transducer to the deepest part of the screen (Fig. 2). For B-lines that were wide or confluent, the score was determined by assessing the percentage of the rib space occupied by B-lines and dividing it by ten [10].

According to the study of Gargani et al. the B-lines score is suggestive of CHF when it is ≥ 15 [15]. The probability of CHF was also expressed according to the following ordinal scale: unlikely if B-lines score < 15, likely if B-lines score is between 16 and 29, and very likely if B-lines score ≥ 30. The operator also had to assess the presence or absence of B-profile pattern which is suggestive of CHF according to Lichtenstein criteria [8]. B-profile pattern was defined as such if two or more lung zones per side were positive. A lung zone was positive if three or more B-lines were identified. The final leading diagnosis of dyspnea was assessed by two independent senior EM physicians after reviewing the entire medical record of each patient it was based on: (1) the clinical presentation (severe shortness of breath, worsening dyspnea, orthopnea, paroxysmal nocturnal dyspnea, coughing up or wheezing with white or pink blood-tinged phlegm, foamy mucus), and the physical exam findings (pulmonary congestion and/or peripheral edema, rales, crackles); (2) the diagnostic tests' results including chest X-ray (pulmonary venous congestion, pleural effusion, interstitial or alveolar edema and cardiomegaly), echocardiography (structural or functional cardiac abnormalities), brain natriuretic peptide (BNP > 300 pg/mL, or NT-proBNP > 1200 pg/mL), the saved images of LUS study, treatment, and outcome [4]. In case of a disagreement, a third senior physician was consulted and adjudicated the case. All senior physicians participating in the study were masked to LUS results. Informed consent was obtained in all the patients before the start of the protocol.

Statistical analysis

Prior to enrollment, a power analysis was performed to determine the sample size needed. Assuming an alpha of 0.05 and a desired precision of 0.07, we calculated a sample size of 502 patients required if we considered that the estimated prevalence of CHF is 25% and the targeted sensitivity and specificity would both be 0.80.

After analysis of normality distribution, variables were expressed by the arithmetic mean and standard deviation (SD) or the median and the 95% confidence interval (or interquartile range). Comparison between patients with CHF (HF group) and those without CHF (non-HF group) was performed by Student's t-test for continuous variables and Chi-2 test for categorical variables. The difference was considered statistically significant for values of $p \leq 0.05$. Discrimination power of the assessed models was studied by the area under the receiver operating characteristic (ROC) curve. An area under curve (AUC) = 1 represents a perfect test; an area of 0.5 represents a worthless test (random prediction), and an area greater than 0.70 means that accuracy of the diagnostic test is at least fair. For the assessment of diagnostic accuracy of B-lines, the scanning order was randomly determined according to an electronic randomization. Agreement between residents' interpretation was assessed by kappa agreement index for qualitative indices (B-lines score as ordinal scale, and B-profile pattern recorded dichotomously as present or absent). Agreement was considered "low" when kappa value was less 0.40, "fair" from 0.41 to 0.60, "good" from 0.61 to 0.80 and "excellent" from 0.81 to 1. For the B-lines score, the Bland and Altman plot was constructed. A good match was defined when the differences between B-lines score pairs is around the average line and between the lines of −2 and +2 SD. The data obtained in this study were collected, recorded and analyzed using SPSS computer software version 18.0 (Chicago, IL).

Results

During the study period, 1024 patients with acute dyspnea were screened. Two hundred forty-two patients were excluded for one or more predefined exclusion criteria; additional 64 patients were excluded for blind protocol violation, and 18 declined or were unable to tolerate a complete examination (Fig. 3). The characteristics of the remaining 700 patients are outlined in Table 1. Four hundred twelve patients (58.8%) were men with a mean age of 68 years (±12.6). Heart failure was the final diagnosis in 53% of dyspneic patients (HF group, $n=371$).

The most common etiology of dyspnea in non-HF group ($n=329$) was chronic obstructive pulmonary disease exacerbation ($n=149$), pneumonia ($n=57$), pulmonary embolism ($n=19$), and acute asthma ($n=12$). The mean B-lines score was 29 ± 9 in HF group and 8 ± 3 in non-HF group. The difference was statistically significant ($p<0.001$). In HF group, the B-lines score was suggestive of CHF (B-lines score ≥ 15) in 325 patients (87.6%). In the same group, B-profile pattern was present in 306 patients (82.5%). The difference in patients' distribution between HF and non-HF groups according to B-profile and B-lines classes is summarized in Fig. 4. This difference was statistically significant ($p<0.001$). The discriminating power of B-lines score and B-profile pattern was good as assessed by area under ROC curve of 0.86 (95% CI 0.83–0.89) and 0.83 (95% CI 0.80–0.86), respectively, for B-lines score and B-profile pattern ($p=0.91$) (Fig. 5). Performance of B-lines score at a cut-off $=15$ showed that sensitivity, specificity, negative predictive value and positive predictive value of the two models were similar with trends to a moderately higher sensitivity for B-lines score compared to B-profile pattern (87.6% versus 82.5%) and lower specificity (74.7% versus 83.9%) (Table 2). Agreement between residents in the determination of CHF diagnosis was excellent for both models as demonstrated by kappa agreement index value of 0.81 and 0.85, respectively, for B-lines score and B-profile pattern. For B-lines scoring, there is a good agreement between residents' interpretation as shown in the Bland and Altman plot (mean differences between B-lines scores $=0.49\pm0.22$, p: not significant) (Fig. 6).

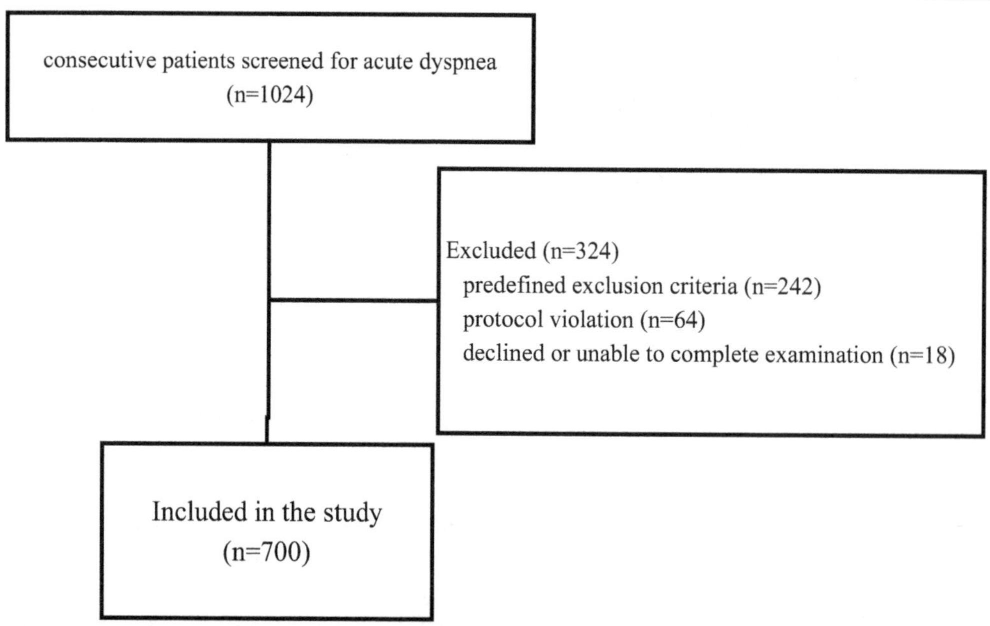

Fig. 3 Summary of patients' selection

Table 1 Characteristics of study population

	Total $n=700$	HF group $n=371$	Non-HF group $n=329$	p
Age (years), mean(SD)	68 (20)	70(24)	65(20)	<0.001
Sex ratio (male/female)	1.43	1.13	1.90	<0.001
Past medical History, n (%)				
COPD	151 (21.6)	44 (11.8)	107 (32.5)	<0.001
Asthma	21 (3)	10 (2.7)	11 (3.3)	0.47
Hypertension	346 (49.4)	225 (60.6)	121(36.7)	<0.001
Diabetes mellitus	287 (41)	188 (50.6)	99 (30)	<0.001
Chronic heart Failure	175 (25)	128 (34.5)	47 (14.2)	<0.001
Coronary artery disease	133 (19)	98 (26.4)	35 (10.6)	<0.001
Treatments				
Angiotensin converting enzyme (ACE) inhibitors	193 (27.5)	176 (47.6)	17 (5.2)	<0.001
Diuretics	167 (23.8)	158 (42.7)	9 (2.6)	<0.001
Beta blockers	50 (7.1)	42 (11.3)	8 (2.4)	<0.001
β 2 mimetics	102 (14.5)	64 (17.2)	38 (11.7)	0.03
Steroids (inhaled)	53 (7.5)	23 (6.3)	30 (9)	0.14
Aspirin	124 (17.7)	89 (23.9)	35 (10.7)	<0.001
Chest X-ray, n (%)				
Cardiomegaly[a]	368 (52.5)	253 (68.2)	115 (35)	<0.001
Interstitial edema	484 (69)	279 (75.2)	205 (62)	0.004
Vascular pulmonary redistribution	290 (41.4)	208 (56)	82 (25)	<0.001
Pleural effusion	227 (32.5)	144 (39)	81 (25)	0.003
Atrial fibrillation	154 (22)	98 (26.4)	56 (17)	0.003
LV ejection fraction, mean (SD)	51 (14)	44 (13)	59 (10)	<0.001
BNP, pg/ml, median [IQR]	216 [68–548]	458[215–771]	62[25–162]	<0.001

HF heart failure, *IQR* interquartile range, *COPD* chronic obstructive pulmonary disease, *LV* left ventricle, *BNP* brain natriuretic peptide

[a] Cardiomegaly: cardiothoracic ratio > 0.5

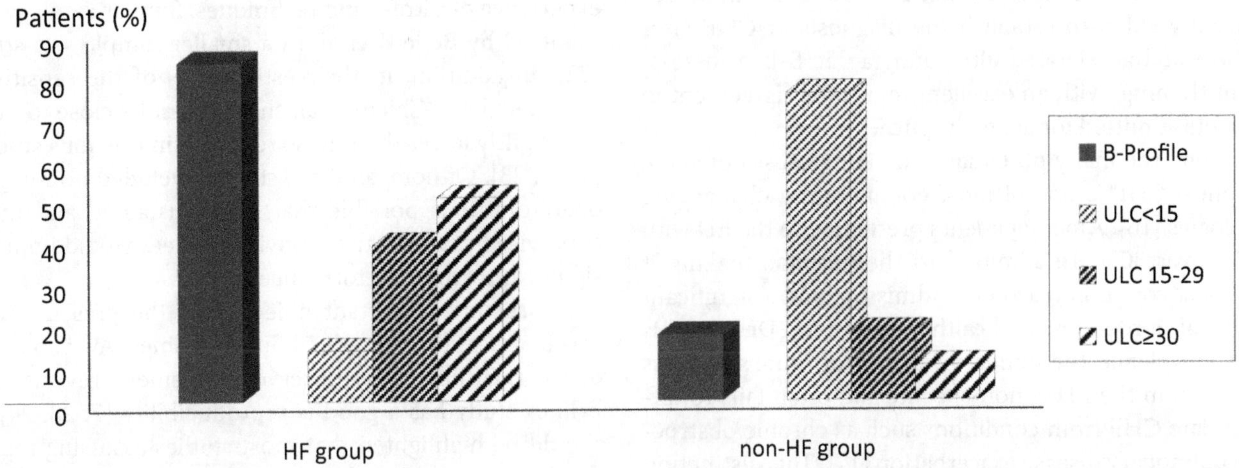

Fig. 4 Distribution of B-profile pattern and ultrasound lung comets (ULC) score between the heart failure (HF) and non-HF groups. *$p<0.001$ *between HF and non-HF groups for B-profile pattern*; **p value <0.001 *between HF and non-HF groups for ULC score*

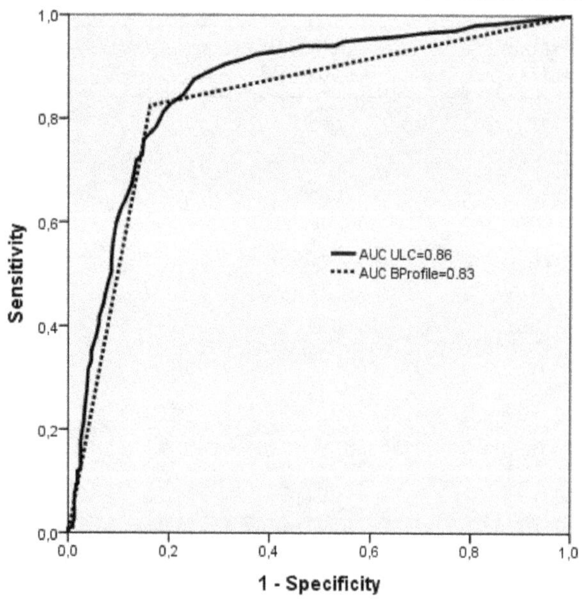

Fig. 5 Receiver operating characteristic (ROC) curve for ultrasound lung comets (ULC) score and B-profile pattern

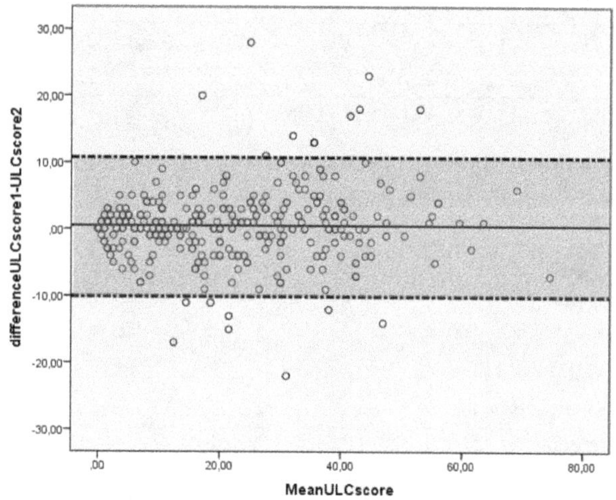

Fig. 6 Bland and Altman plot for ultrasound lung comets score. ULCscore1 denotes ultrasound lung comets score measured by the first operator; ULCscore2 denotes ultrasound Lung comets score measured by the second operator of the same pair of sonographers; shaded area denotes agreement limits

Table 2 Ultrasound lung comets (ULC) score and B-profile pattern accuracy

	ULC score[a]	B-profile pattern
	%[95% confidence interval]	
Sensitivity	87.6 [83.8–90.6]	82.5 [78.3–86]
Specificity	75.1 [70.1–79.4]	83.9 [79.5–87.5]
Positive predictive value	79.9 [76–83.7]	85.2 [81.6–88.9]
Negative predictive value	84.3 [80.1–88.5]	80.9 [76.8–85.1]
Positive likelihood ratio	3.51 [2.90–4.25]	5.12 [3.98–6.58]
Negative likelihood ratio	0.165[0.12–0.21]	0.20 [0.16–0.26]

[a] Cut-off = 15

Discussion

Our study has shown study that EM residents can be significantly aided to establish the diagnosis of CHF after a short and accelerated ultrasonographic B-lines assessment training, with an excellent inter-rater agreement in patients admitted for acute dyspnea.

Among the many potential underlying causes of acute dyspnea, CHF is one of most common and challenging etiologies [16]. Among patients presenting to the ED with CHF, over 80% are admitted to the hospital, making it the most common reason for admission and a significant financial burden on the health care system. Despite this high prevalence, the standard workup for acute shortness of breath in the ED is non-specific and often fails to differentiate CHF from conditions such as chronic obstructive pulmonary disease exacerbation [17]. This distinction is essential as inappropriate management has been shown to affect negatively the morbidity and mortality. Overall, approximately 20% of patients presenting to the ED with dyspnea are misdiagnosed and treated inappropriately [18]. In fact, substantial diagnostic uncertainty is inevitable when relying only on traditional clinical findings [19]. Lung ultrasonography, once considered inconceivable, is increasingly considered as a bedside imaging tool for evaluating pulmonary congestion [20]. A recent systematic review showed that B-lines study is highly accurate in the diagnosis of acute heart failure with an area under ROC of 0.91, a sensitivity of 0.90 and a specificity of 0.93 [21]. Of note, many of the studies included in this review had small sample sizes and were performed in settings other than EDs, even though our results are consistent with the findings of this meta-analysis. Importantly, our study is the largest in demonstrating the accuracy of B-lines study performed by residents with no previous experience of ultrasound techniques. Similar results were reported by Bedetti et al. in a smaller sample size study [22]. In addition, in their estimations of the sensitivity and specificity, Chiem et al. showed results close to ours, but slightly lower than those reported in previous studies [5, 12, 23]. Of note, all these studies included non-expert operators. It is possible that, with sustained and more supervised practice, these novice trainees would improve significantly their performance.

The second important objective of the present study was to assess the reproducibility of B-lines. Available evidence regarding inter-observer agreement reveals that B-lines study has a good is reproducibility [7, 23, 24]. It should be highlighted that most studies assessing reproducibility were based on retrospective LUS imaging review performed longtime after the first LUS testing.

B-lines is a dynamic phenomenon that can be influenced with number of technical and pathologic factors [25]. Consequently, reproducibility should be assessed without delay between pairs of LUS examinations and ideally in the same conditions. In the present study, we minimized this time between each pair of operators testing (one immediately followed the other). Moreover, we demonstrated the excellent inter-observer agreement of B-lines study by using two different models, the B-lines scoring system and the B-profile pattern which reinforces the validity of the results.

Limitations

Our study has some limitations. First, the study was conducted in academic EDs and the same evaluation in another setting may show different results. Second, since only hospitalized patients were considered eligible for the study purpose, a selection bias could not be excluded and our results may not be applicable to patients with milder symptoms. Third, some of our patients received specific heart failure treatment (intravenous diuretics, nitrates, CPAP) before undergoing LUS test, which could improve lung congestion, B-lines number would be reduced and this would probably underestimate the sensitivity of B-lines testing. Lastly, it is not clear whether introduction of LUS in routine clinical practice would influence medical decision-making and change patients' prognosis? It is not possible for us to give a clear answer to this question; it is above the scope of the present study. Nonetheless, the fact that LUS can help to identify rapidly the diagnosis of CHF, this would give to physicians more confidence in choosing the most appropriate and effective treatment. Fourth, the training course of residents is limited in our study to 2 h; this could be insufficient to be comfortable to practice LUS. However, according to a recent meta-analysis in clinical lung ultrasound, the learning time spent in the different included studies ranged from 30 min sessions to 2.5 h sessions [26]. Similar brief durations reported by Noble et al. (1 h) resulted in a significant improvement of image recognition skills for physicians without previous ultrasound experience. Moreover, a recent study by Gargani et al. showed that even web-based training in lung ultrasound can be a highly effective approach for training inexperienced operators [27].

In summary, the present study demonstrated that point-of-care B-lines study in the hand of non-expert residents is a reliable and reproducible technique. It can improve the identification of CHF in ED patients with undifferentiated dyspnea. Our results, if confirmed by other larger prospective high-quality studies, have potentially significant clinical implications. Being a rapid technique with high accuracy in the diagnosis of cardiogenic dyspnea, B-lines study could be suitable in departments with lack of technical and human resources.

Abbreviations

ED: Emergency Department; CHF: Congestive heart failure; M/F: Male/female; LUS: Lung ultrasound; SD: Standard deviation; IQR: OR interquartile range; HF: Heart failure; LR: Likelihood ratios; AUC: Area under curve.

Acknowledgements

The authors acknowledge all of our Research Laboratory LR12SP18 University of Monastir members who contributed greatly to this study.

Authors' contributions

SN, MAM, MM and AS were responsible for study design and writing of the paper. MM, WC, KBHA, IG, and IT undertook recruitment of patients and managed the data, including quality control. WB, AB, and KBHA performed statistical analysis. MHG, KB, KL and ZD supervised the conduct of the trial and were responsible for data collection and took part in data management and analysis. RB and MM made critical revision of the manuscript for key intellectual content. SN takes the responsibility for the paper as a whole. All authors read and approved the final manuscript.

Author details

[1] Emergency Department, Fattouma Bourguiba University Hospital, 5000 Monastir, Tunisia. [2] Emergency Department, Sahloul University Hospital, 4011 Sousse, Tunisia. [3] Research Laboratory LR12SP18, University of Monastir, 5019 Monastir, Tunisia. [4] Cardiology Department, Fattouma Bourguiba University Hospital, 5000 Monastir, Tunisia. [5] Department of Preventive Medicine, Fattouma Bourguiba University Hospital, 5000 Monastir, Tunisia. [6] Emergency Department, Farhat Hached University Hospital, 4031 Sousse, Tunisia.

References

1. Mebazaa A, Tolppanen H, Mueller C et al (2016) Acute heart failure and cardiogenic shock: a multidisciplinary practical guidance. Intensive Care Med 42:147–163. https://doi.org/10.1007/s00134-015-4041-5
2. Stevenson LW, Perloff JK (1989) The limited reliability of physical signs for estimating hemodynamics in chronic heart failure. JAMA 261:884–888
3. Mulrow CD, Lucey CR, Farnett LE (1993) Discriminating causes of dyspnea through clinical examination. J Gen Intern Med 8:383–392. https://doi.org/10.1007/BF02600079
4. Ponikowski P, Voors AA, Anker SD et al (2016) 2016 ESC Guidelines for the diagnosis and treatment of acute and chronic heart failure: the Task Force for the diagnosis and treatment of acute and chronic heart failure of the European Society of Cardiology (ESC)Developed with the special contribution of the Heart Failure Association (HFA) of the ESC. Eur Heart J 37:2129–2200. https://doi.org/10.1093/eurheartj/ehw128
5. Gallard E, Redonnet J-P, Bourcier J-E et al (2015) Diagnostic performance of cardiopulmonary ultrasound performed by the emergency physician in the management of acute dyspnea. Am J Emerg Med 33:352–358. https://doi.org/10.1016/j.ajem.2014.12.003
6. Price S, Platz E, Cullen L et al (2017) Expert consensus document: Echocardiography and lung ultrasonography for the assessment and management of acute heart failure. Nat Rev Cardiol 14:427–440. https://doi.org/10.1038/nrcardio.2017.56
7. Gullett J, Donnelly JP, Sinert R et al (2015) Interobserver agreement in the evaluation of B-lines using bedside ultrasound. J Crit Care 30:1395–1399. https://doi.org/10.1016/j.jcrc.2015.08.021
8. Lichtenstein DA, Mezière GA (2008) Relevance of lung ultrasound in the diagnosis of acute respiratory failure: the BLUE protocol. Chest 134:117–125. https://doi.org/10.1378/chest.07-2800
9. Gargani L (2011) Lung ultrasound: a new tool for the cardiologist. Cardiovasc Ultrasound 9:6. https://doi.org/10.1186/1476-7120-9-6
10. Volpicelli G, Elbarbary M, Blaivas M et al (2012) International evidence-based recommendations for point-of-care lung ultrasound. Intensive Care Med 38:577–591. https://doi.org/10.1007/s00134-012-2513-4
11. Wang Y, Shen Z, Lu X et al (2018) Sensitivity and specificity of ultrasound for the diagnosis of acute pulmonary edema: a systematic review and meta-analysis. Med Ultrason 1:32–36. https://doi.org/10.11152/mu-1223

12. Chiem AT, Chan CH, Ander DS et al (2015) Comparison of expert and novice sonographers' performance in focused lung ultrasonography in dyspnea (FLUID) to diagnose patients with acute heart failure syndrome. Acad Emerg Med 22:564–573. https://doi.org/10.1111/acem.12651
13. Al Deeb M, Barbic S, Featherstone R et al (2014) Point-of-care ultrasonography for the diagnosis of acute cardiogenic pulmonary edema in patients presenting with acute dyspnea: a systematic review and meta-analysis. Acad Emerg Med 21:843–852. https://doi.org/10.1111/acem.12435
14. Frassi F, Gargani L, Tesorio P et al (2007) Prognostic value of extravascular lung water assessed with ultrasound lung comets by chest sonography in patients with dyspnea and/or chest pain. J Card Fail 13:830–835. https://doi.org/10.1016/j.cardfail.2007.07.003
15. Gargani L, Frassi F, Soldati G et al (2008) Ultrasound lung comets for the differential diagnosis of acute cardiogenic dyspnoea: a comparison with natriuretic peptides. Eur J Heart Fail 10:70–77. https://doi.org/10.1016/j.ejheart.2007.10.009
16. Maisel AS, Krishnaswamy P, Nowak RM et al (2002) Rapid measurement of B-type natriuretic peptide in the emergency diagnosis of heart failure. N Engl J Med 347:161–167. https://doi.org/10.1056/NEJMoa020233
17. Wang CS, FitzGerald JM, Schulzer M et al (2005) Does this dyspneic patient in the emergency department have congestive heart failure? JAMA 294:1944–1956. https://doi.org/10.1001/jama.294.15.1944
18. Collins SP, Peacock WF, Lindsell CJ et al (2009) S3 detection as a diagnostic and prognostic aid in emergency department patients with acute dyspnea. Ann Emerg Med 53:748–757. https://doi.org/10.1016/j.annemergmed.2008.12.029
19. Badgett RG, Lucey CR, Mulrow CD (1997) Can the clinical examination diagnose left-sided heart failure in adults? JAMA 277:1712–1719
20. Cardinale L, Volpicelli G, Binello F et al (2009) Clinical application of lung ultrasound in patients with acute dyspnea: differential diagnosis between cardiogenic and pulmonary causes. Radiol Med 114:1053–1064. https://doi.org/10.1007/s11547-009-0451-1
21. Staub LJ, Mazzali Biscaro RR, Kaszubowski E, Maurici R (2019) Lung ultrasound for the emergency diagnosis of pneumonia, acute heart failure, and exacerbations of chronic obstructive pulmonary disease/asthma in adults: a systematic review and meta-analysis. J Emerg Med 56:53–69. https://doi.org/10.1016/j.jemermed.2018.09.009
22. Bedetti G, Gargani L, Corbisiero A et al (2006) Evaluation of ultrasound lung comets by hand-held echocardiography. Cardiovasc Ultrasound 4:34. https://doi.org/10.1186/1476-7120-4-34
23. Pivetta E, Goffi A, Lupia E et al (2015) Lung ultrasound-implemented diagnosis of acute decompensated heart failure in the ED: a SIMEU multicenter study. Chest 148:202–210. https://doi.org/10.1378/chest.14-2608
24. Liteplo AS, Marill KA, Villen T et al (2009) Emergency thoracic ultrasound in the differentiation of the etiology of shortness of breath (ETUDES): sonographic B-lines and N-terminal pro-brain-type natriuretic peptide in diagnosing congestive heart failure. Acad Emerg Med 16:201–210. https://doi.org/10.1111/j.1553-2712.2008.00347.x
25. Pivetta E, Baldassa F, Masellis S et al (2018) Sources of variability in the detection of B-Lines, using lung ultrasound. Ultrasound Med Biol 44:1212–1216. https://doi.org/10.1016/j.ultrasmedbio.2018.02.018
26. Pietersen PI, Madsen KR, Graumann O et al (2018) Lung ultrasound training: a systematic review of published literature in clinical lung ultrasound training. Crit Ultrasound J. https://doi.org/10.1186/s13089-018-0103-6
27. Efficacy of a remote web-based lung ultrasound training for nephrologists and cardiologists: a LUST trial sub-project | Nephrology Dialysis Transplantation | Oxford Academic. https://academic.oup.com/ndt/article/31/12/1982/2661710. Accessed 26 Jan 2021

19

Sonographic assessment of pediatric chest wall thickness and width of the intercostal space: correlation with anthropometric data and implications for needle decompression

Tom Terboven[1], Ivette Betka[1], Christel Weiss[2], Marcus Rudolph[1,3], Tim Viergutz[1], Georg Leonhard[1] and Michael Schöler[1*]

Abstract

Background: Emergent needle decompression in children is a rare event for emergency medicine and critical care providers. Hereby, risk of injury of intrathoracic structures is high and knowledge of age-specific values of chest wall thickness and width of the intercostal space (ICS) is crucial to avoid injuries. Investigation of the correlation of chest wall thickness and width of the intercostal space with age and body dimension like weight and height could provide guidance on depth of insertion and choice of the needle.

Methods: We performed a prospective observational clinical trial in a pediatric surgery operating room that included a convenient sample of children aged 0–10 years undergoing elective surgery. Chest wall thickness and width of the intercostal space were measured with ultrasound at 2nd ICS midclavicular line (MCL) and 4th ICS anterior axillary line (AAL). Correlation of these measures with age, height, weight, BMI and Broselow color was calculated. Furthermore, intra-class correlation coefficient was calculated as a measure of reproducibility and the presence of vital structures (e.g., heart, thymus gland, large pulmonary vessels) at the possible insertion sites for needle decompression was investigated.

Results: Of 410 potentially eligible patients, 300 were included in the study. Correlation of chest wall thickness was moderate with weight (2nd ICS MCL: $r=0.57$; 4th ICS MCL: $r=0.64$) and BMI ($r=0.44$ and $r=0.6$) and was lower with age ($r=0.38$ for both intercostal spaces), height ($r=0.42$ and $r=0.40$) and Broselow color ($r=0.42$ and $r=0.38$). Correlation of width of the ICS with anthropometric data was generally stronger, with height showing the strongest, albeit not really strong, correlation ($r=0.71$ and $r=0.62$). Intra-class correlation was excellent with an ICC of 0.93. Vital structures were significantly more often present at 2nd ICS MCL then at 4th ICS AAL (14 vs. 2 patients; $p=0.0042$).

Conclusions: Correlation of chest wall thickness and width of the intercostal space with anthropometric data is at most moderate. Insertion depth and width of the intercostal space can therefore not be predicted accurately from anthropometric data. Ultrasound assessment of the thoracic wall appears to be a reliable technique and could therefore assist in reducing the risk of injury and increasing decompression success.

*Correspondence: Michael.schoeler@umm.de
[1] Department of Anaesthesiology and Intensive Care Medicine, University Medical Center Mannheim, Theodor-Kutzer-Ufer 1-3, 68167 Mannheim, Germany
Full list of author information is available at the end of the article

Keywords: Tension pneumothorax, Chest wall thickness, Needle decompression, Risk of injury, Sonography, Pediatric

Background

Decompression of tension pneumothorax in children is a potentially life-saving but rather infrequent event in pediatric emergency and critical care medicine. Due to lack of training and experience in mini-thoracostomy, a procedure that requires surgical dissection of tissues, a physician experienced in this technique will mostly be required. Needle decompression appears to be less invasive and easier to perform and therefore still plays a role in high urgency situations, especially when a pediatric surgeon is not immediately available or when wire-guided chest drains are placed. Whereas in adults failure of the procedure, due to chest wall thickness (CWT) exceeding the length of the catheter used for decompression, is a common problem, needle length usually is not the problem in children [1, 2]. The chest wall is thin and the pleural space can easily be reached with common needles. In contrast to adults, intrathoracic structures like the heart, large vessels or the thymus gland are in close proximity to the insertion sites and can therefore be injured during needle decompression [3–5]. Laceration of the intercostal vessels by the decompression needle is a complication that has been described several times in adults and is even much more likely in the tiny intercostal spaces (ICS) in children [6–8]. Therefore, risk of injury by needle decompression appears to be a concern in children. Age-specific values for CWT and width of the ICS have been investigated before and showed a large variability within age groups [2, 3]. Knowing the amount of correlation of these measures with anthropometric data like age, height, weight and BMI could assist in predicting required insertion depth of the needle and choosing the appropriate needle size in an individual child. This correlation has not been studied extensively [2, 9].

We therefore assessed CWT and width of the ICS in children using ultrasound and tested for correlation of these measurements with age, height and weight. We furthermore investigated intra-rater reliability and assessed the presence of vital structures within the ultrasound window at the commonly recommended insertion sites.

Methods

This was a prospective study performed at a pediatric surgery operating room with a planned sample size of 300. All children aged 0–10 years presenting for elective surgery were eligible for inclusion and patients were recruited from February 15th 2019 to August 21st 2019 as a convenience sample without a fixed allocation to age groups. Parent's written informed consent was obtained on the eve of surgery or prior to entering the operating room facilities. Patients with large intrathoracic pathologies, with an asymmetrical thorax or with previous intrathoracic surgery/thoracotomy or surgery of the chest wall were excluded. All measurements were performed and data collected immediately after induction of anesthesia and securing the airway. Chest wall thickness and width of the intercostal space were measured at the 2nd intercostal space at the midclavicular line (MCL) and at the 4th ICS at the anterior axillary line (AAL) on both sides of the thorax. The intercostal spaces were identified by palpation. When in doubt, identification of the correct site was confirmed via ultrasound. Width of the ICS was measured from the inferior border of the superior rib to the superior edge of the inferior rib (Fig. 1). The ultrasound probe was orientated cranio-caudally, perpendicular to the ribs. As a non-perpendicular orientation would lead to false-high values for width of the ICS, the probe was slightly rotated to find the minimal width of the ICS at the investigated insertion sites. Chest wall thickness was measured from skin surface to the pleural line at the superior edge of the inferior rib (Fig. 1). Compression of the subcutaneous tissue by force exerted via the ultrasound probe was recognized as a potential bias and was avoided as possible. All measurements were performed using the 12L linear probe (5–13 MHz) of a GE Healthcare (Solingen, Germany) Vivid S5 ultrasound machine. The investigations were performed by five investigators.

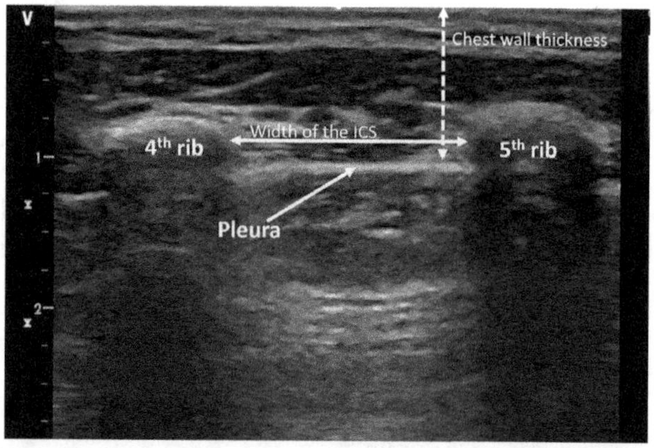

Fig. 1 Ultrasound measurement of "chest wall thickness" and "width of the intercostal space"

All investigators are consultant anesthesiologists and licensed prehospital emergency medicine physicians experienced in ground-based and air rescue missions. They have successfully completed a basic emergency ultrasound course and have at least performed >100 emergency ultrasound investigations of the chest prior to the start of the study. Moreover, they have received an additional 2-h hands-on training in sonography of the chest prior to the study by an instructor for emergency ultrasound who has performed >5000 emergency ultrasound investigations and was one the investigators himself.

Children's height and weight were extracted from the patients' preoperative records as reported by the parents or measured at the ward. Body mass index (BMI) was calculated as weight (kilograms)/height^2 (square meters). Additionally, the children were grouped into different categories based upon the Broselow length-based tape. Primary outcome was the evaluation of the correlation of CWT and width of the ICS with age, height, weight, BMI and Broselow category. Furthermore, the influence of each the mentioned variables on CWT and width of the ICS was tested using multivariable regression analysis and the presence of vital structures (thymus gland/heart/large pulmonary vessels) in the ultrasound window was assessed at the investigated insertion sites. Vital structures were only assessed as "seen" or "not seen" on the screen during evaluation of the chest wall. The distance to the pleura was not measured. As the human thorax, in the absence of pathologies, is symmetrical, we used the measured values at each side of the thorax to assess intra-rater reproducibility of the measured results.

Data were analyzed using SAS, release 9.4 (SAS Institute Inc., Cary, North Carolina, USA). Continuous variables are presented as mean ± standard deviation. Pearson's correlation coefficient was used to test the correlation of CWT and width of the intercostal space with age, height, weight, BMI and Broselow category. The sample size of 300 enables to ensure a correlation between two quantitative variables assuming a Pearson's correlation coefficient of 0.20 (with a power of 0.94). A binominal test was used to test for significance of differences of vital structures at the insertion sites. A test result with a p-value less than 0.05 was considered as statistically significant.

The study was registered at the German Clinical Trials Register (ID: DRKS00014973).

Results

Of 410 patients that were potentially eligible, 110 were not included for various reasons (Additional file 1: Figure S1, Additional file 2: Table S1). The patients were examined by five different investigators with two investigators performing five investigations each, one performing 24 investigations, one performing 108 and one 158 investigations. Mean age of the study participants was 3.7 ± 3.0 years (range 0–10 years), 236 patients (78.7%) were male. Detailed demographic data and results of the ultrasound measurements of chest wall thickness and width of the ICS are shown in supplemental Additional file 3: Table S2 and Additional file 4: Table S3.

Correlation of chest wall thickness with the investigated body dimensions was moderate. The strongest correlation was found for weight of the children (2nd ICS $r=0.57$, 4th ICS $r=0.64$). BMI also showed a rather strong correlation at 4th ICS ($r=0.60$) but not at 2nd ICS ($r=0.44$). Age, height and Broselow categories showed a weaker relationship to chest wall thickness. Detailed results are shown in Table 1.

In multivariable regression analysis, weight was the variable which had the greatest influence on chest wall thickness at all insertion sites (partial $R^2=0.31$–0.40). This influence was greater at the 4th ICS AAL (left: partial $R^2=0.4$; right: partial $R^2=0.39$) than at the 2nd ICS MCL (left and right: partial $R^2=0.31$). The influence of height was also greater at 4th ICS AAL (left: partial $R^2=0.22$; right: partial $R^2=0.25$) than at 2nd ICS MCL (left: partial $R^2=0.08$; right: partial $R^2=$ not significant). Age, sex and Broselow category had statistically significant but very small influence. Detailed results are shown in Table 2.

Regarding width of the intercostal space, the strongest correlation was found for height (2nd ICS MCL $r=0.71$, 4th ICS AAL $r=0.62$). Broselow color, age and weight showed similar correlations. No correlation was found with BMI. Detailed results are shown in Table 3.

In multivariable regression analysis for width of the ICS, height was the only variable that met the significance level for entry into the model at the four investigated insertion sites. Influence of height was stronger at 2nd ICS MCL (right: $R^2=0.5$; left: $R^2=0.47$) than at 4th ICS AAL (right: $R^2=0.37$; left: $R^2=0.31$) (Tab. 4).

Table 1 Correlation of "Chest wall thickness" with anthropometric data (Pearson's correlation coefficient; each $p<0.0001$)

	2nd ICS MCL	4th ICS AAL
Age (years)	0.38	0.38
Weight	0.57	0.64
Height	0.42	0.40
BMI	0.44	0.60
Broselow	0.42	0.38

Table 2 Multivariable regression analysis of factors influencing chest wall thickness (*$p < 0.05$)

Insertion site	Variable	Partial R^2	Model R^2
2nd ICS MCL $_{left}$	Weight	0.31*	0.31*
	Height	0.08*	0.39*
	Broselow	0.02*	0.41*
	Sex	0.01*	0.42*
2nd ICS MCL $_{right}$	Weight	0.31*	0.31*
	Age	0.10*	0.41*
	Sex	0.01*	0.42*
4th ICS AAL $_{left}$	Weight	0.40*	0.40*
	Height	0.22*	0.62*
	Age	0.01*	0.63*
4th ICS AAL $_{right}$	Weight	0.39*	0.39*
	Height	0.25*	0.64*
	Age	0.01*	0.66*

Table 3 Correlation of "width of the intercostal space" with anthropometric data (Pearson`s correlation coefficient; each $p < 0.0001$ if not otherwise specified)

	2nd ICS MCL	4th ICS AAL
Age (years)	0.67	0.58
Weight	0.64	0.58
Height	0.71	0.62
BMI	0.03†	0.06††
Broselow	0.68	0.59

† $p = 0.57$; †† $p = 0.29$

Table 4 Multivariable regression analysis of factors influencing "width of the intercostal space" (*$p < 0.05$)

Insertion site	Variable	Partial R^2	Model R^2
2nd ICS MCL $_{left}$	Height	0.47*	0.47*
2nd ICS MCL $_{right}$	Height	0.50*	0.50*
4th ICS AAL $_{left}$	Height	0.31*	0.31*
4th ICS AAL $_{right}$	Height	0.37*	0.37*

Intra-rater agreement

Overall intra-rater agreement was excellent with an ICC of 0.93 (CI 0.92–0.94). The lowest ICC for a single investigator was 0.75 (CI 0.47–0.89), the highest 0.99 (CI 0.97–0.99). The mean intra-rater difference for "Width of the ICS" was only 0.13 mm with a 95% confidence interval ranging from 0 to 0.34 at 2nd ICS MCL and 0.39 mm (CI 0.21–0.58) at 4th ICS AAL. For "chest wall thickness" mean intra-rater difference was 0.59 mm (CI 0.29–0.89) at 2nd ICS MCL and 0.04 mm (CI 0–0.24) at 4th ICS AAL.

Table 5 Number of children with vital structures visible by ultrasound at the investigated sites

	Left	Right
2nd ICS MCL	12 (4.0%)	2 (0.7%)
4th ICS AAL	2 (0.7%)	0 (0%)

Table 6 Characteristics of patients with vital structures at insertion sites

Age	Weight (kg)	Vital structure	Insertion site
1 month	3.6	Thymus gland	2nd ICS MCL right
1 month	4.1	Heart	2nd ICS MCL left
3 months	6.1	Heart	2nd ICS MCL left
6 months	7.2	Thymus gland	2nd ICS MCL left
6 months	7.2	Thymus gland	2nd ICS MCL right
6 months	8.6	Heart	2nd ICS MCL left
12 months	11	Heart	4th ICS AAL left
12 months	11	Thymus gland	2nd ICS MCL left
1 year 3 months	11.7	Heart	2nd ICS MCL left
1 year 6 months	13.8	Heart	2nd ICS MCL left
1 year 7 months	12.7	Heart	2nd ICS MCL left
1 year 10 months	11.6	Heart	2nd ICS MCL left
3 years 5 months	11.8	Heart	2nd ICS MCL left
3 years 8 months	16	Heart	2nd ICS MCL left
3 years 8 months	16	Heart	2nd ICS MCL left
4 years 7 months	22	Heart	4th ICS AAL left

Vital structures

In 16 children, a vital structure was visible in the ultrasound window at one of the four investigated sites. Table 5 shows the distribution of the structures. Compared to 4th ICS AAL, vital structures were found significantly more often at the 2nd ICS MCL ($p = 0.0042$). A detailed description of patient characteristics and vital structures is shown in Table 6.

Discussion

Decompression of tension pneumothorax in children is a rare but life-saving procedure that usually has to be performed under pressure. Due to the tiny spatial relationships, it carries a significant risk of injury to intrathoracic structures, especially in smaller children. Knowledge of chest wall thickness and width of the intercostal space enables the provider to choose the optimal decompression needle regarding length and bore but has only been investigated by few studies so far [2–4, 9]. Especially the correlation of age and body dimensions with these values has not been well investigated. Knowledge of these correlations could therefore assist in predicting the needed depth of insertion for decompression and minimize the risk of injury to intrathoracic structures and the intercostal vessels and nerve.

Chest wall thickness and width of the intercostal space

In this study, we only found moderate correlations between measures of the chest wall relevant for needle decompression and body dimensions like age, weight and height. For chest wall thickness, the highest correlation was found with weight of the children (2nd ICS MCL $r=0.57$, 4th ICS AAL $r=0.64$). BMI also correlated well with CWT at 4th ICS AAL ($r=0.60$) but not at 2nd ICS MCL ($r=0.44$). Correlation for Broselow categories (2nd ICS MCL $r=0.42$, 4th ICS AAL $r=0.38$) and height (2nd ICS MCL $r=0.42$, 4th ICS AAL $r=0.40$) were lower and the lowest correlation was found for age ($r=0.38$ at both insertion sites). Hossain et al. investigated CWT in a convenience sample of children presenting to the emergency department using ultrasound. Their results for correlation of CWT with weight (2nd ICS MCL: $r=0.55$; 4th ICS AAL: $r=0.58$) are comparable to ours. Correlation of CWT with age, height, BMI and Broselow color, however, was not investigated. Mandt et al. in a CT-based evaluation, also found the highest correlation between chest wall thickness and weight (2nd ICS-MCL: $r=0.53$; 4th ICS-AAL: $r=0.45$) and reported a lower correlation with height-based Broselow categories [2]. In most adult studies however, BMI, followed by weight, showed the strongest correlation with chest wall thickness [10–12]. In multivariable regression analysis in this present pediatric study, weight had the greatest influence on the children's CWT, with a more pronounced influence at 4th ICS AAL. However, the effect size was low with a partial R^2 ranging from 0.31 to 0.4. Both our own previous data as well as Mandt's data showed a large variability of CWT within an age group [2, 3]. Given the at most moderate correlation of CWT with anthropometric data, the low effect size in multivariable regression analysis and the large variability within age groups, one seems to be able to roughly guess CWT from patient characteristics, but accurate prediction of the required insertion depth does not seem possible.

One of the many possible complications of needle thoracostomy that has previously been described in adults is laceration of the intercostal vessels [13]. The width of the intercostal space has, to the knowledge of the authors, not received any attention in adult studies and, even though injury appears much more likely in pediatric needle thoracostomy, was only investigated in one pediatric CT-based study [3]. The results of this study match very well with the results of the ultrasound measurements presented here. Previously recommended bore sizes for decompression in infants vary from 22 to 14G. The margin of safety the provider has when using a 14G needle in an infant is extremely small. One might even encounter an infant in which the use of a 14G needle unavoidably leads to laceration of the intercostal vessels. The mean diameter of the 4th ICS at AAL was 5.3 mm in this study, the outer diameter of a common 14G needle is 2 mm. This leaves a mean safety margin of 3.2 mm. Even a slight deviation from the correct angle of insertion in direction towards the upper rib might therefore lead to vessel injury. With an 18G or 22G needle the difference between the outer diameter of the needle and the width of the ICS is still small with 4 mm and 4.4 mm but increases by 25% or 37.5% compared to the 14G needle. Width of the ICS was moderately correlated with age, weight, height and Broselow color ($r=0.58–0.71$). There was no correlation with BMI. For all variables, except BMI, correlation was higher at 2nd ICS then at 4th ICS. Multivariable regression analysis showed height being the only factor with significant influence on width of the ICS. This influence was more pronounced at 2nd ICS ($R^2=0.47–0.50$) then at 4th ICS ($R^2=0.31–0.37$). To our knowledge, there are no other studies investigating influences on width of the ICS in children or adults to which these findings could be compared.

Reproducibility of the measurements

We found an excellent intra-rater agreement with an overall ICC of 0.93 (0.92–0.94). Mean intra-rater difference between left- and right-sided measurements was remarkably small (< 1 mm) at all insertion sites. To our best knowledge, no other studies examining intra-rater reliability of measurements of CWT or width of the ICS exist. Nanikawa et al. assessed intra-rater reliability of sonographic measurements of the thickness of the lateral abdominal wall muscles and found normal to excellent reliability of the measurements (ICC = 0.74–0.96) [14]. Keshwani et al. reported ICCs > 0.9 in measurements of inter-rectus distance in women with rectus diastasis [15]. These reports of high reliability of ultrasound measurements of the abdominal wall match well with our findings of good to excellent intra-rater agreement of sonographic assessment of CWT and width of the ICS.

Vital structures

Vital structures were only detected in children younger than 5 years of age and significantly more often at the 2nd compared to the 4th ICS. The only structures identified by ultrasound were the heart and the thymus gland, large vessel were not detected. In children, different from adults, risk of injury to intrathoracic structures by the decompression needle seems to be a clearly bigger concern compared to insufficient needle length for decompression [1, 3, 16]. Nevertheless, failure of the procedure remains a problem. Quinn et al. report on 10 needle thoracocenteses performed prehospitally, of which 30% failed [17]. If this was due to inadequate insertion depth or other reasons like kinking of the catheters remains unclear. In their further course, all children required mini-thoracostomies for sufficient relieve of tension physiology. The authors therefore question the use of needle decompression in general and favor mini-thoracostomies [17, 18]. Up to the age of 10 years the intercostal width hardly exceeds 10 mm in the AAL [4]. Due to the small intercostal spaces, finger thoracostomy seems to be difficult in children, so a modified technique, e.g., with forceps, has to be used. It will however be hard to establish widespread sufficient training for this in children quite demanding procedure. Needle decompression therefore remains the technique of choice for many providers. The data from this study show that neither CWT nor width of the ICS can be accurately predicted from patient characteristics like age, weight or height. The rather high periprocedural risk of needle decompression in children in combination with the paucity of data has, in recent years, led to studies investigating this topic. As a result, current pediatric trauma guidelines recommend the 4th or 5th ICS AAL as the preferred insertion site together with the use of age appropriate decompression needles to reduce the risk of injury to vital structures [19]. Another possibility to reduce risk of injury and increase decompression success is using ultrasound. Extended Focused Abdominal Sonography for Trauma (eFAST) is an easy to learn and nowadays standard investigation in trauma care in all age groups and includes assessment of pleural sliding to rule out pneumothorax [20, 21]. Measurement of CWT and width of the ICS as well as recognition of vital structures close to the insertion site can easily be incorporated into ultrasound assessment of respiratory failure and preprocedural planning. One can then tailor the choice of needle size, especially diameter, and insertion depth to the individual patient and thereby increase decompression success and reduce risk of injury.

When ultrasound is not available, the provider has to keep in mind that age and height are rather poor predictors of CWT. The best, yet only moderate correlation was found for weight. As a rule of thumb, CWT only increases very little in the first 5 years of life and is slightly bigger at the anterior insertion site. Width of the intercostal space shows a more linear increase and is also bigger at 2nd ICS MCL.

Limitations

There are several limitations to our study. It was a single-center study with a convenience sample of patients. This led to an uneven distribution of patients regarding age and sex. Furthermore, height and weight were extracted from the children's medical records. We did not assess if these data were reported by the parents or measured by nurses. Because of this, they might differ from true values to a certain extent. In an emergency situation however, weight is usually reported by parents, guessed by the provider or extrapolated with the help of a pediatric tape and therefore will always deviate from true values to a certain degree. The study was conducted in an elective inpatient setting, not in emergency situations, and the measurements were performed after induction of anesthesia. Measuring the sometimes small distances might be more inaccurate in an awake and troubled or anxious child. This might have influence on the external validity of the presented data. Of note, the depth setting of the ultrasound probe was set at 3 cm as a starting point, but could be varied by the investigator. The excellent intra-rater agreement might have been influenced by the fact that the investigators were not blinded regarding the results of their initial measurements on the contralateral side. Inter-rater agreement was not assessed. Intrapleural pathology might distort anatomy and in case of tension pneumothorax move vital structures away from the insertion site. Lastly, there were two investigators that only performed 5 examinations each. These two investigators however are advanced and well trained in emergency sonography at all ages and their measurements were therefore included in this study.

Conclusions

Weight had the greatest influence on chest wall thickness and height the greatest influence on width of the intercostal space. The correlation of chest wall thickness and width of the intercostal space with anthropometric data, however, was at most moderate and an accurate prediction of these measures therefore is hard. Sonography could prove to be helpful in choice of needle bore to minimize the risk of injury to the intercostal vessels and assess the required insertion depth to reach the pleural space for decompression.

Abbreviations

ICS: Intercostal space; MCL: Midclavicular line; AAL: Anterior axillary line; CWT: Chest wall thickness; BMI: Body mass index; eFAST: Extended Focused Abdominal Sonography for Trauma.

Supplementary Information

Additional file 1: Figure S1. Flowchart of patient recruitment and exclusion.

Additional file 2: Table S1. Reasons for exclusion.

Additional file 3: Table S2. Anthropometric data.

Additional file 4: Table S3. Chest wall thickness and width of the intercostal space (mm; mean ± standard deviation).

Acknowledgements
Not applicable.

Authors' contributions
MS and TT designed the study, recruited patients, performed measurements, interpreted the data and wrote the manuscript. IB assisted in planning the study, recruited patients, performed measurements and collected, analyzed and interpreted the data. MR assisted in recruiting patients, performed measurements, interpreted the data and assisted in writing the manuscript. TV and GL assisted in planning the study, interpreting the data and writing the manuscript. CW assisted in planning the study, conducted the statistical analysis and assisted in interpreting the data. All authors read and approved the final manuscript.

Author details
[1]Department of Anaesthesiology and Intensive Care Medicine, University Medical Center Mannheim, Theodor-Kutzer-Ufer 1-3, 68167 Mannheim, Germany. [2]Department of Medical Statistics, University Medical Center Mannheim, Theodor-Kutzer-Ufer 1-3, 68167 Mannheim, Germany. [3]DRF Stiftung Luftrettung gemeinnützige AG, Filderstadt, Germany.

References

1. Laan D, Vu T, Thiels CA, Pandian TK, Schiller HJ, Murad MH, Aho JM (2016) Chest wall thickness and decompression failure: a systematic review and meta-analysis comparing anatomic locations in needle thoracostomy. Injury 47:797–804
2. Mandt MJ, Hayes K, Severyn F, Adelgais K (2019) Appropriate needle length for emergent pediatric needle thoracostomy utilizing computed tomography. Prehosp Emerg Care. https://doi.org/10.1080/10903127.2019.1566422
3. Terboven T, Leonhard G, Wessel L, Viergutz T, Rudolph M, Schöler M, Weis M, Haubenreisser H (2019) Chest wall thickness and depth to vital structures in paediatric patients – implications for prehospital needle decompression of tension pneumothorax. Scand J Trauma Resusc Emerg Med. https://doi.org/10.1186/s13049-019-0623-5
4. Leonhard G, Overhoff D, Wessel L, Viergutz T, Rudolph M, Schöler M, Haubenreisser H, Terboven T (2019) Determining optimal needle size for decompression of tension pneumothorax in children - a CT-based study. Scand J Trauma Resusc Emerg Med. https://doi.org/10.1186/s13049-019-0671-x
5. Terboven T, Felcht J, Zahn K, Rudolph M, Schoeler M (2020) Verletzung der A. pulmonalis im Rahmen einer Nadeldekompression bei einem 5-jährigen Mädchen. Notfall und Rettungsmedizin. https://doi.org/10.1007/s10049-020-00706-7
6. Kanai M, Sekiguchi H (2015) Avoiding vessel laceration in thoracentesis: a role of vascular ultrasound with color Doppler. Chest 147:e5–e7
7. Psallidas I, Helm EJ, Maskell NA, Yarmus L, Feller-Kopman DJ, Gleeson FV, Rahman NM (2015) Latrogenic injury to the intercostal artery: Aetiology, diagnosis and therapeutic intervention. Thorax 70:802–804
8. Mansour W, Samaha G, El Bitar S, Esper Z, Maroun R (2017) Intercostal artery laceration: rare complication of thoracentesis and role of ultrasound in early detection. Case Rep Pulmonol 2017:1–4
9. Hossain R, Qadri U, Dembowski N, Garcia A, Chen L, Cicero MRA (2020) Sound and air: ultrasonographic measurements of pediatric chest wall thickness and implications for needle decompression of tension Pneumothorax. Pediatr Emerg Care. https://doi.org/10.1097/PEC.0000000000002112
10. Hecker M, Hegenscheid K, Völzke H et al (2016) Needle decompression of tension pneumothorax: population-based epidemiologic approach to adequate needle length in healthy volunteers in Northeast Germany. J Trauma Acute Care Surg 80:119–124
11. Wax DB, Leibowitz AB (2007) Radiologic assessment of potential sites for needle decompression of a tension pneumothorax. Anesth Analg 105:1385–1388
12. Powers WF, Clancy TV, Adams A, West TC, Kotwall CA, Hope WW (2014) Proper catheter selection for needle thoracostomy: a height and weight-based criteria. Injury 45:107–111
13. Yacovone ML, Kartan R, Bautista M (2010) Intercostal artery laceration following thoracentesis. Respir Care 55:1495–1498
14. Nanikawa W, Miyazaki J (2019) Examination of the intrarater reliability of ultrasound measurements of the thickness of the lumbar and lateral abdominal muscles in the prone position. J Phys Ther Sci 31:645–648
15. Keshwani N, McLean L (2015) Ultrasound imaging in postpartum women with diastasis recti: intrarater between-session reliability. J Orthop Sports Phys Ther 45:713–718
16. Chang SJ, Ross SW, Kiefer DJ, Anderson WE, Rogers AT, Sing RF, Callaway DW (2014) Evaluation of 8.0-cm needle at the fourth anterior axillary line for needle chest decompression of tension pneumothorax. J Trauma Acute Care Surg. 76:1029–1034
17. Quinn N, Palmer CS, Bernard S, Noonan M, Teague WJ (2019) Thoracostomy in children with severe trauma: an overview of the paediatric experience in Victoria, Australia. Emerg Med Australas. https://doi.org/10.1111/1742-6723.13392
18. Teague W, Amarakone K, Quinn N (2019) Rule of 4's: Safe and effective pleural decompression and chest drain insertion in severely injured children. Emerg Med Australas. https://doi.org/10.1111/1742-6723.13299
19. Lehner M, Jung P, Olivieri M, Schmittenbecher PP (2021) Multiple trauma care in childhood — practical and pragmatic summary of the new guideline. Notfall und Rettungsmedizin 24:32–42
20. Vasquez DG, Berg GM, Srour SG, Ali K (2020) Lung ultrasound for detecting pneumothorax in injured children: preliminary experience at a community-based Level II pediatric trauma center. Pediatr Radiol 50:329–337
21. Brooke M, Walton J, Scutt D, Connolly J, Jarman B (2012) Acquisition and interpretation of focused diagnostic ultrasound images by ultrasound-naive advanced paramedics: Trialling a PHUS education programme. Emerg Med J 29:322–326

Development of supraspinatus imaging guidance for primary care physicians with a focus on patient selection

Anurag Dalai[1*], Leanne Langford[1], Cole Beavis[2] and Haron Obaid[1]

Abstract

Background: Primary care physicians frequently encounter patients with supraspinatus pathology and face a difficult task of managing this subset of patients using limited imaging resources. The purpose of this study was to develop a guidance that could help primary care physicians choose appropriate imaging tests judiciously for patients with suspected supraspinatus pathology.

Methods: The imaging reports of one hundred patients who underwent ultrasound and MRI for suspected supraspinatus tendinopathy were retrospectively assessed. The supraspinatus tendon was recorded as intact, partial tear (articular or bursal), or full-thickness tear (focal or complete width). The agreement between imaging modalities was then evaluated using factors such as pathology type and age.

Results: There was agreement between modalities in 48/100 patients (Kappa statistic = 0.30). The consistency varied with type of pathology: intact tendons by ultrasound had 55.8% agreement with MRI, partial sided bursal tears 50%, partial sided articular tears 25%, and full-thickness focal tears 33.3%. Full-thickness complete-width tears had a much better agreement with MRI at 90.9%. Age was also significant, with increased disagreement between ultrasound and MRI in patients over 50 years old.

Conclusions: Our data showed that ultrasound findings correlated well with MRI in patients under 50 years of age and also in patients with full-thickness supraspinatus tears. We recommend that primary care physicians may consider using ultrasound as the initial test in younger patients and in patients with suspected full supraspinatus tears, based on clinical exam, with MRI as an option for further evaluation to quantify supraspinatus muscle atrophy. These patient selection recommendations will help promote mindful utilization of scarce resources.

Keywords: Rotator cuff tendinopathy, Supraspinatus tendinopathy, MRI, Ultrasound, Musculoskeletal

Background

Shoulder pain is commonly reported in primary care and affects people of all ages [1]. Although the rotator cuff comprises four distinct muscles, tendinopathy in this region most commonly involves the supraspinatus tendon [1]. Proper diagnosis of supraspinatus tendinopathy subsequently allows timely and accurate management. The purpose of this study was to ascertain patient features that will help primary care physicians choose imaging investigations judiciously when considering supraspinatus tendinopathy by evaluating ultrasound and MRI finding agreement.

Primary care physicians rely on history and a complete physical exam to guide further investigation and management. A meta-analysis and systematic review support the incorporation of a thorough history and each of the physical exam components to increase positive predictive value [2]. However, these predictive values can be limited with studies showing varying sensitivity, specificity and

*Correspondence: and837@mail.usask.ca
[1] Department of Radiology, College of Medicine, University of Saskatchewan, 103 Hospital Drive, Saskatoon, SK S7N 0W8, Canada
Full list of author information is available at the end of the article

positive predictive values regarding individual history and physical exam components [2]. Therefore, clinicians should have a low threshold for diagnostic imaging such as ultrasound and MRI [2]. There is currently no widely agreed upon patient metrics which allow for accurate and timely supraspinatus tendinopathy diagnosis and efficient use of resources [2]. One study showed that a higher age and positive Neer test were important predictors of rotator cuff tear, although the sample size was small [3]. Another study showed certain aspects of the physical exam and history in combination led to the accurate detection of a rotator cuff tear, although only X-ray and ultrasound were used as the imaging modalities [4].

As supraspinatus pathology is extremely common, imaging studies are frequently ordered, causing significant utilization of the healthcare system and its resources. Magnetic resonance imaging (MRI) and ultrasound are both used in the diagnosis of supraspinatus tendinopathy. Previous studies comparing MRI with ultrasound in their diagnostic performance of supraspinatus tears have yielded variable results. A 2013 Cochrane review assessing diagnostic tests in patients with suspected rotator cuff tears in addition to the current American College of Radiology (ACR) appropriateness criteria for suspected rotator cuff tear recommend either ultrasound or MRI as the imaging of choice [5, 6]. Other studies recommend using MRI, with ultrasound as a reasonable initial investigation [7, 8].

Ultrasound studies are generally considered as preliminary tests with MRI follow-up suggested if the initial ultrasound is equivocal or if surgical intervention is being considered [9]. Ultrasound is a very appealing first-line imaging modality for evaluation of tendon pathology as it is widely available, non-invasive, inexpensive, dynamic and has no radiation risk [10, 11]. Recognizing these benefits, it would be helpful for clinicians to have more evidence to choose ultrasound as the initial imaging modality using patient features.

Methods

Approval for this study was obtained from the research ethics board of our university, and operational approval was granted from our local health region. The study was then carried out in accordance with the approved protocol. The requirement for patient consent was waived during ethical review. This study focused on evaluating diagnostic agreement between ultrasound and MRI for potential supraspinatus tendinopathy and inferring patient characteristics that may aid clinicians in choosing one modality over another. We were unable to compare the accuracy of either ultrasound or MRI studies to operative reports as not all types of supraspinatus tendinopathies are managed surgically.

A retrospective study of 100 patients age 25 and over with suspected rotator cuff pathology who had an MRI of the shoulders in the Department of Radiology at the University of Saskatchewan was performed. The inclusion criteria were any suspected rotator cuff pathology with an ultrasound performed within 3 months of the MRI. The exclusion criteria included a failed exam, previous rotator cuff surgery or the absence of an ultrasound within 3 months of the MRI. One author, a radiology resident, reviewed the ultrasound and MRI reports and categorized the results based on the indicated findings. These reports were reviewed in a retrospective, sequential manner, until a convenience sample of 100 subjects was reached. Images were taken during the period of June 18, 2015 to March 15, 2016. All ultrasound studies were performed by experienced community sonographers and reported by board certified radiologists. These reports were found on the Picture Archiving Communication System (PACS) or through local radiology clinic databases. Findings of each modality focused on the supraspinatus tendon. Results were classified as: intact, partial tear articular, partial tear bursal, full-thickness tear focal or full-thickness tear complete width.

Statistical analyses provided descriptive statistics (means with standard deviations [SD] and frequencies with proportions), both overall and within groups that, respectively, did and did not have agreement between ultrasound and MRI diagnoses. As a goal of the study was to evaluate ultrasound's ability to predict the MRI result, ultrasound findings and MRI findings were initially cross-classified and the proportions of ultrasounds with an agreeing MRI result were determined, both overall and within each of the five ultrasound diagnostic categories. Kappa statistic was calculated to quantify overall agreement, and Fisher's exact test was used to determine the presence of differences in agreeing proportions between ultrasound categories. Pairwise comparisons with Bonferroni adjusted p-values were subsequently undertaken to identify differing categories. Categories with few cases were combined for additional analysis were clinically and statistically similar, although individual patients were still only deemed to have agreement if the specific ultrasound and MRI diagnoses matched. Comparing characteristics between subjects that did and did not have agreement, age in continuous format was evaluated using the t-test; categorical variables were assessed using Chi-square test or Fisher's exact test. Characteristics were further assessed both individually and combined in respective unadjusted and multivariable logistic regression models to evaluate their ability to predict agreement. Only statistically significant terms ($p < 0.05$) were retained in the final multivariable model. SAS software, version 9.4 (SAS Institute Inc. Cary, NC, USA) was utilized for analysis.

Results

The ages of the 100 patients included in the study ranged from 25 to 65 years, with an average age of 49.2 years (SD = 10.2 years). The male-to-female ratio was 68 to 32. The MRI results were distributed as 19 full-thickness tears, complete width; 11 full-thickness tears, focal; 13 partial tears, bursal side; 22 partial tears, articular side; and 35 no tear.

There was agreement in the findings between ultrasound and MRI in only 48 out of 100 patients (95% confidence interval 38%, 58%), with a kappa statistic of 0.30. Fisher's exact testing detected differences in the consistency of agreement between ultrasound and MRI specifically based on the type of pathology identified on ultrasound ($p = 0.002$). Among the 43 patients with the most common ultrasound result, an intact supraspinatus tendon, 24 had the same finding on MRI (24/43 = 55%). Agreement was least consistent for ultrasound-identified partial tears on the articular aspect (7/25 = 25%). In contrast to complete-width, full-thickness tears were nearly all congruent with MRI (10/11 = 90.9%). Agreement proportions for full thickness but focal tears and bursal sided, partial tears were more intermediate and are available in Table 1. Pairwise comparison showed significant differences in agreement when ultrasound diagnosis was a focal, full-thickness tear or an articular sided, partial tear compared to complete width, full-thickness tears ($p = 0.046$ and $p = 0.002$, respectively).

Given that data on bursal sided, partial tears and focal, full-thickness tears was relatively sparse and did not convincingly suggest different proportions of agreement between them (Table 1), these patients were further combined with those who experienced articular sided, partial tears to create a larger category of incomplete tears. An ultrasound diagnosis of incomplete tear was again less likely to agree with MRI when compared to complete full-thickness tears (30.4% versus 90.9%, $p = 0.0008$) and also when compared to those viewed as intact on ultrasound (30.4% versus 55.8%, $p = 0.047$).

On univariate assessment (Table 2), agreement of MRI findings with observed ultrasound findings did not significantly differ by sex, although age at or exceeding 50 years and involvement of the right shoulder were initially found to be associated with a greater frequency of disagreement (p-value = 0.07 and 0.04, respectively). However, it was also noted that left-sided studies in the sample had ultrasound diagnoses that, as suggested in Table 1, may tend towards better agreement with MRI (i.e. more intact diagnoses and bursal sided, partial tear diagnoses). The right side, in contrast, had more ultrasound articular

Table 2 Comparison of subjects with and without agreement between imaging modalities

	Ultrasound agreement with MRI findings		*p*-value
	Yes, *n* = 48	No, *n* = 52	
Age, mean (SD)	47.9 (10.7)	50.4 (9.6)	0.21
Age, *n* (%)			
Less than 50 years	29 (60.4)	22 (42.3)	0.07
50 years or older	19 (39.6)	30 (57.7)	
Sex			
Male	34 (70.8)	34 (65.4)	0.56
Female	14 (29.2)	18 (34.6)	
Laterality			
Right	20 (42.6)	33 (63.5)	0.04
Left	27 (57.4)	19 (36.5)	
Ultrasound finding			
Intact	24 (50.0)	19 (36.5)	0.0006
Incomplete tear[a]	14 (29.2)	32 (61.5)	
Full-thickness tear, complete width	10 (20.8)	1 (1.9)	

MRI magnetic resonance imaging, *SD* standard deviation

[a] Partial thickness tear or full-thickness tear, but focal

Table 1 Distribution of ultrasound results by corresponding MRI findings

Corresponding MRI results	Ultrasound result, *n* (%)					Total
	Intact	Partial tear, articular side	Partial tear, bursal side	Full-thickness tear, focal	Full-thickness tear, complete	
	n = 43	*n* = 28	*n* = 6	*n* = 12	*n* = 11	*n* = 100
Intact	*24 (55.8)*	7 (25.0)	2 (33.3)	2 (16.7)	0 (0.0)	35 (35.0)
Partial tear, articular side	12 (27.9)	*7 (25.0)*	0 (0.0)	2 (16.7)	1 (9.1)	22 (22.0)
Partial tear, bursal side	4 (9.3)	5 (17.9)	*3 (50.0)*	1 (8.3)	0 (0.0)	13 (13.0)
Full-thickness tear, focal	2 (4.7)	5 (17.9)	0 (0.0)	*4 (33.3)*	0 (0.0)	11 (11.0)
Full-thickness tear, complete	1 (2.3)	4 (14.3)	1 (16.7)	3 (25.0)	*10 (90.9)*	19 (19.0)

Italicized values highlight agreement

sided, partial tear diagnoses, the ultrasound diagnosis with the least MRI agreement. Once differences in the type of pathology were controlled for in the multiple regression model, this association became non-significant; laterality was deleted from the final model.

Notably, a statistically significant difference in diagnostic agreement based on age remained in the adjusted model (Table 3). In older patients, the ultrasound result was less likely to correlate with the MRI study. On average, those 50 years of age and older were 64% (95% CI 12%, 85%) less likely to have their ultrasound result agree with their MRI result compared to younger patients, even after adjustment for type of ultrasound-determined pathology. Agreement as a function of patient age, stratified by type of ultrasound finding, is presented in Fig. 1. Similarly, type of ultrasound finding suggested varying degrees of agreement with MRI depending on the diagnosis, even after adjustment for differences in age. An ultrasound assessment showing an incomplete tear (either partial thickness or complete thickness but focal) was on average 70% (95% CI 26%, 88%) less likely to have the specific corresponding diagnosis on MRI compared to a tendon deemed intact on ultrasound. In contrast, ultrasound-detected full-thickness tears were considerably more likely to have a congruent MRI result (OR – 10.2, 95% CI 1.16, 89.7).

Table 3 Simple and multiple logistic regression models predicting ultrasound and MRI agreement

Predictors, simple regression	OR	95% CI	*p*-value
Age, years	0.975	0.937, 1.014	0.21
Age (reference: < 50 years)	0.48	0.22, 1.07	0.07
Sex (reference: female)	1.29	0.55, 3.0	0.56
Laterality (reference: right)	2.3	1.05, 5.3	0.04
Ultrasound finding (reference: intact)			
Incomplete tear[a]	0.35	0.15, 0.83	0.02
Full thickness	7.9	0.93, 67.4	0.06
Predictors, multiple regression			
Age (reference: < 50 years)	0.36	0.15, 0.88	0.03
Ultrasound finding (reference: intact)			
Incomplete tear[a]	0.30	0.12, 0.74	0.009
Full thickness	10.2	1.16, 89.7	0.04

MRI magnetic resonance imaging, *OR* odds ratio, *CI* confidence interval

[a] Partial thickness tear or full-thickness tear, but focal

Discussion

Imaging plays a vital role in diagnosing musculoskeletal disease or injury. Currently there are various modalities that can help a clinician such as ultrasound, MRI, plain film, fluoroscopy, and CT. With regard to rotator cuff injuries, ultrasound and MRI imaging are the two most commonly used modalities. When rotator cuff pathology is suspected an ultrasound is most often the first choice whether in the community or in the hospital depending on the acuity [9]. A systematic review by Liang et al. concluded that ultrasound is highly efficient in assessing supraspinatus tears due to its high sensitivity, specificity and accuracy [12]. However, a network meta-analysis by

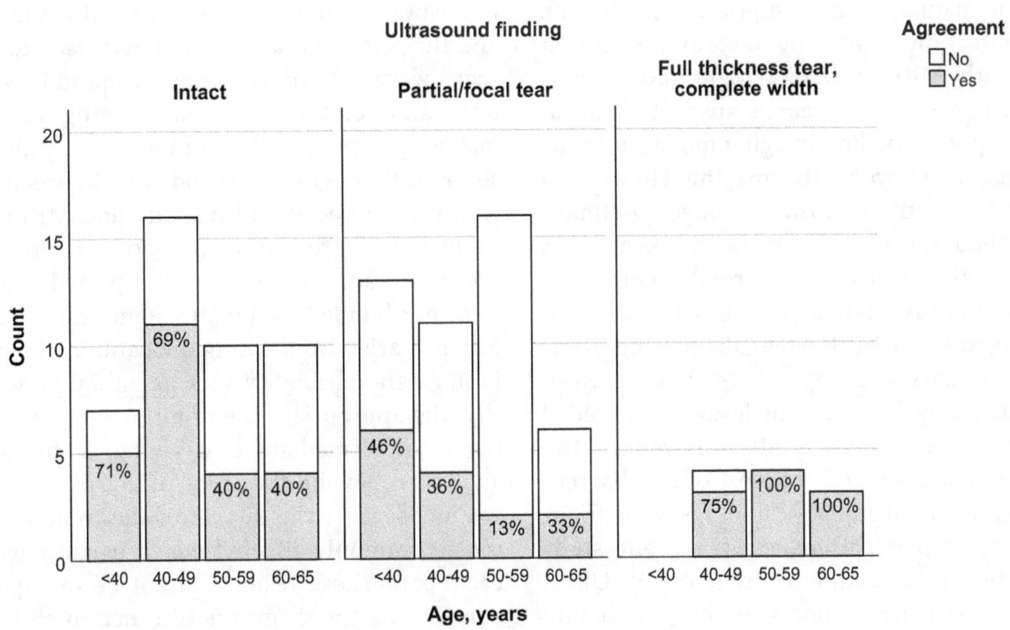

Fig. 1 Proportion of patients with agreement by age, stratified by type of ultrasound finding

Liu compared the diagnostic values of MRA, MRI and ultrasound which showed that high-field MRA had the highest diagnostic value [13]. The decision to proceed to MR imaging usually depends on whether the ultrasound result is equivocal or if the clinical history and exam suggest further investigation or if surgery is being considered [9].

The results of this study showed that the agreement between ultrasound and MRI regarding supraspinatus tendinopathy evaluation varied. Despite the general variability in modality correlation, ultrasound diagnosis with full-thickness complete-width tears had the best agreement at 90.9% with MRI. The next best agreement, an ultrasound diagnosis of intact tendon, shared only 55.8% agreement with MRI. This is in keeping with the literature which showed that both ultrasound and MRI have excellent diagnostic accuracies regarding full-thickness tears (sensitivity of 92% and 94%, respectively, and specificity of 93%) [14]. The evaluative agreement also appeared less consistent with increasing age, at least among ultrasound findings of intact tendons and partial tears. This may, in part, be related to older patients' inability to cooperate with ultrasound scan techniques due to restricted range of shoulder motion in this patient population.

Based on our data, there was only fair agreement between the two modalities. Our results showed that ultrasound findings generally had poor correlation with MRI findings across most types of supraspinatus tendinopathy which contradicts many studies including a systematic review that stated ultrasound correlates with MRI 95% of the time for rotator cuff tendinopathy [15]. Our study's sample size may be in part a reason for this. An example of this discrepancy from our study was in one patient where a supraspinatus tendon appears to be intact on an ultrasound study, but further investigation with MRI showed a high-grade partial thickness tear. If a complete tear is suspected, ultrasound may be a good first-line imaging modality as the findings correlated well with MRI imaging. However, if the ultrasound is negative and there is ongoing clinical concern, MRI should be considered which is keeping in line with current algorithms used for rotator cuff imaging [8]. Although ultrasound has similar sensitivity and specificity compared to MRI when diagnosing some types of supraspinatus tendinopathy, MRI is shown to be better at accurately depicting the lesion size, medial retraction and degree of muscle fatty infiltration [16]. Partial thickness tears were where most of the discrepancy between ultrasound and MRI findings were in our study. Pertaining to partial thickness tears, one study showed that MRI is not completely reliable [2]. Ultrasound and MRI both have poor sensitivity (52% and 74%, respectively) in diagnosing partial thickness tears, but otherwise have no statistically significant difference in diagnosing total ruptures [17]. These findings are similar in re-current tears [18]. In order to improve the diagnosis of partial thickness tears, dynamic ultrasound in combination with MRI was suggested [2].

When it comes to patient and clinical factors, there is currently little in the literature discussing the correlation of rotator cuff physical exam findings with findings on various imaging modalities or arthroscopy and eventual diagnosis. Therefore, it can be difficult for a clinician to choose between ultrasound and MRI. One study with a small sample size showed that clinical patient shoulder examinations had moderate diagnostic value for diagnosing rotator cuff tendinopathy when compared to the patient's respective magnetic resonance arthrogram (MRA) studies [2]. Higher age and a positive Neer test were found to be the most important predictors of rotator cuff tears [2]. Another study found combinations of certain aspects of the history and physical exam led to a greater diagnostic accuracy of rotator cuff tears [3]. Neither of these studies, however, used both ultrasound and MRI nor were components of the physical exam or history found to help guide clinicians in choosing one imaging modality over another.

There were a few limitations to this study. Firstly, the study is retrospective in nature, and included only those individuals who underwent both forms of imaging. However, our convenience sample was sequential and included all patients who met our inclusion and exclusion criteria during a relatively long period of observation; thus, we believe our findings to be adequately representative of this specific group. The noted associations require further confirmation via prospective work. Secondly, the types of ultrasound machines and the settings that sonographers used to conduct the scans were not analysed as ultrasound is widely known to be an operator-dependent imaging test and settings may vary between different operators. Thirdly, interobserver differences that could exist between radiologists who interpreted the ultrasound and MRI could not be evaluated due to the retrospective nature of the study. Fourthly, radiologists who interpreted the MRI scans were not blinded to the ultrasound reports. Fifthly, our findings arise from a single location, which potentially limits generalizability. Sixth, although we anticipate that the appropriate use of ultrasound over MRI would result in immediate cost-saving, a full cost–benefit analysis is beyond the scope of this paper. Furthermore, we focused on the supraspinatus tendon as it is the most commonly affected which usually requires surgical repair. These results cannot be extrapolated when considering the diagnosis of other rotator cuff tendon injuries.

Conclusion

There was considerable variability between ultrasound and MRI in the assessment of supraspinatus tears. Our data showed that ultrasound studies among younger patients correlate better with MRI than patients over 50 years of age where disagreement increases. Primary care physicians can confidently consider using ultrasound as the initial test in younger patients and in patients with suspected full supraspinatus tears or intact tendons based on clinical exam with MRI as an option for further evaluation if necessary. In the case of older patients or in patients with physical exam findings that are equivocal that may not suggest a complete tear nor intact tendon, ultrasound or MRI may be preferred. However, with studies suggesting that neither ultrasound and MRI are particularly reliable nor sensitive for partial tears, ultrasound may serve as a reasonable first step for economic and patient accessibility reasons. These patient selection recommendations would help promote mindful resource utilization, keeping in mind the economic benefits of ultrasound over MRI.

Acknowledgements
Rhonda Bryce MD and Hyun Lim Ph.D. for help with data analysis. Saskatoon Health Region (SHR), College of Medicine, University of Saskatchewan.

Authors' contributions
HO is the principal investigator helped conceive the project and design the analysis in addition to editing the final manuscript. CB also helped conceive the research project and design the analysis. LL helped conceive the project and design the analysis and in addition collected, sorted and helped analyse the patient data from the PACS system. AD carried out the literature search, data analysis and constructed the final manuscript. All authors read and approved the final manuscript.

Author details
[1] Department of Radiology, College of Medicine, University of Saskatchewan, 103 Hospital Drive, Saskatoon, SK S7N 0W8, Canada. [2] Department of Orthopedic Surgery, College of Medicine, University of Saskatchewan, Saskatoon, Canada.

References
1. Gückel C, Nidecker A (1997) Diagnosis of tears in rotator-cuff-injuries. Eur J Radiol 25(3):168–176
2. van Kampen D, van den Berg T, van der Woude H, Castelein R, Scholtes V, Terwee C (2014) The diagnostic value of the combination of patient characteristics, history, and clinical shoulder tests for the diagnosis of rotator cuff tear. J Orthop Surg Res. https://doi.org/10.1186/s13018-014-0070-y
3. Mathiasen R, Hogrefe C (2018) Evaluation and management of rotator cuff tears: a primary care perspective. Curr Rev Musculoskelet Med 11:72–76. https://doi.org/10.1007/s12178-018-9471-6
4. Cadogan A, McNair P, Laslett M, Hing W, Taylor S (2013) Diagnostic accuracy of clinical examination features for identifying large rotator cuff tears in primary health care. J Man Manip Ther 21:148–159. https://doi.org/10.1179/2042618612y.0000000020
5. American College of Radiology ACR Appropriateness Criteria® Shoulder Pain–Traumatic. American College of Radiology. https://acsearch.acr.org/docs/69433/Narrative/. Accessed 17 Sept 2018.
6. Lenza M, Buchbinder R, Takwoingi Y, Johnston RV, Hanchard NC, Faloppa F (2013) Magnetic resonance imaging, magnetic resonance arthrography and ultrasonography for assessing rotator cuff tears in people with shoulder pain for whom surgery is being considered. Cochrane Database Syst Rev. https://doi.org/10.1002/14651858.CD009020.pub2
7. Martín-Hervás C, Romero J, Navas-Acién A, Reboiras JJ, Munuera L (2001) Ultrasonographic and magnetic resonance images of rotator cuff lesions compared with arthroscopy or open surgery findings. J Shoulder Elbow Surg 10(5):410–415
8. Ferrari F, Governi S, Burresi F, Vigni F, Stefani P (2001) Supraspinatus tendon tears: comparison of US and MR arthrography with surgical correlation. Eur Radiol 12(5):1211–1217
9. Nazarian L, Jacobson J, Benson C, Bancroft LW, Bedi A, McShane JM et al (2013) Imaging algorithms for evaluating suspected rotator cuff disease: society of radiologists in ultrasound consensus conference statement. Radiology 267(2):589–595
10. Lento P, Primack S (2007) Advances and utility of diagnostic ultrasound in musculoskeletal medicine. Curr Rev Musculoskelet Med 1(1):24–31
11. Jacobson J (2002) Ultrasound in sports medicine. Radiol Clin N Am 40(2):363–386
12. Liang W, Wu H, Dong F, Tian H, Xu J (2020) Diagnostic performance of ultrasound for rotator cuff tears: a systematic review and meta-analysis. Med Ultrason 22(2):197–202
13. Liu F, Dong J, Shen WJ, Kang Q, Zhou D, Xiong F (2020) Detecting rotator cuff tears: a network meta-analysis of 144 diagnostic studies. Orthop J Sports Med 8(2):2325967119900356
14. Brockmeyer M, Schmitt C, Haupert A, Kohn D, Lorbach O (2017) Limited diagnostic accuracy of magnetic resonance imaging and clinical tests for detecting partial-thickness tears of the rotator cuff. Arch Orthop Trauma Surg 137:1719–1724. https://doi.org/10.1007/s00402-017-2799-3
15. Dinnes J, Loveman E, McIntyre L, Waugh N (2003) The effectiveness of diagnostic tests for the assessment of shoulder pain due to soft tissue disorders: a systematic review. Health Technol Assess. https://doi.org/10.3310/hta7290
16. Okoroha K, Mehran N, Duncan J, Washington T, Spiering T, Bey M (2016) Characterization of rotator cuff tears: ultrasound versus magnetic resonance imaging. Orthopedics 40(1):e124–e130. https://doi.org/10.3928/01477447-20161013-04
17. Lenza M, Buchbinder R, Takwoingi Y, Johnston RV, Hanchard NC, Faloppa F (2013) Magnetic resonance imaging, magnetic resonance arthrography and ultrasonography for assessing rotator cuff tears in people with shoulder pain for whom surgery is being considered. Cochrane Database Syst Rev. https://doi.org/10.1002/14651858.cd009020.pub2
18. Gilat R, Atoun E, Cohen O, Tsvieli O, Rath E, Lakstein D (2018) Recurrent rotator cuff tear: is ultrasound imaging reliable? J Shoulder Elbow Surg 27(7):1263–1267. https://doi.org/10.1016/j.jse.2017.12.017

21

Renal resistive index is associated with acute kidney injury in COVID-19 patients treated in the intensive care unit

Mårten Renberg[1,2*], Olof Jonmarker[3], Naima Kilhamn[1], Claire Rimes-Stigare[1,2], Max Bell[1,2] and Daniel Hertzberg[1,2]

Abstract

Background: Renal resistive index (RRI) is a promising tool for the assessment of acute kidney injury (AKI) in critically ill patients in general, but its role and association to AKI among patients with Coronavirus disease 2019 (COVID-19) is not known.

Objective: The aim of this study was to describe the pattern of RRI in relation to AKI in patients with COVID-19 treated in the intensive care unit.

Methods: In this observational cohort study, RRI was measured in COVID-19 patients in six intensive care units at two sites of a Swedish University Hospital. AKI was defined by the creatinine criteria in the Kidney Disease Improving Global Outcomes classification. We investigated the association between RRI and AKI diagnosis, different AKI stages and urine output.

Results: RRI was measured in 51 patients, of which 23 patients (45%) had AKI at the time of measurement. Median RRI in patients with AKI was 0.80 (IQR 0.71–0.85) compared to 0.72 (IQR 0.67–0.78) in patients without AKI ($p=0.004$). Compared to patients without AKI, RRI was higher in patients with AKI stage 3 (median 0.83, IQR 0.71–0.85, $p=0.006$) but not in patients with AKI stage 1 (median 0.76, IQR 0.71–0.83, $p=0.347$) or AKI stage 2 (median 0.79, min/max 0.79/0.80, $n=2$, $p=0.134$). RRI was higher in patients with an ongoing AKI episode compared to patients who never developed AKI (median 0.72, IQR 0.69–0.78, $p=0.015$) or patients who developed AKI but had recovered at the time of measurement (median 0.68, IQR 0.67–0.81, $p=0.021$). Oliguric patients had higher RRI (median 0.84, IQR 0.83–0.85) compared to non-oliguric patients (median 0.74, IQR 0.69–0.81) ($p=0.009$). After multivariable adjustment, RRI was independently associated with AKI (OR for 0.01 increments of RRI 1.22, 95% CI 1.07–1.41).

Conclusions: Critically ill COVID-19 patients with AKI have higher RRI compared to those without AKI, and elevated RRI may have a role in identifying severe and oliguric AKI at the bedside in these patients.

Keywords: Renal resistive index, Point-of-care ultrasound, Ultrasonography, Renal Doppler, Acute kidney injury, COVID-19

Background

The Coronavirus disease 2019 (COVID-19) pandemic is causing great suffering and is placing strain on health care systems worldwide. Acute kidney injury (AKI) is a common complication in critically ill patients with COVID-19. Initial studies have reported an incidence from 20 to almost 90% among patients admitted to the

*Correspondence: marten.renberg@sll.se
[1] Department of Perioperative Medicine and Intensive Care, Karolinska University Hospital, Solna, 171 76 Stockholm, Sweden
Full list of author information is available at the end of the article

intensive care unit (ICU) or in need of mechanical ventilation [1–4], of which up to one-third have been treated with renal replacement therapy (RRT) [5, 6]. COVID-19 patients who develop AKI may have a 13-fold increased risk of death compared to those who do not develop AKI [4, 7, 8].

Renal resistive index (RRI) is an ultrasonographic Doppler measurement of flow velocities in intraparenchymal renal arteries. Normal values are around 0.60 [9, 10] with 0.70 considered the upper normal threshold in adults [11]. Elevated RRI has shown promise in early detection and prognostication of AKI in mixed ICU populations [12–16], and the method seems feasible within the scope of point-of-care ultrasonography (POCUS) [17].

As thromboembolism and renal microangiopathy have gained interest as possible mechanisms giving rise to AKI in COVID-19 [18, 19], RRI may show to be an especially helpful tool to guide diagnosis and treatment of AKI in these patients. In a recent case–control study, reduced renal perfusion and substantially elevated RRI were described in ten COVID-19 patients with severe AKI [20]. However, RRI has not been described in larger populations of COVID-19 patients and its role in these patients remains unclear. The aim of this study was to describe the pattern of RRI in relation to AKI in patients with COVID-19 treated in the ICU. We specifically investigated if there was an association between RRI and AKI diagnosis, different AKI stages and urine output.

Methods

Study population

This was an observational cohort study conducted in six ICUs designated for COVID-19 patients (COVID-ICUs) at the Karolinska University Hospital, Stockholm, Sweden. Four ICUs were at one of two sites, and two at the other site. On specific dates, patients in each COVID-ICU were screened for participation. Inclusion criteria were infection with Severe Acute Respiratory Syndrome Coronavirus 2 (SARS-CoV-2) detected by a positive reverse transcriptase-polymerase chain reaction taken from upper or lower airways, admission to a COVID-ICU, and age ≥ 18 years. Exclusion criteria were end-stage renal disease (ESRD) before ICU admission, palliative phase of intensive care, ongoing irregular cardiac rhythm or treatment with extracorporeal membrane oxygenation (ECMO).

The study complied with the Declaration of Helsinki and was approved by the Swedish Ethical Review Authority. Requirement for signed informed consent was waived. A printed information sheet was sent to each patient or next of kin with the opportunity to retrospectively withdraw participation.

Definitions

AKI was defined according to the Kidney Disease Improving Global Outcomes (KDIGO) classification as an increase in serum creatinine concentration (sCr) and categorized into three stages [21]. The highest sCr from ICU admission to the day of RRI measurement was compared to baseline sCr. Baseline sCr was defined as the last known value measured in a disease-free phase before admission. When no previous sCr value existed, hospital admission sCr was used. The AKI stages were defined as the following: stage 1, ≥ 1.5- to 1.9-fold increase or an absolute increase ≥ 26 μmol/l; stage 2, ≥ 2.0- to 2.9-fold increase; stage 3, ≥ 3.0-fold increase or an absolute increase > 354 μmol/l or initiation of RRT. The KDIGO urine output criteria were not used since hourly urine output was not always registered in the medical records. If the sCr elevation occurred more than 7 days before the RRI measurement and its value had returned to < 1.5-fold or < 26 μmol/l higher than from baseline, the patient was evaluated as having recovered from an AKI episode and was classified into the no AKI group. Oliguria at the time of RRI measurement was defined as urine output < 0.5 ml/kg ideal body weight/hour for 24 h regardless of diuretic drug administration [22]. Ideal body weight was calculated using the gender-specific Acute Respiratory Distress Syndrome Network formula [23]. Chronic kidney disease (CKD) was defined as estimated glomerular filtration rate (eGFR) < 60 mL/min/1.73 m^2, ESRD was defined as eGFR < 15 mL/min/1.73 m^2, and eGFR was calculated using the Chronic Kidney Disease Epidemiology Collaboration (CKD-EPI) equation [24]. For this, baseline sCr was used when classifying patients as having CKD or ESRD, and a combination of sCr and cystatin C was used when calculating eGFR at the time of RRI measurement. Comorbidities were considered present if documented in the patient's medical record or if the patient was prescribed medication for the current state. The cardiovascular disease group included patients with cardiac failure, atrial arrhythmia, prior myocardial infarction or prior cardiac surgery.

RRI measurements

All RRI measurements were performed by one of two operators (MR and OJ). Both operators had more than one year's clinical experience of the RRI method. For each site a designated ultrasound device with a curvilinear probe of 1.0–6.0 MHz was used (GE Vivid S70N, US and GE Logiq E10, US at the two sites, respectively). The patients were examined in their ICU bed in supine or prone position depending on their respiratory requirements. Both kidneys were examined, and measurements were made on both or the most accessible side since the difference in RRI values between the right and left kidney has been shown to be negligible both in healthy and critically ill patients [9, 12, 17]. After obtaining a complete view of the kidney, color-Doppler was applied to visualize the global organization of intrarenal blood vessels. Pulse waved Doppler at the smallest possible width between 2 and 5 mm was used to measure flow velocities in an interlobular or arcuate artery in the upper, middle and lower kidney pole. The Doppler gain was set to obtain a clear outline of flow waves with minimal background noise. The pulse waved Doppler spectrum was considered optimal when at least three consecutive similar-looking waveforms for each pole were visualized. RRI was calculated for each pole as [(peak systolic velocity–end-diastolic velocity)/peak systolic velocity]. From the pole RRI values, a mean RRI was computed.

Data collection

The following clinical data were collected for each patient at the time of RRI measurement: hemodynamic parameters, vasopressor requirements, sedatives dose and ventilator settings if mechanically ventilated. Severity of illness was graded on the day of measurement using the Sequential Organ Failure Assessment (SOFA) (originally the Sepsis-related Organ Failure Assessment) score [25]. Information on comorbidities, regular and current medication and laboratory data were collected from medical records.

Statistical analysis

Patient characteristics and variables are presented using frequencies and percentages for categorical data, and medians with interquartile range (IQR) and minimum/maximum (min/max) values for continuous data. Clinical characteristics of patients with or without AKI were compared using Fisher's exact test for dichotomous variables and Wilcoxon rank-sum test for continuous variables. Median RRI between different groups were compared using the Wilcoxon rank-sum test. To elucidate potential confounding of the association between RRI and AKI, a multivariable logistic regression model was performed including RRI as a continuous and AKI as a dichotomous variable. Variables in our dataset that were associated with AKI with a p-value < 0.2 in bivariate logistic regression were selected for a manual forward selection procedure. Variables with the strongest association with AKI were included first, and variables that no longer were associated with AKI (p-value > 0.2) during forward selection were excluded. Remaining variables constituted the final model. Odds ratios (OR) and 95% confidence intervals (CI) were calculated. Goodness-of-fit of the model was assessed using the Hosmer–Lemeshow test. For all analyses a p-value < 0.05 was considered significant. The following variables had missing data: hospital admission sCr ($n = 7$ [14%]) and urine output at the day of RRI measurement ($n = 2$ [4%]). Missing data on height ($n = 1$ [2%]) were substituted with the median value according to sex. Statistical analyses were performed using Stata version 15.1 (StataCorp, College Station, US).

Results

Between April 15 and May 15 in 2020, the six COVID-ICUs were screened on specific dates for each ICU when at least one of the operators was available and able to perform measurements. Out of 71 screened patients, 20 were excluded, and a total of 51 patients were analyzed (Fig. 1).

Patient characteristics of the study population are presented in Table 1. Median age was 63 (IQR 57–67, min/max 29/74) and 88% were male. At the time of RRI measurement 23 patients (45%) had AKI (stage 1, $n = 4$ (8%); stage 2, $n = 2$ (4%); stage 3, $n = 17$ (33%) with $n = 13$ (25%) treated with continuous RRT [CRRT]). Among the 28 patients (55%) who did not have AKI, 11 patients (22%) previously during the ICU course had an AKI episode but had recovered (recovered from stage 1, $n = 7$ (14%); from stage 2, $n = 2$ (4%); from stage 3, $n = 2$ [4%]) and 17 patients (33%) never had AKI. Compared to patients without AKI, the AKI patients had a higher body mass index (BMI) and a lower incidence of cardiovascular disease. At the time of RRI measurement, AKI patients had a higher SOFA score, a higher incidence of mechanical ventilation and vasopressor use, lower eGFR and were more often oliguric compared to patients without AKI.

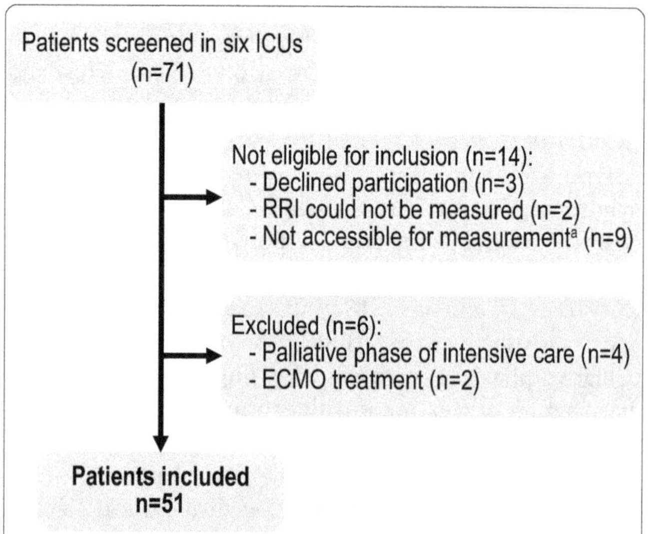

Fig. 1 Selection of the study population. ICU, intensive care unit; ECMO, extracorporeal membrane oxygenation. [a] Not accessible due to ongoing resuscitation, delirium/agitation, ongoing long period of mobilization/physiotherapy or unknown reason

Table 1 Patient characteristics of all patients and those with and without AKI

	All patients ($n=51$)	No AKI ($n=28$)	AKI ($n=23$)	p-value no AKI vs AKI
Age, median (IQR)	63 (57–67)	63 (58–68)	64 (53–65)	0.48
Sex, *n* (%)				0.027
Male	45 (88)	22 (79)	23 (100)	
Female	6 (12)	6 (21)	0 (0)	
BMI, median (IQR)	28.7 (25.2–31.2)	26.8 (24.6–29.9)	30.9 (27.0–34.7)	0.012
Risk factors for AKI, *n* (%)				
Hypertension	29 (57)	15 (54)	14 (61)	0.78
Diabetes	10 (20)	5 (18)	5 (22)	0.74
Chronic lung disease	11 (22)	7 (25)	4 (17)	0.73
Cardiovascular disease	6 (12)	6 (21)	0 (0)	0.027
Chronic kidney disease[a, c]	6 (12)	1 (4)	5 (22)	0.079
End-stage renal disease[b, c]	0 (0)			
No risk factor[d]	15 (29)	7 (25)	8 (35)	0.54
Data at RRI measurement				
ICU day, median (IQR)	18 (6–29)	16 (6–26)	19 (10–31)	0.19
SOFA score, median (IQR)	5 (4–8)	4 (3–7)	7 (5–10)	0.003
Mechanical ventilation, *n* (%)	38 (75)	17 (61)	21 (91)	0.022
Prone position, *n* (%)	9 (18)	5 (18)	4 (17)	1.00
Vasopressors, *n* (%)	26 (51)	10 (36)	16 (70)	0.025
eGFR[c], median (IQR)	58 (41–75)	70 (52–80)	26 (13–41)	< 0.001
Oliguria[e], *n* (%)	5 (24)	0 (0)	5 (24)	0.011
RRT, *n* (%)				
Continuous RRT	13 (25)	0 (0)	13 (57)	< 0.001
Intermittent HD	0 (0)			
Treatment in ICU[f], *n* (%)				
Mechanical ventilation	49 (96)	26 (93)	23 (100)	0.49
Vasopressors	49 (96)	26 (93)	23 (100)	0.49
RRT				
Continuous RRT	13 (25)	0 (0)	13 (57)	< 0.001
Intermittent HD	1 (2)	0 (0)	1 (4)	0.45
Diuretics	48 (94)	25 (89)	23 (100)	0.24
Anti-inflammatory drugs				
Corticosteroids	37 (73)	21 (75)	16 (70)	0.76
Tocilizumab	3 (6)	3 (11)	0 (0)	0.24
Antiviral drugs				
Chloroquine phosphate	1 (2)	0 (0)	1 (4)	0.45
Remdesivir	2 (4)	2 (7)	0 (0)	0.49
Anticoagulation drugs				
LMWH	51 (100)	28 (100)	23 (100)	
Antiplatelets	33 (65)	21 (75)	12 (52)	0.14
Episode of thrombolysis	4 (8)	1 (4)	3 (13)	0.32

AKI acute kidney injury, *BMI* body mass index (kg/m^2), *RRI* renal resistive index, *ICU* intensive care unit, *SOFA score* Sequential Organ Failure Assessment score, *eGFR* estimated glomerular filtration rate (ml/min/1.73 m^2), *RRT* renal replacement therapy, *HD* hemodialysis, *LMWH* low-molecular-weight heparin

[a] Chronic kidney disease was defined as eGFR before ICU admission < 60 ml/min/1.73 m^2

[b] End-stage renal disease was defined as eGFR before ICU admission < 15 ml/min/1.73 m^2

[c] eGFR was calculated using the CKD-EPI equation using serum creatinine for classification of chronic kidney disease and end-stage renal disease, and a combination of serum creatinine and cystatin C at the time of RRI measurement

[d] Patients without history of smoking, chronic diagnoses or regular medications at hospital admission

[e] Oliguria was defined as urine output < 0.5 ml/kg ideal body weight/hour for 24 h

[f] Treatment from ICU admission to RRI measurement

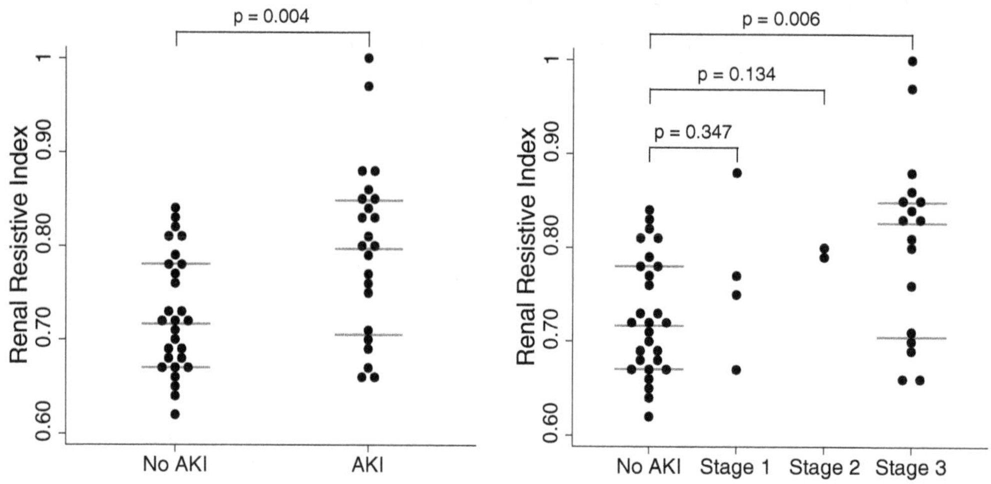

Fig. 2 Dot plot illustrating the association between renal resistive index and acute kidney injury (AKI) in patients with or without AKI (left) and patients with different stages of AKI (right). Each dot represents a patient. The horizontal lines represent the median, upper and lower quartiles

RRI was measured most often in the third week of the ICU and hospital course (median ICU day 18, IQR 6–29, min/max 0/37; median hospital day 20, IQR 10–30, min/max 2/37) and 4 weeks from symptom debut of COVID-19 (median 28, IQR 22–40, min/max 7/72). In 27 patients (53%) RRI was calculated from measurements in the right kidney, in 12 patients (23,5%) from measurements in the left kidney and in 12 patients (23,5%) from measurements in both kidneys. Forty-two patients (82%) were examined in supine and nine patients (18%) in prone position.

RRI in relation to AKI and AKI stage

Median RRI in the study population was 0.76 (IQR 0.69–0.82, min/max 0.62/1.0). One patient had completely diminished end-diastolic blood flow resulting in an RRI of 1.0. Median RRI in patients with AKI was 0.80 (IQR 0.71–0.85, min/max 0.66/1.0) compared to 0.72 (IQR 0.67–0.78, min/max 0.62/0.84) in patients without AKI ($p=0.004$) (Fig. 2). There was no difference in RRI between AKI stage 1 (median 0.76, IQR 0.71–0.83, min/max 0.67/0.88) or AKI stage 2 (median 0.79, min/max 0.79/0.80, $n=2$) compared to no AKI ($p=0.347$ and 0.134, respectively), but RRI was higher in patients with AKI stage 3 (median 0.83, IQR 0.71–0.85, min/max 0.66/1.0) compared to patients without AKI ($p=0.006$) (Fig. 2).

RRI in relation to non-AKI, recovered AKI and ongoing AKI

RRI did not differ within the no AKI group when comparing patients who never had AKI (median 0.72, IQR 0.69–0.78, min/max 0.62/0.83) to patients with recovered AKI (median 0.68, IQR 0.67–0.81, min/max 0.65/0.84) ($p=0.621$), but RRI was higher in the AKI group compared to both these groups ($p=0.015$ and 0.021, respectively) (Fig. 3).

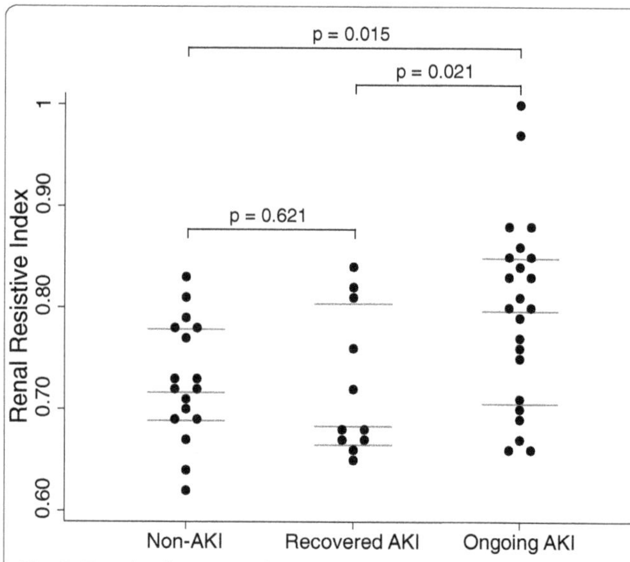

Fig. 3 Dot plot illustrating the association between renal resistive index and acute kidney injury (AKI) in patients who did not develop AKI, developed AKI but recovered, and had an ongoing AKI episode at the time of measurement. Each dot represents a patient. The horizontal lines represent the median, upper and lower quartiles

RRI in relation to oliguria

RRI was higher in oliguric patients (median 0.84, IQR 0.83–0.85, min/max 0.80/0.97) compared to non-oliguric patients (median 0.74, IQR 0.69–0.81, min/max 0.62/1.0) ($p=0.009$) (Fig. 4).

Multivariable analysis

Bivariate and multivariable logistic regression analysis is presented in Table 2. Possible confounders eligible for inclusion in the multivariable model are all variables presented in Table 1 except those that could be influenced by

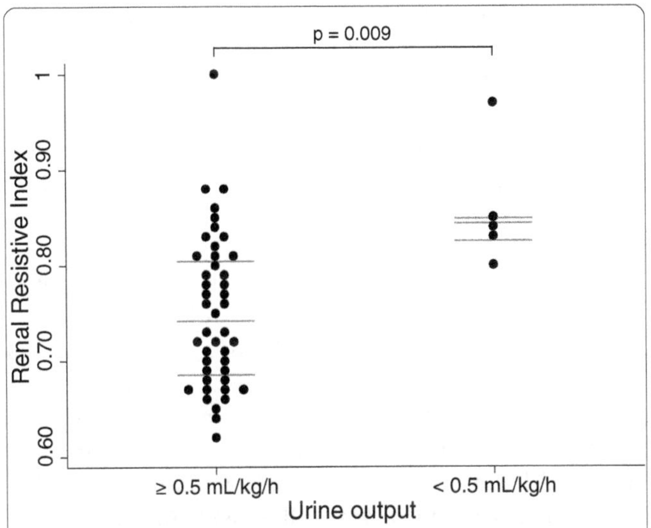

Fig. 4 Dot plot illustrating the association between renal resistive index and oliguria defined as urine output < 0.5 ml/kg ideal body weight/hour for 24 h. Each dot represents a patient. The horizontal lines represent the median, upper and lower quartiles

AKI and hence be part of a causal chain (ICU day, SOFA score, eGFR, oliguria, RRT, administration of diuretics). The following variables were omitted due to perfect prediction in the AKI groups (sex, cardiovascular disease, mechanical ventilation during ICU course, vasopressors during ICU course, tocilizumab, chloroquine phosphate, remdesivir, low-molecular-weight heparin). Variables included in the final model were RRI, BMI, CKD, vasopressors at measurement and administration of antiplatelet drugs. After multivariable adjustment, RRI was independently associated with AKI (OR for 0.01 increments of RRI 1.22, 95% CI 1.07–1.41). Goodness-of-fit had $p = 0.705$.

Discussion

This study presents novel findings of the pattern of RRI in critically ill patients with COVID-19. RRI was higher in patients with AKI compared to patients without AKI, and the difference was significant in patients with AKI stage 3 but not in patients with AKI stage 1 or 2. RRI was higher in patients with an ongoing AKI episode compared to

Table 2 Bivariate and multivariable analysis showing the association with AKI

	Bivariate analysis		Multivariable analysis[a]	
	OR (95% CI)	*p*-value	OR (95% CI)	*p*-value
RRI (0.01 unit step)	1.13 (1.04–1.23)	0.005	1.22[b] (1.07–1.41)	0.004
Age	0.97 (0.91–1.03)	0.296		
BMI	1.11 (0.99–1.23)	0.067	1.23 (1.02–1.48)	0.031
Risk factors for AKI				
Hypertension	1.35 (0.44–4.13)	0.601		
Diabetes	1.28 (0.32–5.10)	0.729		
Chronic lung disease	0.63 (0.16–2.50)	0.513		
Chronic kidney disease[c]	7.50 (0.81–70)	0.076	175 (3.72–8281)	0.009
No risk factor[d]	1.60 (0.48–5.37)	0.447		
Data at RRI measurement				
Mechanical ventilation	6.79 (1.32–35)	0.022	[f]	
Prone position	0.97 (0.23–4.12)	0.965		
Vasopressors	4.11 (1.27–13)	0.019	27 (2.68–268)	0.005
Treatment in ICU[e]				
Anti-inflammatory drugs				
Corticosteroids	0.76 (0.22–2.61)	0.666		
Anticoagulation drugs				
Antiplatelets	0.36 (0.11–1.19)	0.094	0.18 (0.03–1.17)	0.073
Episode of thrombolysis	4.05 (0.39–42)	0.241		

AKI acute kidney injury, *OR* odds ratio, *CI* confidence interval, *RRI* renal resistive index, *BMI* body mass index (kg/m^2), *ICU* intensive care unit

[a] Goodness-of-fit $p = 0.705$

[b] An increase of 0.01 in RRI increased the risk of having AKI at measurement by 22%

[c] Chronic kidney disease was defined as eGFR before ICU admission < 60 ml/min/1.73 m^2

[d] Patients without history of smoking, chronic diagnoses or regular medications at hospital admission

[e] Treatment from ICU admission to RRI measurement

[f] Variable excluded from multivariable logistic regression model during forward selection

patients who had recovered from AKI earlier during the ICU course. Oliguric patients had higher RRI compared to non-oliguric patients. The association between RRI and AKI remained significant after adjustment for possible confounding.

Our results are in line with previous studies on mixed or septic ICU patients instead designed to investigate the role of RRI to predict and prognosticate AKI [12, 13, 16, 26, 27]. These studies have suggested RRI to be able to distinguish severe or persistent AKI from no or transient AKI, with optimal cut-off values for this discrimination varying from 0.69 to 0.80. The median RRI of 0.80 in patients with AKI in our population must be considered high in comparison, but may partly be due to the large proportion of patients with AKI stage 3. This is in line with the results of a recent case–control study which presented higher RRI in ten COVID-19 patients with AKI stage 3 compared to ten patients with AKI from septic shock [20]. Notably, also patients without AKI in our study had higher RRI (median 0.72) compared to non-AKI patients in ICU populations without COVID-19 where reported values typically are lower than 0.65 [12, 14, 28]. It is not clear if elevated RRI in patients without AKI but infected with SARS-CoV-2 is specifically related to the infection itself, or if it reflects severity of illness as indicated by the long length of ICU stay as well as the high incidence of mechanical ventilation and vasopressor use in our population.

There is growing evidence of reduced renal microperfusion in patients with COVID-19-related AKI, both from contrast enhanced ultrasonographic measurements in patients with severe AKI [20] as well as from post-mortem findings of microvascular obstruction [29]. In addition, numerous studies have reported high rates of thrombotic complications in hospitalized COVID-19 patients in general [30–32], and thrombi in the renal microcirculation has been mentioned as a possible mechanism contributing to AKI in these patients [2]. Even if several renal and extrarenal factors influence the final profile of the RRI flow wave and value [33], it is conceivable that renal microcirculatory disturbances further contributed to the generally high RRI values observed in our population.

Previous studies on critically ill patients without COVID-19 have in general focused on prediction of AKI from RRI measurements performed within the first day of ICU admission [12, 14–16, 26]. However, the ability of early RRI measurements to predict short-term AKI reversibility within 3 days recently has been challenged [34, 35]. Our finding of higher RRI in COVID-19 patients with an ongoing AKI episode compared to patients who had recovered from an AKI episode earlier during the ICU course suggests that RRI values decrease with recovered renal function. This indicates that RRI also might have a role later in the ICU or hospital course, but its exact role for prediction of renal recovery or progression towards CKD while the patient still is in hospital needs to be investigated in properly designed studies. In outpatients with already established CKD, RRI $\geq$ 0.70 notably has shown to be predictive of both CKD progression [36, 37] and mortality [38].

Our finding of elevated RRI in COVID-19-related AKI indicates that RRI may have a role in the assessment of this new and unique disease. Further, RRI has shown potential as a precocious ICU monitoring tool for detecting progression of shock states [39, 40], and together with Doppler assessments of other splanchnic organs RRI can expand the bedside monitoring window for hypoperfusion in critically ill patients in general [41]. As a non-invasive and repeatable method that has been demonstrated to be fast to learn also for non-experienced sonographers [17, 42], RRI should be applicable within POCUS protocols for ICU clinicians and thereby contributing as a valuable tool in the present resource scarce times of a pandemic.

Our study has several limitations. First, our study population was small and although we were still able to adjust our analysis for a number of possible confounders, the results should therefore be interpreted with caution. The small number of patients with AKI stage 1 and 2 further makes it difficult to draw conclusions on the association between RRI and AKI in these specific subgroups. Second, due to the challenges of conducting clinical research during a pandemic, RRI measurements were performed at different time points in different patients and most of the measurements were made late in the ICU course. The Karolinska University Hospital is a tertiary referral hospital, and many patients were transferred to its ICUs from other hospitals when they had already received several days of intensive care. This meant there was a delay from ICU admission to accessibility in some of the patients, and we were therefore not able to perform early measurements to investigate the ability of RRI as an early predictor of subsequent AKI development. Third, intra- and inter-observer variability for the operators were not investigated. Our group has previously shown that RRI measurements by inexperienced sonographers were reliable, accurate and precise compared to an expert after only a brief training session [17], and both operators in our study were experienced with the RRI method. Lastly, our study was affected by some of the well-known pitfalls in AKI research. The use of hospital admission sCr as baseline level in patients in whom pre-admission sCr was missing might have resulted in an underestimation of the AKI incidence. Further, using sCr decline to define recovery from an AKI episode could in patients with muscle wasting during a prolonged ICU course lead to overestimation of renal function recovery [43]. However, we used eGFR calculations based on a combination of sCr and cystatin C at the time of RRI measurement and still observed a difference in estimated renal function between patients classified with or without AKI, suggesting any such misclassification was negligible.

Conclusion

Critically ill COVID-19 patients with AKI have higher RRI compared to those without AKI, and elevated RRI may have a role in identifying severe and oliguric AKI at the bedside in these patients. The exact role of RRI as a POCUS application for AKI assessment and monitoring of ICU patients with COVID-19 should be established in further studies.

Abbreviations

COVID-19: Coronavirus disease 2019; AKI: Acute kidney injury; ICU: Intensive care unit; RRT: Renal replacement therapy; RRI: Renal resistive index; POCUS: Point-of-care ultrasonography; COVID-ICU: Intensive care unit designated for care of COVID-19 patients; SARS-CoV-2: Severe acute respiratory syndrome coronavirus 2; ESRD: End-stage renal disease; ECMO: Extracorporeal membrane oxygenation; KDIGO: Kidney Disease Improving Global Outcomes; sCr: Serum creatinine concentration; eGFR: Estimated glomerular filtration rate; CKD-EPI: Chronic Kidney Disease Epidemiology Collaboration; CKD: Chronic kidney disease; SOFA: Sequential Organ Failure Assessment; IQR: Interquartile range; min/max: Minimum/maximum; OR: Odds ratio; CI: Confidence interval; CRRT: Continuous renal replacement therapy; BMI: Body mass index.

Acknowledgements

We would like to thank all ICU health care workers that made measurements and data collection possible with their flexibility during a stressful time.

Authors' contributions

MR, DH, MB, and CRS conceived the study. MR, OJ and NK performed the data collection. MR and DH conducted the analyses and interpretation of the data. MR drafted the manuscript. DH, MB, CRS, OJ and NK substantially revised the manuscript. DH and MB supervised the process. All authors read and approved the final manuscript.

Author details

[1] Department of Perioperative Medicine and Intensive Care, Karolinska University Hospital, Solna, 171 76 Stockholm, Sweden. [2] Department of Physiology and Pharmacology, Karolinska Institutet, Stockholm, Sweden. [3] Department of Radiology, Karolinska University Hospital, Huddinge, Stockholm, Sweden.

References

1. Yang X, Jin Y, Li R, Zhang Z, Sun R, Chen D (2020) Prevalence and impact of acute renal impairment on COVID-19: a systematic review and meta-analysis. Crit Care 24:356. https://doi.org/10.1186/s13054-020-03065-4
2. Gabarre P, Dumas G, Dupont T, Darmon M, Azoulay E, Zafrani L (2020) Acute kidney injury in critically ill patients with COVID-19. Intensive Care Med 46:1339–1348. https://doi.org/10.1007/s00134-020-06153-9
3. Hirsch JS, Ng JH, Ross DW, Sharma P, Shah HH, Barnett RL, Hazzan AD, Fishbane S, Jhaveri KD (2020) Acute kidney injury in patients hospitalized with COVID-19. Kidney Int 98:209–218. https://doi.org/10.1016/j.kint.2020.05.006
4. Hansrivijit P, Qian C, Boonpheng B, Thongprayoon C, Vallabhajosyula S, Cheungpasitporn W, Ghahramani N (2020) Incidence of acute kidney injury and its association with mortality in patients with COVID-19: a meta-analysis. J Investig Med. https://doi.org/10.1136/jim-2020-001407
5. Karagiannidis C, Mostert C, Hentschker C, Voshaar T, Malzahn J, Schillinger G, Klauber J, Janssens U, Marx G, Weber-Carstens S, Kluge S, Pfeifer M, Grabenhenrich L, Welte T, Busse R (2020) Case characteristics, resource use, and outcomes of 10 021 patients with COVID-19 admitted to 920 German hospitals: an observational study. Lancet Respir Med. https://doi.org/10.1016/s2213-2600(20)30316-7
6. Cummings MJ, Baldwin MR, Abrams D, Jacobson SD, Meyer BJ, Balough EM, Aaron JG, Claassen J, Rabbani LE, Hastie J, Hochman BR, Salazar-Schicchi J, Yip NH, Brodie D, O'Donnell MR (2020) Epidemiology, clinical course, and outcomes of critically ill adults with COVID-19 in New York City: a prospective cohort study. Lancet 395:1763–1770. https://doi.org/10.1016/s0140-6736(20)31189-2
7. Cheng Y, Luo R, Wang K, Zhang M, Wang Z, Dong L, Li J, Yao Y, Ge S, Xu G (2020) Kidney disease is associated with in-hospital death of patients with COVID-19. Kidney Int 97:829–838. https://doi.org/10.1016/j.kint.2020.03.005
8. Lim MA, Pranata R, Huang I, Yonas E, Soeroto AY, Supriyadi R (2020) Multiorgan failure with emphasis on acute kidney injury and severity of COVID-19: systematic review and meta-analysis. Can J Kidney Health Dis 7:2054358120938573. https://doi.org/10.1177/2054358120938573
9. Ponte B, Pruijm M, Ackermann D, Vuistiner P, Eisenberger U, Guessous I, Rousson V, Mohaupt MG, Alwan H, Ehret G, Pechere-Bertschi A, Paccaud F, Staessen JA, Vogt B, Burnier M, Martin PY, Bochud M (2014) Reference values and factors associated with renal resistive index in a family-based population study. Hypertension 63:136–142. https://doi.org/10.1161/hypertensionaha.113.02321
10. Keogan MT, Kliewer MA, Hertzberg BS, DeLong DM, Tupler RH, Carroll BA (1996) Renal resistive indexes: variability in Doppler US measurement in a healthy population. Radiology 199:165–169. https://doi.org/10.1148/radiology.199.1.8633141
11. Tublin ME, Bude RO, Platt JF (2003) Review. the resistive index in renal doppler sonography: where do we stand? AJR Am J Roentgenol 180:885–892. https://doi.org/10.2214/ajr.180.4.1800885
12. Haitsma Mulier JLG, Rozemeijer S, Rottgering JG, Spoelstra-de Man AME, Elbers PWG, Tuinman PR, de Waard MC, Oudemans-van Straaten HM (2018) Renal resistive index as an early predictor and discriminator of acute kidney injury in critically ill patients; a prospective observational cohort study. PLoS ONE 13:e0197967. https://doi.org/10.1371/journal.pone.0197967
13. Boddi M, Bonizzoli M, Chiostri M, Begliomini D, Molinaro A, Tadini Buoninsegni L, Gensini GF, Peris A (2016) Renal Resistive Index and mortality in critical patients with acute kidney injury. Eur J Clin Invest 46:242–251. https://doi.org/10.1111/eci.12590
14. Song J, Wu W, He Y, Lin S, Zhu D, Zhong M (2018) Value of the combination of renal resistance index and central venous pressure in the early prediction of sepsis-induced acute kidney injury. J Crit Care 45:204–208. https://doi.org/10.1016/j.jcrc.2018.03.016
15. Lerolle N, Guerot E, Faisy C, Bornstain C, Diehl JL, Fagon JY (2006) Renal failure in septic shock: predictive value of Doppler-based renal arterial resistive index. Intensive Care Med 32:1553–1559. https://doi.org/10.1007/s00134-006-0360-x
16. Garnier F, Daubin D, Larcher R, Bargnoux AS, Platon L, Brunot V, Aarab Y, Besnard N, Dupuy AM, Jung B, Cristol JP, Klouche K (2020) Reversibility of acute kidney injury in medical icu patients: predictability performance of urinary tissue inhibitor of metalloproteinase-2 x Insulin-like growth factor-binding protein 7 and renal resistive index. Crit Care Med. https://doi.org/10.1097/ccm.0000000000004218
17. Renberg M, Kilhamn N, Lund K, Hertzberg D, Rimes-Stigare C, Bell M (2020) Feasibility of renal resistive index measurements performed by an intermediate and novice sonographer in a volunteer population. Ultrasound J 12:28. https://doi.org/10.1186/s13089-020-00175-6
18. Ostermann M, Lumlertgul N, Forni LG, Hoste E (2020) What every Intensivist should know about COVID-19 associated acute kidney injury. J Crit Care 60:91–95. https://doi.org/10.1016/j.jcrc.2020.07.023
19. Batlle D, Soler MJ, Sparks MA, Hiremath S, South AM, Welling PA, Swaminathan S (2020) Acute kidney injury in COVID-19: emerging Evidence of a distinct pathophysiology. J Am Soc Nephrol 31:1380–1383. https://doi.org/10.1681/asn.2020040419
20. Watchorn J, Huang DY, Joslin J, Bramham K, Hutchings SD (2020) Critically ILL COVID-19 patients with acute kidney injury have reduced renal blood

flow and perfusion despite preserved cardiac function. Shock, A Case-Control Study Using Contrast Enhanced Ultrasound. https://doi.org/10.1097/shk.0000000000001659
21. Kidney Disease: Improving Global Outcomes (KDIGO) Acute Kidney Injury Work Group. KDIGO Clinical Practice Guideline for Acute Kidney Injury (2012). Kidney inter, Suppl:1–138
22. Fliser D, Laville M, Covic A, Fouque D, Vanholder R, Juillard L, Van Biesen W (2012) A european renal best practice (ERBP) position statement on the Kidney Disease Improving Global Outcomes (KDIGO) clinical practice guidelines on acute kidney injury: part 1: definitions, conservative management and contrast-induced nephropathy. Nephrol Dial Transplant 27:4263–4272. https://doi.org/10.1093/ndt/gfs375
23. Brower RG, Matthay MA, Morris A, Schoenfeld D, Thompson BT, Wheeler A (2000) Ventilation with lower tidal volumes as compared with traditional tidal volumes for acute lung injury and the acute respiratory distress syndrome. N Engl J Med 342:1301–1308. https://doi.org/10.1056/nejm200005043421801
24. Levey AS, Stevens LA, Schmid CH, Zhang YL, Castro AF 3rd, Feldman HI, Kusek JW, Eggers P, Van Lente F, Greene T, Coresh J (2009) A new equation to estimate glomerular filtration rate. Ann Intern Med 150:604–612. https://doi.org/10.7326/0003-4819-150-9-200905050-00006
25. Vincent JL, Moreno R, Takala J, Willatts S, De Mendonça A, Bruining H, Reinhart CK, Suter PM, Thijs LG (1996) The SOFA (Sepsis-related Organ Failure Assessment) score to describe organ dysfunction/failure. On behalf of the working group on sepsis-related problems of the european society of intensive care medicine. Intensive Care Med 22:707–710. https://doi.org/10.1007/bf01709751
26. Schnell D, Deruddre S, Harrois A, Pottecher J, Cosson C, Adoui N, Benhamou D, Vicaut E, Azoulay E, Duranteau J (2012) Renal resistive index better predicts the occurrence of acute kidney injury than cystatin C. Shock 38:592–597. https://doi.org/10.1097/SHK.0b013e318271a39c
27. Darmon M, Schortgen F, Vargas F, Liazydi A, Schlemmer B, Brun-Buisson C, Brochard L (2011) Diagnostic accuracy of Doppler renal resistive index for reversibility of acute kidney injury in critically ill patients. Intensive Care Med 37:68–76. https://doi.org/10.1007/s00134-010-2050-y
28. Oliveira RAG, Mendes PV, Park M, Taniguchi LU (2019) Factors associated with renal Doppler resistive index in critically ill patients: a prospective cohort study. Ann Intensive Care 9:23. https://doi.org/10.1186/s13613-019-0500-4
29. Su H, Yang M, Wan C, Yi LX, Tang F, Zhu HY, Yi F, Yang HC, Fogo AB, Nie X, Zhang C (2020) Renal histopathological analysis of 26 postmortem findings of patients with COVID-19 in China. Kidney Int 98:219–227. https://doi.org/10.1016/j.kint.2020.04.003
30. Helms J, Tacquard C, Severac F, Leonard-Lorant I, Ohana M, Delabranche X, Merdji H, Clere-Jehl R, Schenck M, Fagot Gandet F, Fafi-Kremer S, Castelain V, Schneider F, Grunebaum L, Anglés-Cano E, Sattler L, Mertes PM, Meziani F (2020) High risk of thrombosis in patients with severe SARS-CoV-2 infection: a multicenter prospective cohort study. Intensive Care Med 46:1089–1098. https://doi.org/10.1007/s00134-020-06062-x
31. Klok FA, Kruip M, van der Meer NJM, Arbous MS, Gommers D, Kant KM, Kaptein FHJ, van Paassen J, Stals MAM, Huisman MV, Endeman H (2020) Confirmation of the high cumulative incidence of thrombotic complications in critically ill ICU patients with COVID-19: An updated analysis. Thromb Res 191:148–150. https://doi.org/10.1016/j.thromres.2020.04.041
32. Bilaloglu S, Aphinyanaphongs Y, Jones S, Iturrate E, Hochman J, Berger JS (2020) Thrombosis in hospitalized patients with COVID-19 in a New York City health system. JAMA. https://doi.org/10.1001/jama.2020.13372
33. Di Nicolo P, Granata A (2019) Renal intraparenchymal resistive index: the ultrasonographic answer to many clinical questions. J Nephrol 32:527–538. https://doi.org/10.1007/s40620-018-00567-x
34. Darmon M, Bourmaud A, Reynaud M, Rouleau S, Meziani F, Boivin A, Benyamina M, Vincent F, Lautrette A, Leroy C, Cohen Y, Legrand M, Morel J, Terreaux J, Schnell D (2018) Performance of Doppler-based resistive index and semi-quantitative renal perfusion in predicting persistent AKI: results of a prospective multicenter study. Intensive Care Med 44:1904–1913. https://doi.org/10.1007/s00134-018-5386-3
35. Wiersema R, Kaufmann T, van der Veen HN, de Haas RJ, Franssen CFM, Koeze J, van der Horst ICC, Keus F (2020) Diagnostic accuracy of arterial and venous renal Doppler assessment for acute kidney injury in critically ill patients: a prospective study. J Crit Care 59:57–62. https://doi.org/10.1016/j.jcrc.2020.05.012
36. Sugiura T, Wada A (2011) Resistive index predicts renal prognosis in chronic kidney disease: results of a 4-year follow-up. Clin Exp Nephrol 15:114–120. https://doi.org/10.1007/s10157-010-0371-3
37. Parolini C, Noce A, Staffolani E, Giarrizzo GF, Costanzi S, Splendiani G (2009) Renal resistive index and long-term outcome in chronic nephropathies. Radiology 252:888–896. https://doi.org/10.1148/radiol.2523080351
38. Toledo C, Thomas G, Schold JD, Arrigain S, Gornik HL, Nally JV, Navaneethan SD (2015) Renal resistive index and mortality in chronic kidney disease. Hypertension 66:382–388. https://doi.org/10.1161/hypertensionaha.115.05536
39. Corradi F, Brusasco C, Vezzani A, Palermo S, Altomonte F, Moscatelli P, Pelosi P (2011) Hemorrhagic shock in polytrauma patients: early detection with renal Doppler resistive index measurements. Radiology 260:112–118. https://doi.org/10.1148/radiol.11102338
40. Anile A, Ferrario S, Campanello L, Orban MA, Castiglione G (2019) Renal resistive index: a new reversible tool for the early diagnosis and evaluation of organ perfusion in critically ill patients: a case report. Ultrasound J 11:23. https://doi.org/10.1186/s13089-019-0138-3
41. Corradi F, Via G, Tavazzi G (2020) What's new in ultrasound-based assessment of organ perfusion in the critically ill: expanding the bedside clinical monitoring window for hypoperfusion in shock. Intensive Care Med 46:775–779. https://doi.org/10.1007/s00134-019-05791-y
42. Schnell D, Reynaud M, Venot M, Le Maho AL, Dinic M, Baulieu M, Ducos G, Terreaux J, Zeni F, Azoulay E, Meziani F, Duranteau J, Darmon M (2014) Resistive Index or color-Doppler semi-quantitative evaluation of renal perfusion by inexperienced physicians: results of a pilot study. Minerva Anestesiol 80:1273–1281
43. Ravn B, Rimes-Stigare C, Bell M, Hansson M, Hansson LO, Martling CR, Larsson A, Mårtensson J (2019) Creatinine versus cystatin C based glomerular filtration rate in critically ill patients. J Crit Care 52:136–140. https://doi.org/10.1016/j.jcrc.2019.04.007

22

Resuscitative transesophageal echocardiography in the diagnosis of post-CABG loculated pericardial clot causing cardiac tamponade

Osman Adi[1*], Azma Haryaty Ahmad[1], Chan Pei Fong[1], Asri Ranga[2] and Nova Panebianco[3]

Abstract

Background: Pericardial effusion is a known complication of post-open cardiac surgery which can progress to life-threatening cardiac tamponade. Classical signs of tamponade such as hypotension and pulsus paradoxus are often absent. Diagnosing acute cardiac tamponade with transthoracic echocardiography (TTE) can be challenging in post-cardiac surgical patients due to distorted anatomy and limited scanning windows by the presence of surgical dressings or scar. Additionally, this patient population is more likely to have a loculated pericardial effusion, or an effusion that is isoechoic in appearance secondary to clotted blood. These findings can be challenging to visualize with traditional TTE. Missed diagnosis of cardiac tamponade due to loculated pericardial clot can result in delayed diagnosis and clinical management.

Case presentation: We report a case series that illustrates the diagnostic challenge and value of resuscitative transesophageal echocardiography (TEE) in the emergency department (ED) for the diagnosis of cardiac tamponade due to posterior loculated pericardial clot in post-surgical coronary artery bypass graft (CABG) patients.

Conclusions: Cardiac tamponade due to loculated posterior pericardial clot post-CABG requires prompt diagnosis and appropriate management to avoid the potential for hemodynamic instability. Transesophageal echocardiography allows a rapid diagnosis, early appropriate referral and an opportunity to institute appropriate therapeutic measures.

Keywords: Resuscitative transesophageal echocardiography, Post-CABG posterior pericardial clot, Cardiac tamponade

Background

Pericardial effusion is a known complication of open cardiac surgery with 1–3% of patients needing intervention [1–3]. Postoperative pericardial effusion secondary to bleeding into the pericardial sac is commonly identified prior to hospital discharge [1]. Delayed pericardial effusion can arise within a week to 6 months post-cardiac surgery [4, 5]. The progression of this collection as a cause of life-threatening cardiac tamponade can be overlooked because of atypical symptoms and absence of classical echocardiography changes [5–7].

Late-onset pericardial effusion is commonly related to post-pericardiotomy syndrome due to inflammation of the pericardium after a cardiac procedure [8]. Loculated effusions are more common in this patient population because of pericardial adhesions or scarring associated with surgery [6, 9]. Inflammation or bleeding may lead to fluid accumulation at the posterior and lateral part of the pericardium, making it difficult to visualize with

*Correspondence: osman.adi@gmail.com
[1] Resuscitation & Emergency Critical Care Unit, Department of Emergency and Trauma, Raja Permaisuri Bainun Hospital, Jalan Raja Ashman (Jalan Hospital), 30400 Ipoh, Perak, Malaysia
Full list of author information is available at the end of the article

transthoracic echocardiogram (TTE) [10, 11]. Transthoracic echocardiogram has been identified as a sensitive modality to evaluate the heart for complications after cardiac surgery [12].

In recent years, the usage of TEE has escalated in the emergency department (ED) and critical care, and this trend is well documented in the literature [13–22]. Focused or resuscitative TEE are terms used to describe the usage of limited TEE views to facilitate early recognition of pathologic processes and to guide clinical decision-making in critically ill patients [13–15]. In contrast to the 20-view conventional TEE in a standard cardiology exam, focused TEE utilizes five important views which are the mid-esophageal four-chamber, mid-esophageal long axis, transgastric short axis, bicaval view, and descending thoracic aorta long axis [16, 17]. Focused TEE in the ED is beneficial in the management of cardiac arrest [17, 18] undifferentiated shock [19] and trauma [20, 21]. The use of TEE by non-cardiologists in the ED and intensive care setting for critically ill patients is safe [22] and extremely useful in resource-limited setting [23]. However, focused TEE does not replace the need for comprehensive TEE when clinical questions exceed the scope of a limited exam.

In this case series, we describe the role of resuscitative TEE in managing patients with loculated cardiac tamponade post-coronary artery bypass grafting (CABG) surgery.

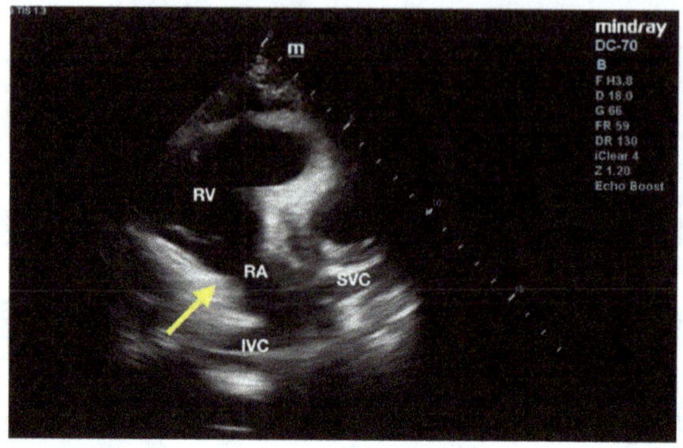

Fig. 1 Transthoracic echocardiogram (TTE) of right ventricle inflow view showed a small and compressed right atrium (yellow arrow). Posterior pericardial clot is not well visualized in this view. *IVC* inferior vena cava, *RA* right atrium, *RV* right ventricle, *SVC* superior vena cava

Case 1

A 52-year-old male patient presented to the ED with dizziness and breathlessness. He was recently discharged after an on-pump CABG for triple vessel disease. His post-operative recovery was uneventful, and his hospital length of stay was 10 days. On representation to the ED, he was in shock with blood pressure (BP) of 84/45 mmHg, afebrile and pulse rate (PR) of 98 beats per minute with no pulsus paradoxus. He was tachypneic with a respiratory rate (RR) of 24 breaths per minute and oxygen spirometry (SpO_2) 97% on room air. On examination, his jugular venous pressure was not elevated. His sternotomy scar was clean and not inflamed. His cardiorespiratory and abdominal examinations were unremarkable. There was no neurological deficit. Echocardiogram showed sinus rhythm without any ischemic changes. Chest X-ray showed cardiomegaly with clear lung fields. His arterial blood gas showed good gas exchange with no metabolic acidosis. The hemoglobin level was 11 g/dL and his coagulation profile was normal. The renal and liver function tests did not show any abnormalities.

The bedside TTE of right ventricle (RV) inflow view showed compression of the right atrium (RA) by a pericardial clot (Fig. 1, Additional file 1: Video S1). Given the TTE findings, TEE was performed by the attending emergency physician and revealed a localized posterior clot measuring 3×5 cm compressing the right atrium (Figs. 2, 3, Additional file 2: Video S2, Additional file 3: Video S3 and Additional file 4: Video S4). He was started on intravenous infusion of noradrenaline 0.3 mcg/kg/min for blood pressure support. The patient was diagnosed with possible cardiac tamponade due to loculated posterior pericardial clot and transferred to his previous managing cardiothoracic surgery team which was 200 km away for definitive surgical intervention after cardiology consultation. He made a complete recovery and was discharged after a week.

Case 2

A 62-year-old obese diabetic male patient presented to the ED complaining of dizziness and syncope 11 days after an on-pump CABG procedure for left main stem disease. On examination, he was drowsy and tachypneic. He was ill appearing with a BP of 75/42 mmHg, PR 88 beats per minute, without pulsus paradoxus, RR 30 breaths per minute and SpO_2 85% on room air. He had a short neck and his neck veins were not prominent. His midline chest wound was well healed. Lung examination showed decreased air entry at the bases. Physical examination of his other systems was unremarkable. Echocardiogram revealed a sinus rhythm without any acute ischemic changes. Cardiomegaly on chest X-ray revealed bilateral basal atelectasis. The patient was intubated for respiratory distress and hemodynamics stabilized with intravenous noradrenaline 0.2 mcg/kg/min. His arterial blood gas showed pH 7.30, PO_2 90 mmHg, PCO_2 57 mmHg, HCO_3 37 mmol/L, and BE 10 mmol/L under a low setting synchronized intermittent mandatory ventilation (SIMV) mode. His complete blood count was normal with hemoglobin of 14 g/dL, white blood count 10

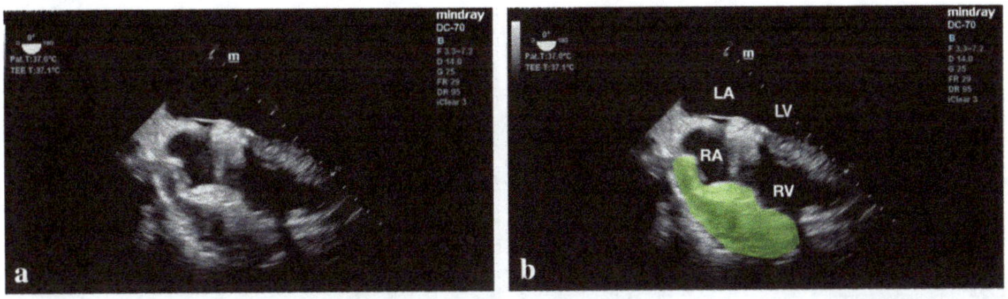

Fig. 2 **a, b** Transesophageal echocardiogram (TEE) at mid-esophageal 4-chamber view with probe rotating to the right showed a compressed right atrium and a posterior pericardial clot measuring about 2 × 5 cm (green watermark). *LA* left atrium, *LV* left ventricle, *RA* right atrium, *RV* right ventricle

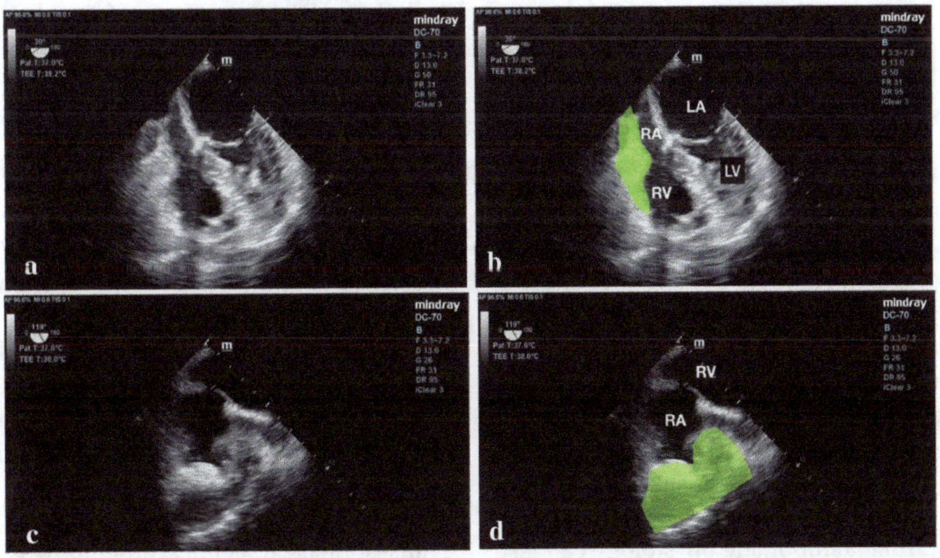

Fig. 3 **a, b** Transesophageal echocardiogram (TEE) mid-esophageal 4-chamber view showed a compressed right atrium and posterior pericardial clot (green watermark). **c, d** TEE bicaval view showed similar findings with right atrium compression by an extrinsic posterior pericardial clot (green watermark). *LA* left atrium, *LV* left ventricle, *RA* right atrium, *RV* right ventricle

X 10^9/L and platelet count of 160×10^9/L. Apart from a mildly raised glucose of 14 mmol/L and a baseline raised creatinine of 120 umol/L, his other blood profile values were within a normal range.

Bedside TTE images were suboptimal except for the subcostal view which showed good bi-ventricular systolic function with trace pericardial effusion (< 1 cm). Other structures could not be evaluated with TTE due to the poor echo window.

Transesophageal echocardiography was performed in ED by attending emergency physician and revealed a large clot localized in the posterior pericardial cavity around the right atrium at the base of the heart (Fig. 4, Additional file 5: Video S5). The clot partially obliterated the right atrium during diastole causing tamponade physiology. The TEE findings were conveyed to an in-house cardiologist. The patient was readmitted to the cardiothoracic surgery for surgical drainage and he made an uneventful recovery.

Discussion

There are several conditions that can cause hemodynamic instability in post-cardiac surgery patients, with their own unique treatment pathways. These conditions include failed graft, sepsis, bleeding, pulmonary embolism, tamponade and cardiac arrhythmias. Therefore, rapid stabilization and diagnosis are crucial for life-saving interventions to be performed. However, assessment of these undifferentiated post-cardiac surgery patients is challenging due to non-specific symptoms and signs as in the cases described earlier.

In the pathophysiology of cardiac tamponade of any cause, increased intrapericardial pressure exceeds the intracardiac pressure causing compression of the

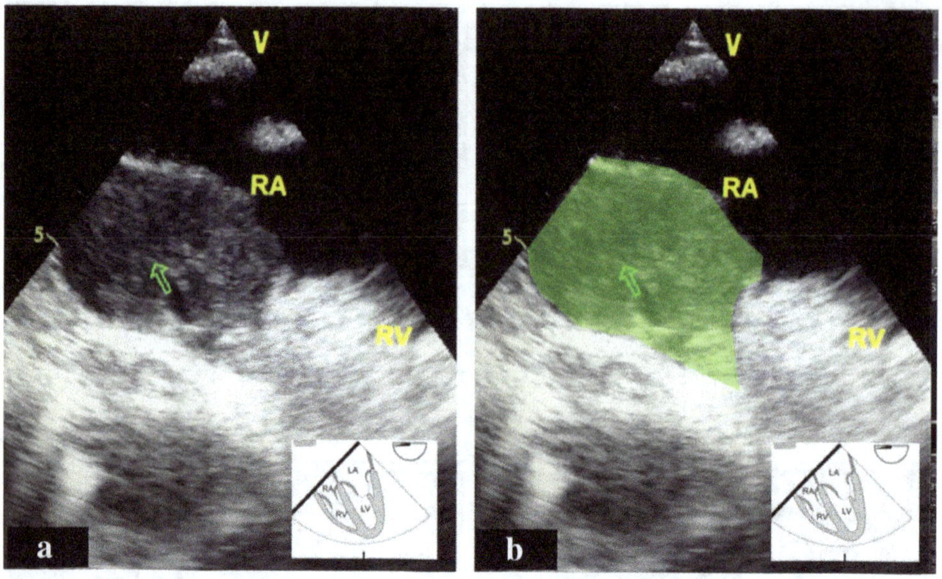

Fig. 4 a, b Transesophageal echocardiogram (TEE) at mid-esophageal 4-chamber view with probe rotating to the right showed a compressed right atrium and a posterior pericardial clot measuring (green watermark). *RA* right atrium, *RV* right ventricle

adjacent cardiac chamber [24]. Pericardial effusion after cardiac surgery may be loculated due to a pericardial adhesion that may lead to selective chamber compression [5]. Constant high left ventricular pressure in the isolated right-sided chamber compression may explain the absence of classical signs of cardiac tamponade such as pulsus paradoxus, transmitral and transtricuspid flow variability [25].

Low-pressure cardiac tamponade physiology can also occur in post-cardiac surgery patients. This is due to medication-induced reduction in filling pressures by the use of diuresis and vasodilators [24]. The suppression of the compensatory sympathetic stimulation by beta-blockers may also contribute to the atypical presentation of these patients.

Both our patients presented more than a week after CABG. Apart from the obvious signs of shock, clinical examination, conventional bedside tests such as electrocardiogram and chest X-ray did not give much clue to the cause of hypotension. Point-of-care ultrasound was used to assess the volume status, determine heart function and exclude the life-threatening diagnosis.

In the first case, the TTE image was inconclusive and showed a small right atrium with posterior hyperechoic structure suggestive of compression from the extracardiac source. With this finding, a high index of suspicion that a localized pericardial effusion was present prompted the decision to proceed with TEE. In the second case, the patient was immediately intubated and stabilized with inotropic support upon arrival at the ED.

Cardiac tamponade is a complication of post-cardiac surgery that may be difficult to assess using TTE [11, 12]. Identifying loculated pericardial effusions and clotted blood in the pericardium can be challenging [12]. Typical ultrasound features found in usual cardiac tamponade cases such as right atrial systolic collapse, right ventricular diastolic collapse, swinging heart and plethoric inferior vena cava may be absent. Transesophageal echocardiography is not limited by chest wall-related barriers and may provide life-saving diagnostic information in this patient cohort.

Conclusion

Cardiac tamponade secondary to loculated posterior pericardial clot is a life-threatening cause of hemodynamic instability in the post-CABG patient. Transesophageal echocardiography may be of limited utility because of patient-level post-surgical variables. Transesophageal echocardiography performed in the ED can allow for a rapid diagnosis, an early referral and an opportunity to institute appropriate therapeutic measures in this challenging patient population.

Abbreviations

BP: Blood pressure; CABG: Coronary artery bypass graft; CT: Computed tomography; ECG: Echocardiogram; ED: Emergency department; Fig.: Figure; FiO_2: Fraction of inspired oxygen; PEEP: Positive end expiratory pressure; PR: Pulse rate; RA: Right atrium; RR: Respiratory rate; RV: Right ventricle; SpO_2: Oxygen spirometry; Supp: Supplementary; TEE: Transesophageal echocardiography; TTE: Transthoracic echocardiography; TV: Tidal volume.

Supplementary Information

Additional file 1: Video S1. Transesophageal echocardiogram (TEE) of right ventricle inflow view showed a small and compressed right atrium. Posterior pericardial clot is not well visualized in this view. IVC: inferior vena cava, RA: right atrium, RV: right ventricle, SVC: superior vena cava.

Additional file 2: Video S2. Transesophageal echocardiogram (TEE) at mid-esophageal 4-chamber view with probe rotating to the right showed a compressed right atrium and a posterior pericardial clot measuring, about 2 × 5 cm (green watermark). LA: left atrium, LV: left ventricle, RA: right atrium, RV: right ventricle.

Additional file 3: Video S3. Transesophageal echocardiogram bicaval view showed right atrium compression by an extrinsic posterior pericardial clot (green watermark). LA: left atrium, LV: left ventricle, RA: right atrium, RV: right ventricle.

Additional file 4: Video S4. Transesophageal echocardiogram mid-esophageal 4-chamber view showed a compressed right atrium and posterior pericardial clot (green watermark).

Additional file 5: Video S5. Transesophageal echocardiogram (TEE) at mid-esophageal 4-chamber view with probe rotating to the right showed a compressed right atrium and a posterior pericardial clot (green watermark). RA: right atrium, RV: right ventricle.

Acknowledgements
We would like to thank Miss Anne John Michael and Ipoh Emergency Critical Care Society (IECCS) for their assistance.

Authors' contributions
OA and NP were involved in the initial conception and drafting of the manuscript. All authors contributed to image interpretation, as well as the writing, revision, and approval of the manuscript. All authors read and approved the final manuscript.

Author details
[1] Resuscitation & Emergency Critical Care Unit, Department of Emergency and Trauma, Raja Permaisuri Bainun Hospital, Jalan Raja Ashman (Jalan Hospital), 30400 Ipoh, Perak, Malaysia. [2] Department of Cardiology, Hospital Serdang, Serdang, Selangor, Malaysia. [3] Division of Emergency Ultrasound, Department of Emergency Medicine, Hospital of the University of Pennsylvania, 3400 Spruce St, Philadelphia, PA 19104, USA.

References

1. Nguyen HS, Nguyen HD, Vu TD (2018) Pericardial effusion following cardiac surgery. A single-center experience. Asian Cardiovasc Thorac Ann 26(1):5–10. https://doi.org/10.1177/0218492317744902
2. Kuvin JT, Harati NA, Pandian NG, Bojar RM, Khabbaz KR (2002) Postoperative cardiac tamponade in the modern surgical era. Ann Thorac Surg 74(4):1148–1153. https://doi.org/10.1016/s0003-4975(02)03837-7
3. Ashikhmina EA, Schaff HV, Sinak LJ, Li Z, Dearani JA, Suri RM, Park SJ, Orszulak TA, Sundt TM 3rd (2010) Pericardial effusion after cardiac surgery: risk factors, patient profiles, and contemporary management. Ann Thorac Surg 89(1):112–118. https://doi.org/10.1016/j.athoracsur.2009.09.026
4. Khan NK, Järvelä KM, Loisa EL, Sutinen JA, Laurikka JO, Khan JA (2017) Incidence, presentation and risk factors of late postoperative pericardial effusions requiring invasive treatment after cardiac surgery. Interact Cardiovasc Thorac Surg 24(6):835–840. https://doi.org/10.1093/icvts/ivx011
5. Russo AM, O'Connor WH, Waxman HL (1993) Atypical presentations and echocardiographic findings in patients with cardiac tamponade occurring early and late after cardiac surgery. Chest 104(1):71–78. https://doi.org/10.1378/chest.104.1.71
6. Chuttani K, Tischler MD, Pandian NG, Lee RT, Mohanty PK (1994) Diagnosis of cardiac tamponade after cardiac surgery: relative value of clinical, echocardiographic, and hemodynamic signs. Am Heart J 127(4 Pt 1):913–918. https://doi.org/10.1016/0002-8703(94)90561-4
7. Price S, Prout J, Jaggar SI, Gibson DG, Pepper JR (2004) "Tamponade" following cardiac surgery: terminology and echocardiography may both mislead. Eur J Cardiothorac Surg 26(6):1156–1160. https://doi.org/10.1016/j.ejcts.2004.08.020
8. Gabaldo K, Sutlić Ž, Miškovic D, Knežević Pravеček M, Prvulović Đ, Vujeva B, Cvitkušic Lukenda K, Hadžibegović I (2019) Postpericardiotomy syndrome incidence, diagnostic and treatment strategies: experience AT two collaborative centers. Acta Clin Croat 58(1):57–62. https://doi.org/10.20471/acc.2019.58.01.08
9. Imazio M, Adler Y (2013) Management of pericardial effusion. Eur Heart J 34(16):1186–1197. https://doi.org/10.1093/eurheartj/ehs372
10. Pepi M, Muratori M, Barbier P, Doria E, Arena V, Berti M, Celeste F, Guazzi M, Tamborini G (1994) Pericardial effusion after cardiac surgery: incidence, site, size, and haemodynamic consequences. Br Heart J 72(4):327–331. https://doi.org/10.1136/hrt.72.4.327
11. Ionescu A, Wilde P, Karsch KR (2001) Localized pericardial tamponade: difficult echocardiographic diagnosis of a rare complication after cardiac surgery. J Am Soc Echocardiogr 14(12):1220–1223. https://doi.org/10.1067/mje.2001.115620
12. Imren Y, Tasoglu I, Oktar GL et al (2008) The importance of transesophageal echocardiography in diagnosis of pericardial tamponade after cardiac surgery. J Card Surg 23(5):450–453. https://doi.org/10.1111/j.1540-8191.2008.00581.x
13. Arntfield R (2019) Lifesaving applications of transesophageal echocardiography in critical and emergency care. ICU Management & Practice 3. https://www.sonosite.com/sites/default/files/Life%20Saving%20Applications%20of%20TEE%20in%20Critical%20and%20Emergency%20Care%2C%20November%202019.pdf. Accessed 9 Mar 2021.
14. O'Neil M, Nagdev A, Teran F (2020) How to perform resuscitative transesophageal echocardiography in the emergency department. ACEP Now, Vol 39-No 07. https://www.intelligentultrasound.com/content/uploads/2020/09/How-to-Perform-Resuscitative-Transesophageal-Echocardiography-in-the-Emergency-Department-ACEP-Now.pdf. Accessed 9 Mar 2021.
15. Heiberg J, El-Ansary D, Royse CF, Royse AG, Alsaddique AA, Canty DJ (2016) Transthoracic and transoesophageal echocardiography: a systematic review of feasibility and impact on diagnosis, management and outcome after cardiac surgery. Anaesthesia 71(10):1210–1221. https://doi.org/10.1111/anae.13545 (**Epub 2016 Jun 25**)
16. Arntfield R, Pace J, McLeod S, Granton J, Hegazy A, Lingard L (2015) Focused transesophageal echocardiography for emergency physicians-description and results from simulation training of a structured four-view examination. Crit Ultrasound J 7(1):27. https://doi.org/10.1186/s13089-015-0027-3 (**Epub 2015 Jun 12**)
17. Fair J, Mallin M, Mallemat H, Zimmerman J, Arntfield R, Kessler R, Bailitz J, Blaivas M (2018) Transesophageal echocardiography: guidelines for point-of-care applications in cardiac arrest resuscitation. Ann Emerg Med 71(2):201–207. https://doi.org/10.1016/j.annemergmed.2017.09.003
18. Teran F, Dean AJ, Centeno C, Panebianco NL, Zeidan AJ, Chan W, Abella BS (2019) Evaluation of out-of-hospital cardiac arrest using transesophageal echocardiography in the emergency department. Resuscitation 137:140–147. https://doi.org/10.1016/j.resuscitation.2019.02.013
19. Arntfield R, Pace J, Hewak M, Thompson D (2016) Focused transesophageal echocardiography by emergency physicians is feasible and clinically influential: Observational results from a novel ultrasound program. J Emerg Med 50(2):286–294. https://doi.org/10.1016/j.jemermed.2015.09.018 (**Epub 2015 Oct 24**)
20. Leichtle SW, Singleton A, Singh M, Griffee MJ, Tobin JM (2017) Transesophageal echocardiography in the evaluation of the trauma patient: A trauma resuscitation transesophageal echocardiography exam. J Crit Care 40:202–206. https://doi.org/10.1016/j.jcrc.2017.04.007
21. Osman A, Fong CP, Wahab SFA, Panebianco N, Teran F (2020) Transesophageal echocardiography at the golden hour: identification of blunt traumatic aortic injuries in the Emergency Department. J Emerg Med 59(3):418–423. https://doi.org/10.1016/j.jemermed.2020.05.003
22. Wray TC, Schmid K, Braude D, Azevedo K, Dettmer T, Tawil I, Boivin M, Marinaro J (2021) Safety of transesophageal echocardiography performed by intensivists and emergency physicians in critically ill patients with coagulopathy and thrombocytopenia: a single-center experience. J Intensive Care Med 36(1):123–130. https://doi.org/10.1177/0885066619887693

23. Raiten J, Ahmed N, Amatya A, Sharma A, Acharya S, Lanahan J, Werlhof H, Ko HA, Tsui C, Reza T, Bajracharya S, Hagen O, Shrestha G (2020) Perioperative point-of-care ultrasound and transesophageal echocardiography in resource-limited settings-a focus on Nepal and Bangladesh. J Cardiothorac Vasc Anesth 34(10):2604–2610. https://doi.org/10.1053/j.jvca.2020.06.017
24. Carmona P, Mateo E, Casanovas I, Peña JJ, Llagunes J, Aguar F, De Andrés J, Errando C (2012) Management of cardiac tamponade after cardiac surgery. J Cardiothorac Vasc Anesth 26(2):302–311. https://doi.org/10.1053/j.jvca.2011.06.007
25. Reddy PS, Curtiss EI, O'Toole JD, Shaver JA (1978) Cardiac tamponade: hemodynamic observations in man. Circulation 58(2):265–272. https://doi.org/10.1161/01.cir.58.2.265

"Sigmoid diverticulitis mimicking cholecystitis" a clinical challenge

Ilaria Pulzato[1*], Enrico Boero[2], Elona Shaipi[3] and Luciano Cardinale[3]

Abstract

Diverticular disease is a common disorder and its incidence increases with ageing. Pathophysiology is multifactorial. Lifestyle, including smoking, alcohol intake, decreased dietary fibres and lack of physical activity, plays a predominant role. Genetics seems also to contribute specifically for right-sided diverticular disease (RSD). The majority of the patients with diverticular disease are asymptomatic. Diverticulitis is the inflammation of the diverticula usually presenting with abdominal pain associated to nausea, vomiting, rectal bleeding, diarrhoea and fever. When the inflammation process affects the diverticula in the ascending colon, the condition represents a clinical challenge as it can be easily misdiagnosed with other acute abdominal emergencies. We reported a case of a 70-year-old female who presented to our Emergency Department (ED) with right upper quadrant pain and an initial clinical suspicion of cholecystitis. Ultrasound (US) and Computed Tomography (CT) demonstrated an anatomical variation of the sigmoid colon diverticulitis. This clinical report demonstrates that ultrasound plays a relevant part as first-step approach to the acute abdominal conditions and its accuracy increases together with other diagnostic tools such as Computer Tomography.

Keywords: Diverticulitis, Ultrasound, Computed Tomography, Colon embryologic abnormalities

Background

Diverticular disease is a common disorder affecting almost 50% of the population over 60 years. Its incidence increases with ageing, reaching up to 80% in the population older than 80 years [1]. Diverticula consist of outpouching from the large intestine wall, occurring mainly in the sigmoid colon. Pathophysiology of diverticulosis is not yet completely understood. Many factors such as colonic hypermobility, micro oral content and visceral hypersensitivity are involved in its development. Lifestyle, including smoking and alcohol intake, decreased dietary fibres and lack of physical activity, plays a predominant role [2]. Genetics seems to be involved specifically in the right-sided diverticular disease (RSD), which has an incidence of approximately 8.5% in the Western and 40% in the Eastern population [3]. Up to 90% of the patients with diverticular disease are asymptomatic. Few of them can develop large intestine carcinoma, whereas solitary diverticulum of the caecum may occur as a congenital lesion [3].

Diverticulitis is the inflammation of the diverticula, which can lead to complications such as abscess or perforation. Presenting symptoms are usually pain, nausea, vomiting, rectal bleeding, diarrhoea and fever. When the inflammation process affects the diverticula in the right-sided large intestine, it becomes a clinical challenge, as it can be easily misdiagnosed with other acute abdominal emergencies, such as appendicitis, cholecystitis, appendagitis [4].

The distinction between these acute abdominal conditions is relevant for the prognosis, as RSD is treated conservatively, and abscess formation is rare.

Case presentation

A 70-year-old female presented to our ED with right upper quadrant abdominal pain of 1-day duration described as sharp in nature, which started suddenly and became constant over time. No nausea, vomiting, melena, hematochezia or hematemesis were reported.

*Correspondence: ilaria.pulzato@gmail.com
[1] Dipartimento di Medicina interna e Specialità mediche, Di.M.I. Università degli Studi di Geniva, Viale Benedetto XV, 10, 16132 Genoa, GE, Italy
Full list of author information is available at the end of the article

The patient's past medical history was irrelevant; she also had no family history of inflammatory bowel disease or gastrointestinal malignancies. Physical examination was unremarkable, apart from right superior quadrant tenderness with localised guarding. Vital parameters were within the normal range. Blood tests results showed elevated white blood cell count (14,500 per microlitre with 79.2% neutrophils), while electrolytes and pancreas function were within the limits.

Management and outcome

In the broad spectrum of differential diagnosis, gallbladder disease, appendicitis, peptic disease and pancreatitis were considered. According to symptom presentation and hospital policy, an abdominal ultrasound was initially performed. This showed normal appearance of the abdominal solid structures (Fig. 1a), apart from a marked segmental large bowel-wall thickening on the right hypochondrium surrounded by hyperechoic, non-compressible fatty tissue and a small fluid collection. According to these findings, the clinical suspicion was either inflammatory bowel disease or diverticulitis. The patient underwent a Computed Tomography (CT) which confirmed wall thickening of the descending and sigmoid colon, diverticular outpouching and stranding of perivisceral fat complicated with localised perforation. Due to the patient's inborn anatomical variant of redundancies of large intestine, also known as dolichocolon condition, her sigmoid colon was displaced on the right-side of the abdomen (Fig. 2a, b). The patient was referred to the surgical team and admitted to the ward for intravenous fluid therapy and antibiotics. She was discharged after a week with clinical follow-up.

Discussion

Diverticula are defined as sac-like protrusions from the large intestine wall due to a combination of anatomical, dietary, motility and structural influences [5]. They are divided in two general anatomical types, true and false. The majority of the colon diverticula are false diverticula (also known as pseudodiverticula), composed of mucosa and submucosa protruding through the muscularis externa, covered only by serosa. They are acquired, multiple and frequently located in the sigmoid colon. True diverticula involve all three layers of the bowel wall (mucosa, submucosa and muscularis externa) as seen in most congenital diverticula such as Meckel's diverticula and in the diverticula of right-sided large intestine [6, 7]. They are mostly congenital and solitary [8].

When infection of the diverticulum occurs, it can manifest with a spectrum of symptoms such as pain, fever, diarrhoea, nausea, vomiting and bloody stools. Right-sided diverticulitis (RSD) may mimic several abdominal emergencies such as cholecystitis, appendicitis or epiploic appendagitis. The distinction between these conditions and RSD is crucial as the latter is treated conservatively and abscess formation is rare [9, 10]. Within the range of possible investigations, US plays its role being the first imaging study modality performed in patients presenting with abdominal pain. It can safely rule out cholecystitis and identify several abdominal conditions such as epiploic appendagitis (EA), appendicitis, colitis, neoplastic lesion and Crohn's disease, each of them characterised by specific sonographic aspects.

The sonographic appearance of the inflamed diverticulum is defined as hypoechoic wall thickening, due to oedema and muscular hypertrophy. US can also reveal

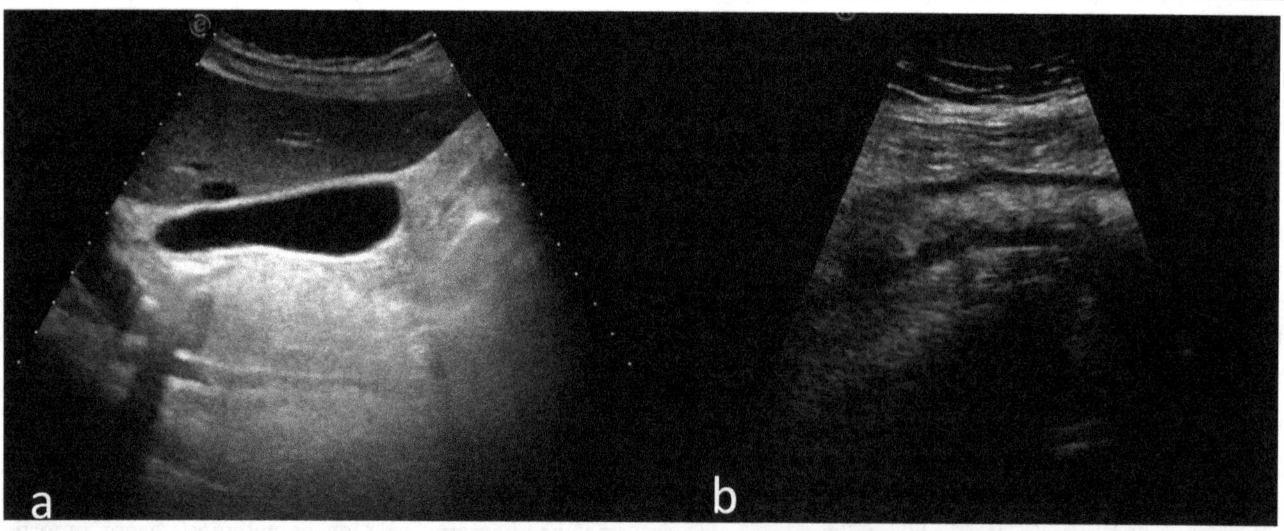

Fig. 1 The ultrasound demonstrated normal liver, spleen, kidneys, no free fluid and normal gall bladder (**a**). A diffuse wall thickening of the bowel in the right upper quadrant (**b**). The impression was of a right-sided inflammatory bowel disease or colon diverticulitis

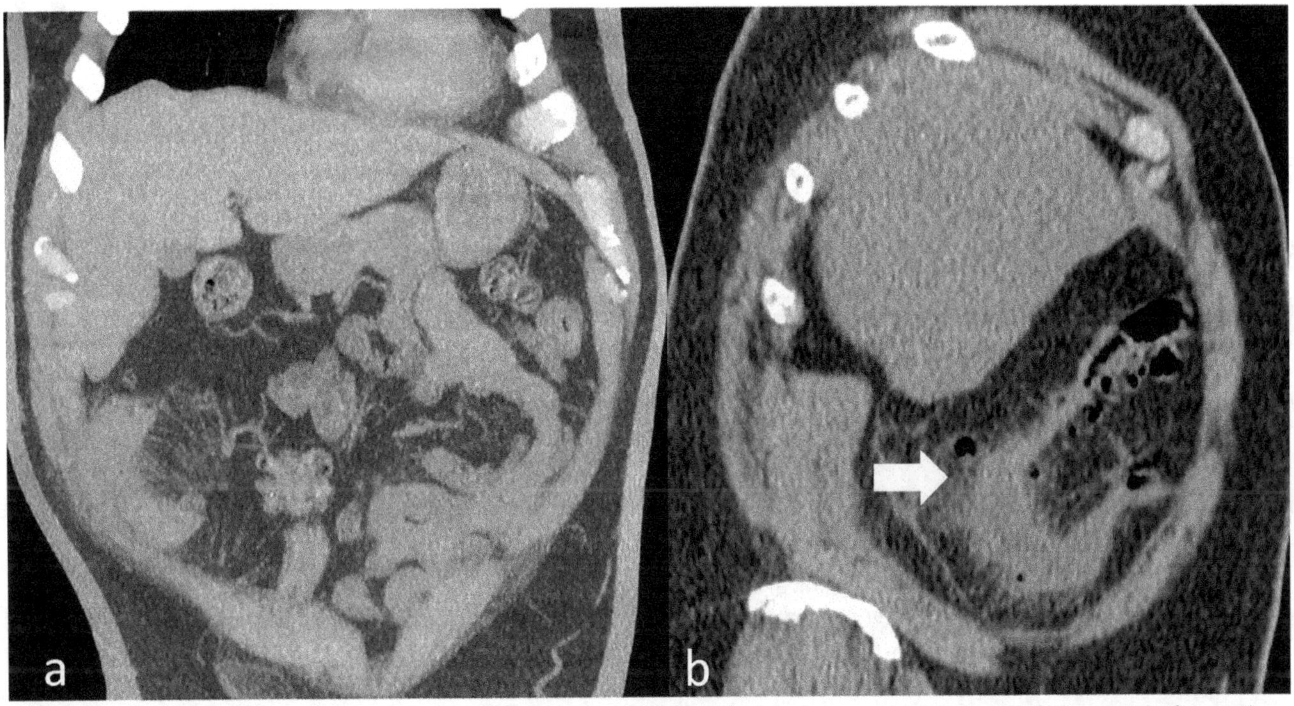

Fig. 2 The CT scan of the abdomen and pelvis without intravenous contrast material. In **a**, the coronal reformat and in **b** the sagittal reformat. The scan showed the wall thickening of the left and sigmoid colon, with diverticular outpouching. Moreover, there was stranding of the perivisceral fat due to perivisceral tissue inflammation complicated with limited perforation and a small free air pocket next it; therefore, the diagnosis favoured was diverticulitis with limited perforation (white arrow). There was no free fluid

complications such as inflammation of the pericolic fat and free fluid collection around the target area. Specifically, the pericolic fat stranding consists of hyperechoic non-compressible mass-like finding whether the free fluid has a hypoechoic ultrasound aspect [11]. Give US its crucial role in the decision-making process, the CT remains the modality of choice in the diagnosis of diverticulitis, due to its ability to identity the anatomical location along the large intestine, the involvement of adjacent organs and the presence of complications such as perforation, abscess and fistula [7]. In summary, ultrasound evaluation of abdominal emergencies is a rapid and useful first-level investigation that may lead the next step in the clinical decision-making process, such as a second-level imaging study, surgical or conservative approach. Both imaging modalities have their advantages and limitations, making their combined use crucial for the best appropriate clinical management of patients.

Abbreviations
ED: Emergency Department; CT: Computed Tomography; RSD: right-sided diverticulitis; US: ultrasound; EA: epiploic appendagitis.

Acknowledgements
Not applicable.

Authors' contributions
All authors read and approved the final manuscript.

Author details
[1] Dipartimento di Medicina interna e Specialità mediche, Di.M.I. Università degli Studi di Geniva, Viale Benedetto XV, 10, 16132 Genoa, GE, Italy. [2] Dipartimento di scienze Chirurgiche, Università degli Studi di Torino, Turin, Italy. [3] SCDU Radiodiagnostica e Medicina Nucleare, Azienda Ospedaliero-Universitaria S.Luigi Gonzaga, Regione Gonzole 10, 10043 Orbassano, TO, Italy.

References
1. Kahveci S, Tokmak TT et al (2013) Acute right-sided colonic diverticulitis mimicking appendicitis: a report of two cases. J Clin Ultrasound 41(4):238–241
2. Radhi JM, Ramsay JA et al (2011) Diverticuar disease of the right colon. BMC Res Notes 4:383
3. Karatepe O, Gulcicek OB et al (2008) Cecal diverticulitis mimicking acute appendicitis: a report of 4 cases. World J Emerg Surg 3(1):16
4. Komaricaand EB, Zvizdic Z et al (2012) Right-sided perforated ascending colonic diverticulum mimicking acute appendicitis. Acta Inform Med 20(4):269–270
5. Monari F, Cervellera M, Pirrera B et al (2017) Right-sided acute diverticulitis: a single Western center experience. Int J Surg 44:128–131. https://doi.org/10.1016/j.ijsu.2017.06.025 **(Epub 2017 Jun 13)**
6. Oudenhoven LF, Koumans RK, Puylaert JB (1998) Right colonic diverticulitis: US and CT findings—new insight about frequency and natural history. Radiology 208:611–618
7. Espinosa J, Sharma R et al (2017) Case report medical approach to right colon diverticulitis with perforation. Case Rep Emerg Med. https://doi.org/10.1155/2017/2563218
8. Beranbaum SL, Zausner J, Lane B (1972) Diverticular disease of the right colon. AJR 115:334–348
9. O'Malley ME, Wilson SR (2003) US of gastrointestinal tract abnormalities with CT correlation. Radiographics 23:59–72

24

Diagnostic value of transcranial ultrasonography for selecting subjects with large vessel occlusion

Daria Antipova[1*], Leila Eadie[1], Ashish Stephen Macaden[2] and Philip Wilson[1]

Abstract

Introduction: A number of pre-hospital clinical assessment tools have been developed to triage subjects with acute stroke due to large vessel occlusion (LVO) to a specialised endovascular centre, but their false negative rates remain high leading to inappropriate and costly emergency transfers. Transcranial ultrasonography may represent a valuable pre-hospital tool for selecting patients with LVO who could benefit from rapid transfer to a dedicated centre.

Methods: Diagnostic accuracy of transcranial ultrasonography in acute stroke was subjected to systematic review. Medline, Embase, PubMed, Scopus, and The Cochrane Library were searched. Published articles reporting diagnostic accuracy of transcranial ultrasonography in comparison to a reference imaging method were selected. Studies reporting estimates of diagnostic accuracy were included in the meta-analysis.

Results: Twenty-seven published articles were selected for the systematic review. Transcranial Doppler findings, such as absent or diminished blood flow signal in a major cerebral artery and asymmetry index ≥ 21% were shown to be suggestive of LVO. It demonstrated sensitivity ranging from 68 to 100% and specificity of 78–99% for detecting acute steno-occlusive lesions. Area under the receiver operating characteristics curve was 0.91. Transcranial ultrasonography can also detect haemorrhagic foci, however, its application is largely restricted by lesion location.

Conclusions: Transcranial ultrasonography might potentially be used for the selection of subjects with acute LVO, to help streamline patient care and allow direct transfer to specialised endovascular centres. It can also assist in detecting haemorrhagic lesions in some cases, however, its applicability here is largely restricted. Additional research should optimize the scanning technique. Further work is required to demonstrate whether this diagnostic approach, possibly combined with clinical assessment, could be used at the pre-hospital stage to justify direct transfer to a regional thrombectomy centre in suitable cases.

Keywords: Large vessel occlusion, Stroke, Acute cerebral ischaemia, Intracerebral haemorrhage, Transcranial ultrasonography, Neuroimaging

Introduction

Rationale

Stroke is the second largest cause of death and one of the most common causes of complex disability in adults worldwide [1]. Mechanical thrombectomy (MT) preceded by intravenous thrombolysis provides optimal care for patients with acute ischaemic stroke due to large vessel occlusion (LVO) [2]. While thrombolysis is offered in many general hospitals, MT can only be performed in specialised endovascular centres with neurointerventional facilities. Earlier initiation of endovascular reperfusion is associated with greatly improved outcome [3, 4]. Therefore, patients with suspected LVO could benefit from direct transfer to a specialised endovascular centre.

A number of clinical assessment tools have been developed to triage subjects, but their false negative rates remain high which means that more than 20% of patients with LVO would be transferred to a centre with no

*Correspondence: daria.antipova@abdn.ac.uk
[1] Centre for Rural Health, University of Aberdeen, Old Perth Road, Inverness IV2 3JH, UK
Full list of author information is available at the end of the article

dedicated facilities available [5]. Furthermore, false positive results can lead to unnecessary and costly emergency transfers. Hence, there is an urgent need to establish a reliable process to select patients with LVO, particularly in areas with long transport times.

Portable transcranial ultrasound (see Glossary for explanations of the different ultrasound types) has emerged as a potential method for rapidly assessing intracranial circulation and brain structures in the pre-hospital and early hospital phase [6]. The evidence base for the diagnostic accuracy of transcranial ultrasonography in acute stroke population appears to be extensive, with more than 150 publications. Up to date, it has not been demonstrated whether ultrasonography can be implemented as part of a triage system for patients with LVO to streamline care. A systematic analysis of the existing data in the field was therefore performed.

Objectives

The following questions are addressed in the current review:

1. What is the diagnostic accuracy of transcranial ultrasonography in detecting occlusion and/or stenosis of cerebral vessels in acute ischaemic stroke population compared with other available diagnostic techniques?
2. Can transcranial ultrasonography be a useful tool to exclude intracranial haemorrhage as one of the contraindications for endovascular reperfusion compared with other available diagnostic techniques?
3. Can transcranial ultrasonography be a useful tool to detect midline shift suggestive of space-occupying stroke compared with other available diagnostic techniques?

Methods

Protocol and registration

The protocol is registered in PROSPERO, International prospective register of systematic reviews, and can be accessed at: https://www.crd.york.ac.uk/prospero/display_record.php?RecordID=75882.

Eligibility criteria

Inclusion and exclusion criteria are listed in Table 1.

Information sources

A systematic search of the literature was conducted during May–June 2017, using a database-specific search strategy for each of the following electronic databases: PubMed, Medline, Embase, Scopus and The Cochrane Library.

Search

The search strategy included a combination of multiple iterations of MeSH and keyword terms relating to each component of the research question as outlined in Additional file 1.

The search was restricted to human studies, English language, and adult participants. There was no restriction for the year of publication.

Study selection

The study selection process is illustrated in Fig. 1.

Eligible papers were tabulated and used in the qualitative synthesis. Studies which reported diagnostic accuracy values such as true positive (TP), false positive (FP), true negative (TN), false negative (FN), and sensitivity and specificity values were included in the quantitative analysis.

Data collection and extraction

A dedicated data extraction form was developed and used to collect relevant information from the included studies. The inclusion of information fields in the data collection form was guided by the review questions. The following components were assessed:

- Study setting.
- Main characteristics of the patient population.
- Number of subjects recruited into the study and included in the study analysis.
- Ethical approval.
- Modality of transcranial ultrasonography being investigated, its technical considerations and qualifications of researchers performing transcranial ultrasound scanning.
- Reference test and technical considerations.
- Blindness of investigators performing and/or interpreting the tests' results.
- Time interval from symptom onset to index and reference tests, time interval between index and reference tests.
- Whether results were presented in the form of diagnostic accuracy (sensitivity, specificity, TP, FP, TN, FN, predictive values), or a narrative.

Two of this review's authors completed the data extraction form for each paper. If authors disagreed, a third author adjudicated. As our analysis concerned only published data, further data from investigators were not sought.

Table 1 Inclusion and exclusion criteria

Domain	Inclusion	Exclusion
Study type	Comparative observational studies	Case reports
	Prospective observational studies	Selected case series
	Cohort studies	Literature review
	Unselected case series	Conference proceedings
		Full text unavailable
Participants	Human	Non-human subjects
	Adults	Exclusively paediatric patients Mixed paediatric and adult populations (where paediatric and adult groups are not possible to identify separately)
	Patients with acute stroke—ischaemic (including patients with a transient ischaemic attack) or haemorrhagic	Patients with non-stroke conditions, such as sickle cell disease, arteriovenous malformation, traumatic brain injury, and cerebral tumour
	Patients with acute spontaneous subarachnoid haemorrhage	
Setting	Any	
Procedure	Transcranial ultrasonography (grey-scale/Doppler/colour-coded sonography) with/without contrast (microbubble) enhancement if the outcomes are reported separately	Transcranial ultrasonography (grey-scale/Doppler/colour-coded sonography) with contrast (microbubble) enhancement as sole ultrasound method, or if the outcomes are not reported separately
	A reference standard diagnostic tool, such as conventional imaging (CT, MRI), cerebral angiography (computed tomography angiography, magnetic resonance angiography, digital subtraction angiography)	No reference test employed
	Maximal time interval between the onset of symptoms and index and reference tests: 72 h	Unknown or more than 72 h'time interval between the symptoms onset and index and/or reference tests
	Maximal time interval between the index and reference tests: 24 h	Unknown or more than 24 h'time interval between the index and reference tests
Aims/outcomes	Detection of signs of acute cerebral ischaemia, acute intracranial haemorrhage, midline shift in space-occupying stroke as measured by both transcranial ultrasonography as index test and reference test	Detection of signs of vasospasm following subarachnoid haemorrhage

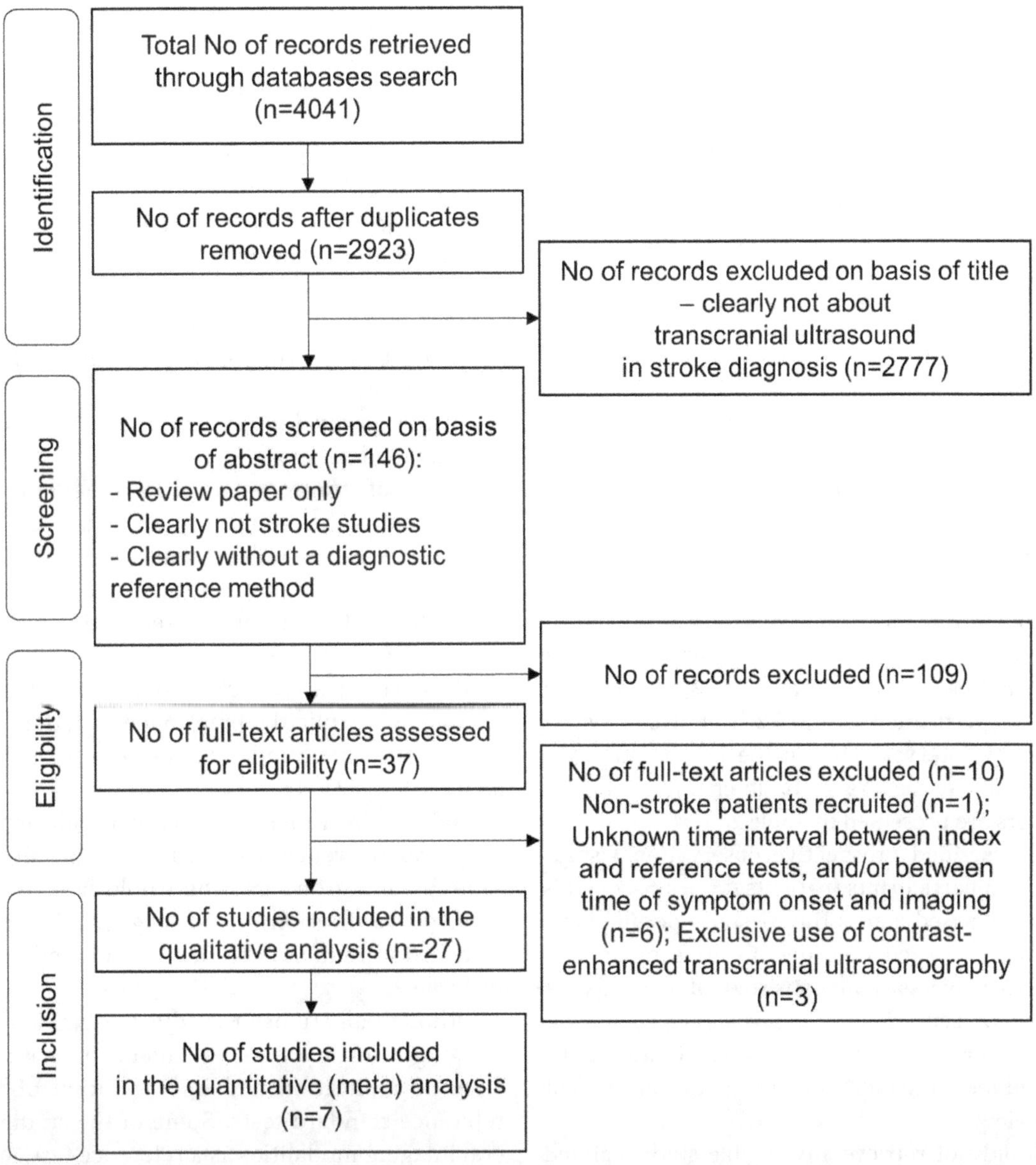

Fig. 1 PRISMA flowchart. Outline of the study selection process using inclusion and exclusion criteria

Risk of bias assessment in individual studies

Included studies were assessed qualitatively for concerns regarding their applicability for each of the four domains: patient selection, index test, reference standard, and flow and timing, in accordance with the QUADAS-2 Tool quality assessment system [7]. The risk of bias and applicability concerns were identified using RevMan 5.3 software and presented as a summary table.

Statistical analysis

The statistical analysis was performed in accordance with the Cochrane guidelines for diagnostic test accuracy reviews [8]. Two-by-two tables were constructed for the transcranial ultrasound results of diagnosis of acute steno-occlusion, intracranial haemorrhage, and detection of midline shift showing the binary test results cross-classified with the binary reference standard. The diagnostic values including the TP, TN, FP, and FN values were entered into RevMan 5.3. The sensitivity and specificity, as well as their 95% confidence intervals, were also calculated in RevMan 5.3. The data from each study were presented graphically by plotting sensitivities and specificities on a coupled forest plot and summary receiver operating characteristics (SROC) plot. Area under the curve for the SROC plot was calculated as a summary value for given sensitivities and specificities using IBM SPSS Statistics 25 package.

Risk of bias assessment across studies

Provided that the number of studies reporting diagnostic accuracy values was ten or above, publication bias assessment with a funnel plot to illustrate the possibility of selective publication of small studies with positive results would be performed.

Results

Study selection

The results of the study selection process are illustrated in Fig. 1.

Study characteristics

Included studies

27 studies in which participants were subjected to both transcranial ultrasonography and gold standard diagnostic imaging for diagnosing acute stroke were eligible for inclusion in the final analysis. In all studies, transcranial ultrasound was performed within 72 h of stroke symptom onset. Time interval between the index and reference tests did not exceed 24 h. Basic characteristics of included papers are presented in Table 2.

All papers described prospective observational studies. In total, 1683 participants (patients $n=1566$, controls $n=117$) were analysed across the 27 study populations. Individual studies varied considerably in sample size, from 4 to 213 subjects, and consisted of participants recruited upon presentation to the hospital or outpatient departments. There were no pre-hospital studies identified that would meet the inclusion criteria for the current systematic review.

The search did not retrieve any eligible studies aimed to assess accuracy of transcranial ultrasonography for detecting signs of subarachnoid haemorrhage (SAH).

Seven papers presented study results reporting quantitative values of the diagnostic accuracy of the transcranial ultrasonography (TP, TN, FP, FN, sensitivity, and specificity), whereas 20 discussed outcomes qualitatively or did not fully report diagnostic accuracy values.

On the basis of their full-text articles, ten studies were not included in the final analysis [9–18]. Principal reasons were unknown or unclear time interval between symptom onset and reference/index imaging and/or between reference and index imaging [9, 10, 12, 14–18], the use of contrast-enhanced transcranial sonography either exclusively or in combination with non-contrast ultrasound without reporting outcomes separately for each group [9, 11, 13], or a non-stroke population [12].

Risk of bias assessment in individual studies

A summary of bias and applicability concerns is presented in Table 3.

Case–control methodologies were employed in three included studies [19–21] in which groups of patients with and without the target condition were identified before the index test was performed.

The papers were also evaluated in regard to the sample size and divided into three groups [22]: low sample size (< 100 participants), intermediate (100–300 participants), and high (> 300 participants). Only six studies had intermediate sample size, whereas in the remaining 21 it was low.

Ethical approval was not reported in 44% ($n=12$) of the included papers.

A list of transcranial ultrasonography modalities used in individual studies as an index test is provided in Table 2. All included studies were assessed against the adequate blinding criterion. In 19, the results of the index test were interpreted without knowledge of the results of the reference standard [19, 23–40]. Two studies [41, 42] were lacking blindness, and in 6 papers it was not explicitly mentioned whether or not the investigator was blinded to the results of the reference standard [20, 21, 43–46].

Studies in which transcranial ultrasound scanning and reference standards were performed on the same patient group and the whole sample should have received verification of the diagnosis by the reference standard were included. The control methods are listed in Table 2.

Although all studies that did not employ a reference imaging modality were excluded, there was inconsistency in application and interpretation of the various reference standard tests. Some of the studies used several imaging modalities as a reference test, and for most articles, it was either computed tomography angiography (CTA), magnetic resonance angiography (MRA), or digital subtraction angiography (DSA) [21, 25, 27, 39]. For example, in the paper by Gerriets et al. [27], the choice of reference test (CTA, MRA, or DSA) was left up to the treating centre.

Diagnostic accuracy of transcranial ultrasonography in acute stroke

The diagnostic accuracy of transcranial ultrasonography in detecting signs of acute steno-occlusive lesions, intracranial haemorrhage and/or midline shift was a primary outcome in all studies. All included studies that specified the type of a probe and frequency of transcranial ultrasonography performed scanning with a sector probe at low frequency (2–4 MHz) (Table 2). Kenton et al. [29] used a curved phase array probe for their study, however,

Table 2 Characteristics of included studies

Reference	Study setting	Condition of interest	Index test	Reference test	Number of patients included in the analysis	Time interval from symptoms onset to index test	Time interval between index test and reference imaging	Experience of the researcher performing transcranial ultrasonography	Type of transducer	Frequency of insonation
Akopov and Whitman [19]	In-hospital	AIS	TCD	MRA, CT	12	Only the results of TCD that was performed within 24 h after ictus were analysed	MRA was performed together with the first TCD examination for seven patients (included in the analysis). For all others, MRA was performed 24–72 h after the ictus and close to the second TCD (not included in the analysis)	Unclear—TCD was performed by the authors	Not specified	2 MHz
Bar et al. [23]	In-hospital	AIS	TCCS ± contrast enhancement	CTA	31	Within 3 h	20 min	Three skilled sonographers with at least 5 years of experience in ultrasound diagnostics	Sector	2–4 MHz
Boddu et al. [24]	Unclear—"in the laboratory"	AIS	TCD	MRA	128	Not specified—within 24 h in 33% of participants and within maximum 29 h in 67% of participants	From 30 to 300 min (median 60 min)	Credentialed neurosonologist	Not specified	2 MHz
Brunser et al. [25]	In-hospital	AIS	TCD (PMD)	CTA	100	Mean 468 min ± SD 343.2 min	Mean 77.8 min ± SD 88.5 min	Experienced sonographer certified by the American Society of Neuroimaging	Not specified	

Table 2 (continued)

Reference	Study setting	Condition of interest	Index test	Reference test	Number of patients included in the analysis	Time interval from symptoms onset to index test	Time interval between index test and reference imaging	Experience of the researcher performing transcranial ultrasonography	Type of transducer	Frequency of insonation
Gerriets et al. [26]	In-hospital	AIS, MLS	TCCS	CT	40	Only results of TCCS examination that were performed 8 ± 3 and 16 ± 3 h from onset were analysed	6 h	Unclear—"three investigators"	Sector	2.5 MHz
Gerriets et al. [27]	In-hospital	AIS	TCCS ± contrast enhancement	CTA, MRA, DSA	58	Immediately on admission, within 6 h from symptom onset (mean 3.4 h)	Mean time difference = 0.8 h in 14 patients; 6.1 in 18 patients	Doctors with at least 1 year of experience in the field of colour-coded duplex sonography of the brain-supplying arteries	Sector	2–2.5 MHz
Goertler et al. [41]	Presumably in-hospital, department of neurology	AIS	TCCS	Contrast-enhanced TCCS	23	Within 5 h	Not specified but both tests performed within 5 h from symptom onset	A sonographer	Sector	2–2.5 MHz
Guan et al. [28]	In-hospital	AIS	TCD	CTA	128	The mean time from symptom onset to admission was 12.3 (10.1) hours The mean time from admission to TCD was 15.5 (SD 10.1) minutes	The mean time interval between both examinations was 89.7 (77.8) min 65% patients—less than 30 min difference between them; 25%, 31–90 min; 15%, more than 90 min but less than 180 min	Experienced sonographer	Not specified	2 MHz

Table 2 (continued)

Reference	Study setting	Condition of interest	Index test	Reference test	Number of patients included in the analysis	Time interval from symptoms onset to index test	Time interval between index test and reference imaging	Experience of the researcher performing transcranial ultrasonography	Type of transducer	Frequency of insonation
Kadimi et al. [43]	Not specified—presumably in-hospital	AIS	TCD	CT	4	Within 6 h	Not specified—both CT and TCD were performed within 6 h of the onset of symptoms	Not specified	Sector	2 MHz
Kenton et al. [29]	In-hospital	AIS	TCCS	MRA	30	Ranged from 4 to 24 h, mean 15.4 h	Within 4 h, range 15 min to 4 h; median, 2 h	Not specified	Curved phase array	2.25 MHz
Kern et al. [30]	In-hospital, stroke unit	ICH	Native transcranial b-mode ultrasound, UPI with contrast enhancement	CT	12	Unclear—on day 1 as soon as possible after admission	4.1 ± 2.5 h on day 1 (CT first)	Sonographers	Sector	2–4 MHz
Kukulska-Pawluczuk et al. [44]	In-hospital	ICH, MLS	TCCS	CT	39	The time between initial symptoms of focal neurologic deficit and hospital admission ranged from 1.5 to 48 h with a median of 5.9 h. Index test was performed not later than 12 h after initial CT which was done directly upon admission	Not more than 12 h	Unknown	Sector	2.5 MHz
Leanyvari et al. [45]	Unclear	AIS	TCD	CT	12	Within 12.5 ± 8 h after stroke onset or not more than 24.5 h	TCD measurements were made before or no more than 4 h after CT	Not specified	Not specified	2 MHz

Table 2 (continued)

Reference	Study setting	Condition of interest	Index test	Reference test	Number of patients included in the analysis	Time interval from symptoms onset to index test	Time interval between index test and reference imaging	Experience of the researcher performing transcranial ultrasonography	Type of transducer	Frequency of insonation
Matsumoto et al. [31]	In-hospital	ICH	TCCS	CT	20	Within 21 h (within 12 h of the CT study which was performed 4.6 ± 4.4 h from symptom onset)	Within 12 h (mean 3.9 ± 4.1 h)	Not specified	Sector	2.5 MHz
Nasr et al. [32]	Outpatient, TIA clinic	AIS	TCCS	MRI-3D-TOF angiography	116	Unclear but presumably within 24 h from the onset	4 h	Unclear	Not specified	
Ovesen [42]	In-hospital	ICH	Transcranial b-mode ultrasound	CT, CTA	25	Within 4.5 h	Mean 61.1 min (SD 26.6)	Unclear ("a single observer")	Sector	1.7–3.1 MHz
Panerai et al. [20]	In-hospital	AIS	TCD	MRI-DWI	11 plus 9 healthy controls	Within 48 h	Median time interval 2 h (range 0.5–8 h)	Unclear—performed "in a dedicated cardiovascular research laboratory"	Not specified	2 MHz
Rathakrishnan et al. [33]	In-hospital	AIS	TCD	CTA	15	Not specified	Within 24 h	Not specified, a stroke neurologist credentialed in cerebrovascular ultrasound interpreted the TCD findings	Not specified	2 MHz
Seidel et al. [34]	In-hospital	AIS, HT	TCCS	CT	32	For the purpose of the current review only TCCS findings which were obtained < 12 and 24 ± 4 h from symptoms onset were analysed	Unclear but before TCCS	Sonographer	Sector	2–4 MHz

Table 2 (continued)

Reference	Study setting	Condition of interest	Index test	Reference test	Number of patients included in the analysis	Time interval from symptoms onset to index test	Time interval between index test and reference imaging	Experience of the researcher performing transcranial ultrasonography	Type of transducer	Frequency of insonation
Seidel et al. [35]	In-hospital	AIS, HT	TCCS	CT, MRI in individual cases	55	Within 32 h (mean time 10.6 h (SD, 7.2; median, 8.5; interquartile range, 6.5 h after stroke symptom onset)	Within mean time of 14 h (CT was performed immediately after stroke symptom onset with mean 3.3 h; SD, 3.0; median, 2.0; interquartile range, 3.75)	The ultrasound investigator	Sector	2 MHz
Stolz et al. [36]	In-hospital	AIS, ICH, MLS	TCCS	CT	61	Unclear, presumably within 24 h	3–12 h	Four sonographers with sufficient experience with the method	Not specified	2–2.5 MHz
Tang et al. [37]	In-hospital, stroke unit	ICH, MLS	TCCS	CT	51	Unclear but presumably within 24 h because time from symptom onset to reference imaging was 4.1 ± 3.7 h	Not more than 12 h, average interval was 5.9 ± 4.0 h	Well-trained and experienced sonographers	Sector	2 MHz
Tsivgoulis et al. [38]	Emergency department	AIS	TCD	CTA	132	Within 24 h	Range 10–130 min (median 35 min)	Experienced sonographers	Not specified	2 MHz
Tsivgoulis et al. [39]	Emergency room	AIS	TCD (PMD)	CTA, MRA, DSA	213	Within 24 h	Presumed 24 h, angiography was performed within 48 h from ictus	Stroke neurologists with specialised training and credentials in cerebrovascular ultrasound	Not specified	2 MHz

Table 2 (continued)

Reference	Study setting	Condition of interest	Index test	Reference test	Number of patients included in the analysis	Time interval from symptoms onset to index test	Time interval between index test and reference imaging	Experience of the researcher performing transcranial ultrasonography	Type of transducer	Frequency of insonation
Viola et al. [21]	In-hospital	AIS	TCD (3D)	MRA, CT	47 plus 67 healthy controls	Within 3–24 h	Unclear, presumably not more than 24 h—both tests were performed 3–24 h from onset	Not specified	Not specified	2 MHz
Wada et al. [40]	Not specified	AIS	TCCS	DSA	40	Within 24 h	Not specified—"immediately before cerebral angiography"	Unclear	Not specified	2–3 MHz, 3700 Hz pulse repetition frequency, low-pass filter was 50 Hz
Zubkov et al. [46]	In-hospital	AIS	TCD	CTA	31	Approximately 30 h after symptom onset	Unclear, presumably within 24 h	Experienced ultrasonographers	Not specified	2 MHz

For the purpose of the current review, terminology used to describe an ultrasound probe has been standardised and phased array, sector and pulsed wave Doppler are referred to as the same type of probe

3D three-dimensional, *AIS* acute ischaemic stroke, *CT* computed tomography, *CTA* computed tomography angiography, *DSA* digital subtraction angiography, *ICH* intracranial haemorrhage, *HT* haemorrhagic transformation, *MRA* magnetic resonance angiography, *MRI-3D-TOF* magnetic resonance three-dimensional time-of-flight imaging, *MRI-DWI* diffusion weighted magnetic resonance imaging; *PMD* power motion-mode, *SD* standard deviation, *TCCS* transcranial colour-coded duplex sonography, *TCD* transcranial Doppler, *UPI* ultrasound perfusion imaging

Table 3 Risk of bias and applicability concerns summary

	Risk of bias				Applicability concerns		
	Patient selection	Index test	Reference standard	Flow and timing	Patient selection	Index test	Reference standard
Akopov and Whitman [19]	High	Low	Unclear	Low	Low	Low	Low
Bar et al. [23][a]	Low	Low	Low	High	Low	Low	Low
Boddu et al. [24]	Low	Low	Low	Low	Low	Low	Low
Brunser et al. [25][a]	Low	Low	Low	Unclear	Low	Low	Low
Gerriets et al. [26]	Low	Low	Low	Low	Low	Low	Low
Gerriets et al. [27]	Low	Low	Low	High	Low	Low	Low
Goertler et al. [41]	Unclear	High	High	Unclear	High	Low	Low
Guan et al. [28][a]	Unclear	Low	Low	Low	Unclear	Low	Low
Kadimi et al. [43]	Unclear	Unclear	Unclear	Low	Low	Low	Low
Kenton et al. [29]	Unclear	Low	Low	High	Low	Low	Low
Kern et al. [30]	Low	Low	Low	Low	Low	Low	Low
Kukulska-Pawluczuk et al. [44]	Unclear	Unclear	Low	High	Low	Low	Low
Leanyvari et al. [45]	High	Low	High	Low	Low	Low	High
Matsumoto et al. [31]	Low	Low	Low	Unclear	Low	Low	Low
Nasr et al. [32]	Low	Low	Low	High	Low	Low	Low
Ovesen et al. [42]	Low	High	Low	High	Low	Low	Low
Panerai et al. [20]	High	High	High	Low	High	Low	High
Rathakrishnan et al. [33][a]	High	Low	Low	Unclear	Low	Low	Low
Seidel et al. [34]	High	Low	Unclear	Low	Low	Low	Low
Seidel et al. [35]	Unclear	Low	Unclear	Low	Low	Low	Low
Stolz et al. [36]	Unclear	Low	Unclear	Low	Low	Low	Low
Tang et al. [37]	Low	Low	Unclear	High	Low	Low	Low
Tsivgoulis et al. [38][a]	Low	Low	Low	Low	Low	Low	Low
Tsivgoulis et al. [39][a]	Unclear	Low	Low	Low	Low	Low	Low
Viola et al. [21]	High	Unclear	High	High	Low	Low	High
Wada et al. [40][a]	Low	Low	Low	Low	Low	Low	Low
Zubkov et al. [46]	Unclear	High	Unclear	High	Low	Unclear	Low

Review author's judgement about each domain for each included study

Studies marked with an "a" were included in the quantitative analysis

this did not seem to provide any additional and/or contradictory information to other reviewed studies.

The majority of included papers (22/27) aimed to evaluate diagnostic accuracy of transcranial Doppler sonography (TCD) in detecting signs of acute occlusion and/or stenosis in acute ischaemic stroke population (Table 2). However, there was marked diversity in diagnostic protocol and criteria for steno-occlusive lesions (Additional files 2 and 3).

Seventeen studies assessed diagnostic value of TCD in identifying occlusion of the cerebral arteries [19, 21, 23, 25, 27–29, 32, 33, 35, 38–41, 43, 45, 46]. Diagnosis of the middle cerebral artery (MCA) mainstem occlusion can be considered when the flow was absent or minimal, blunted, or damped throughout the MCA while the flow in the distal internal carotid artery, anterior and posterior cerebral arteries was diverted [23, 27, 35, 38, 40]. Similarly, anterior cerebral artery occlusion and occlusion in the posterior circulation (vertebral, basilar and posterior cerebral arteries) were defined as the absence of the flow or the presence of minimal, blunted, or dampened flow signals throughout these vessels [38, 39].

The interhemispheric asymmetry index has been used to describe the difference in the blood flow velocity between symptomatic and asymptomatic hemispheres [47]. Asymmetry index ≥ 21% was shown to correlate accurately with clinical presentation and to detect major branch or multiple branch occlusion [21, 23, 29, 35, 41]. In patients with an asymmetry index of < 21%, conventional imaging (CT, MRI) is likely to offer normal appearance or show only very minor changes suggestive of acute brain ischemia [21, 28, 29]. Kadimi et al. [43] reported a

Study	TP	FP	FN	TN	Sensitivity (95% CI)	Specificity (95% CI)
Bar 2010	22	2	0	7	1.00 [0.85, 1.00]	0.78 [0.40, 0.97]
Brunser 2009	30	4	3	63	0.91 [0.76, 0.98]	0.94 [0.85, 0.98]
Guan 2013	35	1	0	92	1.00 [0.90, 1.00]	0.99 [0.94, 1.00]
Rathakrishnan 2008	16	3	5	81	0.76 [0.53, 0.92]	0.96 [0.90, 0.99]
Tsivgoulis 2007	34	5	9	84	0.79 [0.64, 0.90]	0.94 [0.87, 0.98]
Tsivgoulis 2008	17	6	8	182	0.68 [0.46, 0.85]	0.97 [0.93, 0.99]
Wada 2002	3	1	0	86	1.00 [0.29, 1.00]	0.99 [0.94, 1.00]

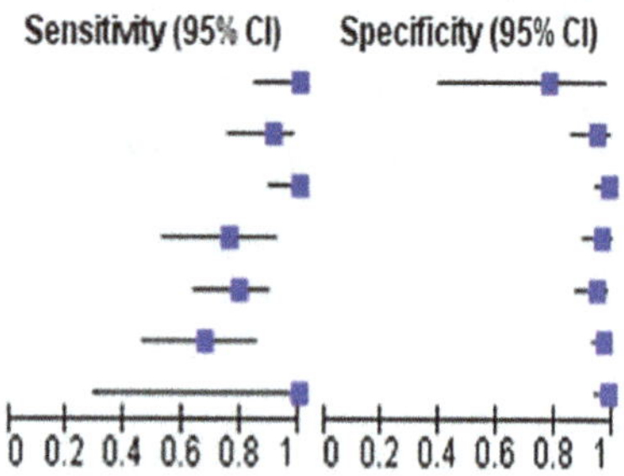

Fig. 2 Forest plot. Estimated diagnostic accuracy of transcranial ultrasonography in detecting steno-occlusive lesions in acute stroke population

hyperechoic appearance of MCA with no Doppler signal or waveform suggestive of a large occlusion, similar to hyperdense MCA on CT. Occlusion of one or two terminal branches of the MCA presenting as lacunar stroke has been reported to be "insufficient" to cause changes detectable with TCD [47].

Diagnostic accuracy values for the detection of cerebral steno-occlusive lesions in comparison to angiography as the reference test (CTA [23, 25, 28, 33, 38], CTA/MRA/DSA [39], DSA [40]) are presented in the forest plot (Fig. 2) and SROC plot (Fig. 3).

In general, there was a good correlation between TCD and reference standard findings in the acute ischaemic stroke population, with the sensitivity ranging from 68 to 100% and the specificity 78–99%. The area under the SROC curve was 0.91. However, TCD appeared to be more sensitive in detecting MCA steno-occlusive lesions when compared to assessment of the posterior cerebral circulation but was less specific (Additional file 4) [33, 38],

Transcranial ultrasonography can also provide evidence of intracranial haemorrhage in some cases. Acute haemorrhagic foci are usually seen on ultrasound images as homogenous hyperechogenic structures that are well distinguished from surrounding tissues. Transcranial ultrasound has been shown to detect 52.9% of haemorrhagic foci in deep cerebral structures, such as basal ganglia, whereas cortico-subcortical lobar lesions were missed in about 67% of cases, mainly in the temporal and frontal lobes [30, 34, 44], There was a good correlation between the volumes of haemorrhagic foci measured by transcranial ultrasound and CT [31, 42, 44]. It revealed haemorrhagic foci with volumes as small as 0.47 mm^3 and as large as 234 mm^3 [44].

Although transcranial ultrasonography has been shown to identify haemorrhage in supratentorial and infratentorial locations, and intraventricular haemorrhages [42], echogenicity of haemorrhage appears to be similar to that of the cerebellar tentorium and calcifications within choroid plexuses. Cerebral tumours, vascular malformations and cerebral microangiopathies may also appear as hyperechogenic areas mimicking haemorrhagic lesions [44, 48].

Transcranial ultrasound has been demonstrated to be a useful diagnostic tool in detecting midline shift in space-occupying haemorrhagic or ischaemic stroke lesions [42]. There was a good consistency between the studies in the technique used to measure midline shift as a deviation from the presumed midline ipsilaterally and contralaterally to the focus as a distance between the source of the ultrasound beam and the centre of the third ventricle.

There was an excellent correlation between transcranial ultrasonography and CT measurements of the midline shift with a coefficient of about 0.9 [26, 36, 37, 44]. Midline shift has been reported to be the most sensitive indicator of intracranial haemorrhage with a significant correlation between haemorrhagic focus volume and midline shift [37, 44].

Ultrasound window availability

One of the technical limitations of transcranial ultrasonography is the inability to visualise brain structures of interest in patients who have an inadequate temporal bone acoustic window.

The average incidence of temporal acoustic window failure in the included studies was 19.7%, which led to false negative results in a number of cases [27]. Notably, in the study by Matsumoto et al. [31], the majority of patients were Asian, and there was a higher reported rate of temporal window failure of 56.3% of cases (27/48).

Risk of bias assessment across studies

Since only seven papers presented study results reporting quantitative values of the diagnostic accuracy of the test, publication bias assessment illustrating the possibility of selective publication of small studies with positive results was not performed.

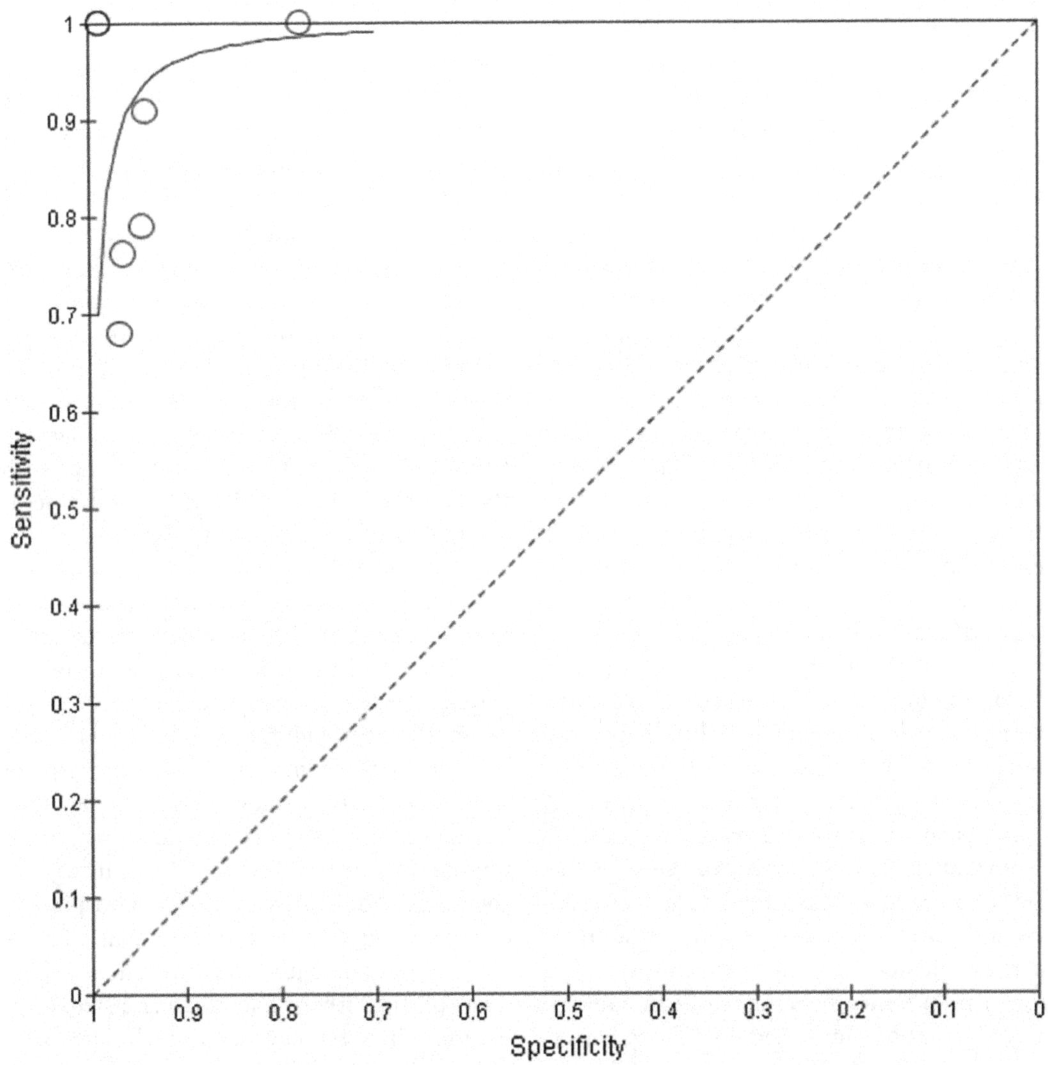

Fig. 3 Summary receiver operating characteristic plot. Each circle represents the sensitivity and specificity estimate from one study

Discussion

There is a substantial number of published diagnostic accuracy evaluations of transcranial ultrasonography in acute stroke population. 27 English-language studies that compared ultrasonography with other conventional imaging tools within 72 h of stroke symptom onset and with not more than 24 h' time difference between the index and reference tests were identified.

Different types of transcranial ultrasonography were used in the studies selected for the final analysis. TCD appeared to be the most commonly employed techniques, which could be explained by the fact that more than 80% of the papers aimed to evaluate cerebral blood flow and to detect signs of acute occlusion and/or stenosis.

Seventeen studies included in the current review evaluated diagnostic value of TCD in identifying patients with acute vessel occlusion. Thus, absent or diminished Doppler signal in the MCA mainstem is suggestive of its occlusion [38]. Asymmetry index equal or higher than 21% is considered indicative of a large branch or multiple branch occlusion. It is less likely to be of diagnostic value in lacunar stroke cases as blood flow abnormalities caused by MCA terminal branch occlusion might not be detected with TCD [21, 29, 47]. A finding of hyperechoic MCA signal is comparable to a hyperdense MCA on CT and suggestive of a large vessel occlusion [43].

The sensitivity and specificity for detecting steno-occlusive lesions in cerebral arteries were 68–100% and 78–99%, respectively, with the highest specificity for MCA lesions. These findings could potentially be used for the selection of subjects with LVO for direct transfer to an endovascular centre. Its application for detection of distal MCA stenosis [46] and steno-occlusive lesions in the posterior cerebral circulation is, however, limited.

This might be explained by a suboptimal angle of insonation which may lead to ambiguous findings [23, 24, 29, 33, 38]. This limitation can be potentially overcome by obtaining angle-corrected flow velocities [24].

There was a significant variation in diagnostic criteria used to detect acute steno-occlusive lesions. The lack of any approved diagnostic protocol for assessing cerebral artery occlusion and stenosis represents a big challenge as the results of studies are not absolutely compatible. There are a few recognised limitations of TCD, such as an inability to visualise anatomical landmarks, and as a consequence, a risk of inaccurate classification of specific blood vessels. Identification of blood vessels usually proceeds on the basis of indirect parameters, in particular: depth of insonation, flow direction and transducer orientation and position.

Differentiation between haemorrhagic and ischemic stroke is an important step in determining patient pathways. Transcranial ultrasonography can be used in some cases to detect intraparenchymal bleeds located in the brain structures that can be easily visualised with ultrasonographic examination, such as the basal ganglia. However, imaging of cortical regions, specifically frontal and parietal lobes, is largely restricted by the low spatial resolution of transcranial ultrasonography in these areas. It has also been reported that trace amounts of blood in the ventricular system may be missed, specifically in the occipital horn of the lateral ventricle [17]. Furthermore, some pathological lesions within the brain structures, such as calcifications, tumours, and vascular malformation can mimic the appearance of intracranial haemorrhage, and therefore may lead to false positive ultrasonographic findings [44, 48]. Midline shift might be used as an indirect parameter suggestive of increased intracranial pressure due to space-occupying stroke lesion [26, 42].

Our search also did not identify any eligible papers assessing diagnostic accuracy of transcranial ultrasonography in detecting signs of spontaneous SAH that have been described elsewhere as a hyperechogenic signal in the basal cisterns [49]. Studies evaluating diagnostic accuracy of transcranial ultrasonography for the detection of vasospasm after SAH were excluded from the current review.

Transcranial ultrasound is a simple, non-invasive and affordable diagnostic tool that can be repeated as many times as required at the patient's bedside and in space-restricted environments, such as ambulances [31, 44, 50, 51]. It takes on average 4.3–13.6 min for the complete examination of cerebral vessels [27, 41]. It can provide useful information complementary to clinical assessment, serving as a "stethoscope for the brain" [28]. A fast-track protocol for contrast-enhanced duplex ultrasound assessment in the Emergency Department has been suggested by Connolly et al. [52]. They demonstrated that the mean time to complete the ultrasound examination reduced on average by 1 min 46 s if performed by more experienced sonographers. As demonstrated previously [50, 51, 53], transcranial ultrasound images can be transferred for expert interpretation from remotely supported ambulances in remote and rural areas.

There are, however, a few limitations that restrict its use from being more widespread: namely the operator-dependent nature of interpretation, and the possibility of patients having inadequate temporal acoustic windows. Temporal bone acoustic window failure has been reported in 8–29% of the general population, and is more commonly seen in women over the age of 50 years and the Asian population [54, 55]. Contrast-enhanced transcranial ultrasonography may be considered as a possible solution, since it has been shown to provide a better visualisation compared with non-enhanced examination [41]. Further research is required for technique optimization of transcranial ultrasonography with the potential application of lower frequency, which may provide greater penetration through the skull into the brain.

Early definitive imaging in patients suspected of having suffered an acute stroke is desirable. However, rapid performance of a CT or angiography is unrealistic in many remote regions of the world requiring expensive and sometimes hazardous transfers to hospital. The gathered evidence suggests that transcranial ultrasound assessment alone currently does not allow an accurate diagnosis particularly in haemorrhagic stroke cases which is the main requirement for this technique to be used in the reliable pre-hospital triage process. However, its diagnostic accuracy might be improved by adding clinical assessment [5] to justify transfer to hospital associated with high costs and risks.

Limitations and bias

Given the highly specific nature of the literature search, almost all of the relevant literature available is believed to have been retrieved. However, papers in languages other than English were not included. Some papers reporting negative results in their evaluation of diagnostic accuracy of transcranial ultrasonography in acute stroke were not included, since they did not meet our inclusion criteria [18, 56]. Thus, Kamal et al. [18] studied cerebral artery stenosis in stroke patients from a South Asian population, and concluded that TCD has poor sensitivity for detection of arterial stenosis when compared to MRA. This study was not included in the qualitative analysis because of the unclear time interval between stroke onset and examinations and between index and reference tests. Suwanwela et al. [56] reported that TCD should not be used as a screening tool for identifying stenotic lesions in MCA territory stroke since a normal TCD examination does not exclude stenosis of the distal MCA branches. This paper was excluded from the final analysis as the time interval between TCD and CTA could exceed 24 h. However, none of the above studies reported findings that would contradict the results of the other reviewed papers.

Three studies that employed case–control methodology to compare transcranial ultrasound findings in patients with acute stroke and a healthy age-matched population were identified. Case–control studies have been shown to report two- or threefold higher estimates of diagnostic accuracy when compared to single series studies (spectrum bias) [57].

Most of the studies were relatively small, with the number of recruited patients being less than 100, and all were conducted in in-hospital settings. This might indicate potential selection bias. The present systematic review was not restricted to studies recruiting consecutive participants, however, a protocol which allows researchers to select individuals for inclusion in the study may also have selection bias.

One source of potential biases in the methodology relating to the reference test involved lack of blinding of investigators performing or interpreting results. This might affect the interpretation of the results potentially leading to either over- or underestimated performance of the reference test.

A time interval of not more than 24 h between the index and reference imaging to ensure minimal discrepancy between studies due to evolution of changes as a result of hypoxia or thrombus propagation, dissolution, or reocclusion [28, 38] was one of the inclusion criteria for the present systematic review. Therefore, this source of bias was not identified in any of the papers. However, the timing of the diagnostic tests was often not specifically reported as within 24 h but, for instance, "on admission".

Some potential biases were identified indicated by inconsistent reporting of important methodological details, such as level of expertise of the person performing the investigation with transcranial ultrasonography and blindness of investigators performing and/or interpreting reference and index tests. In the majority of the studies, ultrasonography investigation was performed by a specialist, reducing the risk of potential diagnostic bias in these cases. It is important to ensure that operators performing or interpreting transcranial ultrasound scans have specialist knowledge and adequate experience in the field if their assessment results are to be used to guide management of acute stroke patients. Inexperienced transcranial ultrasound users might potentially misinterpret findings leading to higher rates of false results and consequent wrong management decisions.

It appears that in most studies the index and reference tests were interpreted independently, without knowledge of the other's findings. About 37% (10/27) of reviewed studies included fewer than 80% of the participants in the analysis of outcomes and results which may introduce bias in the studies if there is some systematic difference between the excluded participants and those included in the final analysis.

In some studies, several imaging modalities were used as reference tests [21, 25, 27, 39]. The choice of imaging modality in acute stroke is guided by different factors, including suspected type of stroke, the time from symptom onset, contraindications for specific diagnostic tool, etc. However, such variability across the study population might lead to misinterpretation of the diagnostic accuracy of the index test.

Currently, a sector (cardiac) probe is most commonly used for the purposes of transcranial ultrasonography, since it has a small footprint and allows scanning at low frequency (2–4 MHz). However, it does not allow a continuous satisfactory visualisation of brain structures within the acoustic window during the scanning due to its poor conformity with temporal bone anatomy. Future work is needed to develop a probe that would be anatomically suitable specifically for transcranial scanning and allows imaging at angles that would allow better coverage of the brain.

Conclusions

This systematic review demonstrates that transcranial ultrasonography might potentially be used for the selection of subjects with acute LVO, to help streamline patient care and allow direct transfer to specialised endovascular centres. It can also assist in detecting haemorrhagic lesions in some cases, however, its applicability here is largely restricted. Further work is needed to establish a formal diagnostic protocol and criteria for detecting signs of acute stroke, to ensure consistency in reporting results. Additional research should optimize the scanning technique at lower frequency with potential for construction of a dedicated probe that would be compatible with anatomical shape of the temporal bone windows. Future work is also required to demonstrate whether this diagnostic approach, possibly combined with clinical assessment, could be used at the pre-hospital stage to justify direct transfer to a regional thrombectomy centre in suitable cases.

Supplementary information

Additional file 1. Search strategy.

Additional file 2. Criteria for the diagnosis of arterial stenosis in individual studies.

Additional file 3. Criteria for the diagnosis of arterial occlusion in individual studies.

Additional file 4. The accuracy parameters of transcranial ultrasonography for detecting cerebral arterial stenosis or occlusion in individual studies.

Abbreviations

CT: computed tomography; CTA: computed tomography angiography; DSA: digital subtraction angiography; FN: false negative value; FP: false positive value; LVO: large vessel occlusion; MCA: middle cerebral artery; MRA: magnetic resonance angiography; MRI: magnetic resonance imaging; MT: mechanical thrombectomy; SAH: subarachnoid haemorrhage; SROC: summary receiver operating characteristics; TCD: transcranial Doppler sonography; TN: true negative value; TP: true positive value.

Acknowledgements

This work is part of a Ph.D. project supported by the University of Aberdeen's Elphinstone Scholarship Programme. LE's work was funded by the European Space Agency SatCare grant. The authors would like to thank Dr. Lorenzo Bandieri for the help with assessing full text of articles for eligibility for the current review.

Authors' contributions

All four authors were involved in the conceptualisation and development of the methodology. DA performed a complete literature search. Assessment of full text of articles for eligibility and data extraction was performed by DA and LE. DA performed a formal analysis of the collected data and writing of the original draft (including all tables and figures). DA finalised all drafts in consultation with LE, AM and PW. LE, AM and PW reviewed the manuscript. All authors read and approved the final manuscript.

Glossary

Transcranial brightness mode (b-mode) sonography	Application of low-frequency ultrasound wave through a thin skull bone to enable a grey-scale visualisation of cerebral structures [58].
Transcranial Doppler sonography (TCD)	A pulsed Doppler system with low transmitter frequency for recording blood flow velocities from basal cerebral arteries on the basis of indirect parameters: the depth of the sample volume, the position of the transducer, and the flow direction [59].
Transcranial colour-coded duplex sonography (TCCS)	A method of ultrasonography that enables the visualisation of the basal cerebral arteries by colour coding of blood flow velocity; a combination of b-mode and Doppler ultrasonography [58].

Author details

[1] Centre for Rural Health, University of Aberdeen, Old Perth Road, Inverness IV2 3JH, UK. [2] Department of Stroke and Rehabilitation Medicine, Raigmore Hospital, NHS Highland, Inverness IV2 3UJ, UK.

References

1. Adamson J, Beswick A, Ebrahim S (2004) Is stroke the most common cause of disability? J Stroke Cerebrovasc Dis 13:171–177
2. Goyal M, Menon BK, van Zwam WH, Dippel DWJ, Mitchell PJ, Demchuk AM et al (2016) Endovascular thrombectomy after large-vessel ischaemic stroke: a meta-analysis of individual patient data from five randomised trials. Lancet 387:1723–1731
3. Saver JL, Goyal M, van der Lugt A, Menon BK, Majoie CBLM, Dippel DW et al (2016) Time to treatment with endovascular thrombectomy and outcomes from ischemic stroke: a meta-analysis. JAMA 316:1279–1288
4. Saver JL, Fonarow GC, Smith EE, Reeves MJ, Grau-Sepulveda MV, Pan W et al (2013) Time to treatment with intravenous tissue plasminogen activator and outcome from acute ischemic stroke. JAMA 309:2480–2488
5. Turc G, Maier B, Naggara O, Seners P, Isabel C, Tisserand M et al (2016) Clinical scales do not reliably identify acute ischemic stroke patients with large-artery occlusion. Stroke 47:1466–1472
6. Martinez-Sanchez P, Serena J, Alexandrov AV, Fuentes B, Fernandez-Dominguez J, Diez-Tejedor E (2009) Update on ultrasound techniques for the diagnosis of cerebral ischemia. Cerebrovasc Dis 27(Suppl 1):9–18
7. Whiting PF, Rutjes AWS, Westwood ME, Mallett S, Deeks JJ, Reitsma JB et al (2011) QUADAS-2: a revised tool for the quality assessment of diagnostic accuracy studies. Ann Intern Med 155:529–536
8. Macaskill P, Gatsonis C, Deeks JJ, Harbord RM, Takwoingi Y (2013) Chapter 10: Analysing and presenting results. In: Deeks JJ, Bossuyt PM, Gatsonis C (eds) Cochrane handbook for systematic reviews of diagnostic test accuracy Version 100. The Cochrane Collaboration. https://srdta.cochrane.org
9. Schlachetzki F, Herzberg M, Holscher T, Ertl M, Zimmermann M, Ittner KP et al (2012) Transcranial ultrasound from diagnosis to early stroke treatment: part 2: prehospital neurosonography in patients with acute stroke: the Regensburg stroke mobile project. Cerebrovasc Dis 33:262–271
10. Saqqur M, Hill MD, Alexandrov AV, Roy J, Schebel M, Krol A et al (2006) Derivation of power M-mode transcranial Doppler criteria for angiographic proven MCA occlusion. J Neuroimaging 16:323–328
11. Ogata T, Kimura K, Nakajima M, Naritomi H, Minematsu K (2005) Diagnosis of middle cerebral artery occlusive lesions with contrast-enhanced transcranial color-coded real-time sonography in acute stroke. Neuroradiology 47:256–262
12. Motuel J, Biette I, Srairi M, Mrozek S, Kurrek MM, Chaynes P et al (2014) Assessment of brain midline shift using sonography in neurosurgical ICU patients. Crit Care 18:676
13. Herzberg M, Boy S, Holscher T, Ertl M, Zimmermann M, Ittner K-P et al (2014) Prehospital stroke diagnostics based on neurological examination and transcranial ultrasound. Crit Ultrasound J 6:3
14. de Bray JM, Missoum A, Dubas F, Emile J, Lhoste P (1997) Detection of vertebrobasilar intracranial stenoses: transcranial Doppler sonography versus angiography. J Ultrasound Med 16:213–218
15. Bertram M, Khoja W, Ringleb P, Schwab S (2000) Transcranial colour-coded sonography for the bedside evaluation of mass effect after stroke. Eur J Neurol 7:639–646
16. Alexandrov AV, Bladin CF, Norris JW (1994) Intracranial blood flow velocities in acute ischemic stroke. Stroke 25:1378–1383
17. Mäurer M, Shambal S, Berg D, Woydt M, Hofmann E, Georgiadis D et al (1998) Differentiation between intracerebral hemorrhage and ischemic stroke by transcranial color-coded duplex-sonography. Stroke 29:2563–2567
18. Kamal AK, Rehman H, Mustafa N, Ahmed B, Jan M, Wadivalla F et al (2015) Diagnostic TCD for intracranial stenosis in acute stroke patients: experience from a tertiary care stroke center in Karachi, Pakistan. BMC Res Notes 8:341
19. Akopov S, Whitman GT (2002) Hemodynamic studies in early ischemic stroke: serial transcranial Doppler and magnetic resonance angiography evaluation. Stroke 33:1274–1279
20. Panerai RB, Jara JL, Saeed NP, Horsfield MA, Robinson TG (2016) Dynamic cerebral autoregulation following acute ischaemic stroke: comparison of transcranial Doppler and magnetic resonance imaging techniques. J Cereb Blood Flow Metab 36:2194–2202
21. Viola S, Tenaglia MG, De Leonardis E, Aquilone L, Gambi D (1993) Acute hemispheric stroke: correlation between three-dimensional transcranial Doppler, MR-angiography, CT and clinical findings. Ital J Neurol Sci 14:225–232

22. Meader N, King K, Llewellyn A, Norman G, Brown J, Rodgers M et al (2014) A checklist designed to aid consistency and reproducibility of GRADE assessments: development and pilot validation. Syst Rev 3:82
23. Bar M, Skoloudik D, Roubec M, Hradilek P, Chmelova J, Czerny D et al (2010) Transcranial duplex sonography and CT angiography in acute stroke patients. J Neuroimaging 20:240–245
24. Boddu DB, Sharma VK, Bandaru VCSS, Jyotsna Y, Padmaja D, Suvarna A et al (2011) Validation of transcranial Doppler with magnetic resonance angiography in acute cerebral ischemia. J Neuroimaging 21:e34–e40
25. Brunser AM, Lavados PM, Hoppe A, Lopez J, Valenzuela M, Rivas R (2009) Accuracy of transcranial Doppler compared with CT angiography in diagnosing arterial obstructions in acute ischemic strokes. Stroke 40:2037–2041
26. Gerriets T, Stolz E, Konig S, Babacan S, Fiss I, Jauss M et al (2001) Sonographic monitoring of midline shift in space-occupying stroke: an early outcome predictor. Stroke 32:442–447
27. Gerriets T, Goertler M, Stolz E, Postert T, Sliwka U, Schlachetzki F et al (2002) Feasibility and validity of transcranial duplex sonography in patients with acute stroke. J Neurol Neurosurg Psychiatry 73:17–20
28. Guan J, Zhou Q, Ouyang H, Zhang S, Lu Z (2013) The diagnostic accuracy of TCD for intracranial arterial stenosis/occlusion in patients with acute ischemic stroke: the importance of time interval between detection of TCD and CTA. Neurol Res 35:930–936
29. Kenton AR, Martin PJ, Abbott RJ, Moody AR (1997) Comparison of transcranial color-coded sonography and magnetic resonance angiography in acute stroke. Stroke 28:1601–1606
30. Kern R, Kablau M, Sallustio F, Fatar M, Stroick M, Hennerici MG et al (2008) Improved detection of intracerebral hemorrhage with transcranial ultrasound perfusion imaging. Cerebrovasc Dis 26:277–283
31. Matsumoto N, Kimura K, Iguchi Y, Aoki J (2011) Evaluation of cerebral hemorrhage volume using transcranial color-coded duplex sonography. J Neuroimaging 21:355–358
32. Nasr N, Ssi-Yan-Kai G, Guidolin B, Bonneville F, Larrue V (2013) Transcranial color-coded sonography to predict recurrent transient ischaemic attack/stroke. Eur J Neurol 20:1212–1217
33. Rathakrishnan R, Berne YI, Quek KK, Hong CS, Ong BK, Chan BP et al (2008) Validation of transcranial Doppler with CT angiography in cerebral ischaemia: a preliminary pilot study in Singapore. Ann Acad Med Singapore 37:402–405
34. Seidel G, Cangur H, Albers T, Meyer-Wiethe K (2005) Transcranial sonographic monitoring of hemorrhagic transformation in patients with acute middle cerebral artery infarction. J Neuroimaging 15:326–330
35. Seidel G, Cangur H, Albers T, Burgemeister A, Meyer-Wiethe K (2009) Sonographic evaluation of hemorrhagic transformation and arterial recanalization in acute hemispheric ischemic stroke. Stroke 40:119–123
36. Stolz E, Gerriets T, Fiss I, Babacan SS, Seidel G, Kaps M (1999) Comparison of transcranial color-coded duplex sonography and cranial CT measurements for determining third ventricle midline shift in space-occupying stroke. Am J Neuroradiol 20:1567–1571
37. Tang SC, Huang SJ, Jeng JS, Yip PK (2006) Third ventricle midline shift due to spontaneous supratentorial intracerebral hemorrhage evaluated by transcranial color-coded sonography. J Ultrasound Med 25:203–209
38. Tsivgoulis G, Sharma VK, Lao AY, Malkoff MD, Alexandrov AV (2007) Validation of transcranial Doppler with computed tomography angiography in acute cerebral ischemia. Stroke 38:1245–1249
39. Tsivgoulis G, Sharma VK, Hoover SL, Lao AY, Ardelt AA, Malkoff MD et al (2008) Applications and advantages of power motion-mode Doppler in acute posterior circulation cerebral ischemia. Stroke 39:1197–1204
40. Wada K, Kimura K, Minematsu K, Yasaka M, Uchino M, Yamaguchi T (2002) Combined carotid and transcranial color-coded sonography in acute ischemic stroke. Eur J Ultrasound 15:101–108
41. Goertler M, Kross R, Baeumer M, Jost S, Grote R, Weber S et al (1998) Diagnostic impact and prognostic relevance of early contrast-enhanced transcranial color-coded duplex sonography in acute stroke. Stroke 29:955–962
42. Ovesen C, Christensen AF, Krieger DW, Rosenbaum S, Havsteen I, Christensen H (2014) Time course of early postadmission hematoma expansion in spontaneous intracerebral hemorrhage. Stroke 45:994–999
43. Kadimi S, Terry JB, Gomez CR (2000) Hyperechoic middle cerebral artery: acute occlusion detected by transcranial duplex ultrasonography. J Neuroimaging 10:228–230
44. Kukulska-Pawluczuk B, Ksiazkiewicz B, Nowaczewska M (2012) Imaging of spontaneous intracerebral hemorrhages by means of transcranial color-coded sonography. Eur J Radiol 81:1253–1258
45. Leanyvari Z, Vastagh I, Fulesdi B, Szirmai I, Lengyel A, Csiba L et al (2002) Computed tomographic and transcranial Doppler sonographic findings in acute and subacute phases of middle cerebral artery strokes. J Clin Ultrasound 30:33–37
46. Zubkov AY, Uschmann H, Rabinstein AA (2008) Rate of arterial occlusion in patients with acute ischemic stroke. Neurol Res 30:835–838
47. Zanette EM, Fieschi C, Bozzao L, Roberti C, Toni D, Argentino C et al (1989) Comparison of cerebral angiography and transcranial Doppler sonography in acute stroke. Stroke 20:899–903
48. Seidel G, Gerriets T, Kaps M, Missler U (1996) Dislocation of the third ventricle due to space-occupying stroke evaluated by transcranial duplex sonography. J Neuroimaging 6:227–230
49. Olatunji RB, Ogbole GI, Atalabi OM, Adeyinka AO, Lagunju I, Oyinlade A et al (2015) Role of transcranial colour-coded duplex sonography in stroke management—review article. West African J Ultrasound 16:33–42
50. Eadie L, Mulhern J, Regan L, Mort A, Shannon H, Macaden A et al (2018) Remotely supported prehospital ultrasound: a feasibility study of real-time image transmission and expert guidance to aid diagnosis in remote and rural communities. J Telemed Telecare 24:616–622
51. Eadie L, Regan L, Mort A, Shannon H, Walker J, MacAden A et al (2015) Telestroke assessment on the move: prehospital streamlining of patient pathways. Stroke 46:e38–e40
52. Connolly F, Rohl J-E, Guthke C, Wengert O, Valdueza JM, Schreiber SJ (2019) Emergency room use of "fast-track" ultrasound in acute stroke: an observational study. Ultrasound Med Biol 45:1103–1111
53. Mort A, Eadie L, Regan L, Macaden A, Heaney D, Bouamrane MM et al (2016) Combining transcranial ultrasound with intelligent communication methods to enhance the remote assessment and management of stroke patients: framework for a technology demonstrator. Health Inform J 22:691–701
54. Maeda H, Matsumoto M, Handa N, Hougaku H, Ogawa S, Itoh T et al (1993) Reactivity of cerebral blood flow to carbon dioxide in various types of ischemic cerebrovascular disease: evaluation by the transcranial Doppler method. Stroke 24:670–675
55. Marinoni M, Ginanneschi A, Forleo P, Amaducci L (1997) Technical limits in transcranial Doppler recording: inadequate acoustic windows. Ultrasound Med Biol 23:1275–1277
56. Suwanwela NC, Suwanwela N, Phanthumchinda K (2000) Comparison of transcranial Doppler ultrasound and computed tomography angiography in symptomatic middle cerebral artery stenosis. Australas Radiol 44:174–177
57. Whiting P, Rutjes AWS, Reitsma JB, Glas AS, Bossuyt PMM, Kleijnen J (2004) Sources of variation and bias in studies of diagnostic accuracy: a systematic review. Ann Intern Med 140:189–202
58. Bartels E (2012) Transcranial color-coded duplex ultrasonography in routine cerebrovascular diagnostics. Perspect Med 1–12:325–330
59. Arnolds BJ, von Reutern G-M (1986) Transcranial Dopplersonography. Examination technique and normal reference values. Ultrasound Med Biol 12:115–123

25

Factors affecting perception of the normal pediatric appendix on sonography

Denise Castro[1], Joseph Yang[2*], Prasan Patel[1], Eric Sauerbrei[1], Wilma Hopman[3], Mila Kolar[4] and Don Soboleski[1]

Abstract

Background: To determine if an inherent perception skill along with sonographer experience, knowledge base, scanning time play a role in the identification of the normal appendix in the pediatric population. This is a retrospective review of pediatric (< 18 years old) patients with a clinical suspicion of acute appendicitis presenting to the emergency department of two affiliated academic tertiary care hospitals over a 1-year time span. All patients had a sonogram performed by 1/15 sonographers or by 1/8 on-call radiology residents. Those with a normal or non-visualized appendix with subsequent discharge from ER were included in the study. Patient demographics, minutes spent scanning, and sonographer years of experience in general abdominal scanning and residents level of training were recorded.

Results: Of the 127 patients included in the study, 51 (40%) were male and 76 (60%) were female, with a mean age of 11.8 ± 4.2 years. Sonographers who failed to see a normal appendix had less experience (median 8 years) than those who did visualize the appendix (median 15 years), $p \leq 0.001$. Longer time spent scanning was also associated with visualizing a normal appendix (20.4 versus 29.1 min, $p = 0.001$). In multivariable logistic regression, more time spent scanning (OR 1.04, 95% CI 1.01, 1.07, $p = 0.012$) and increased sonographer experience (OR 1.07, 95% CI 1.02, 1.13, $p = 0.012$) resulted in greater odds of perceiving the appendix. The top 4 were significantly more likely to visualize the appendix (88.0%) than all of the other combined (20.8%, $p < 0.001$), and they also had substantially more experience (median 15 years versus 8 years, $p < 0.001$). Overall, sonographers were more likely to see a normal appendix (61%) than the residents (14%), $p < 0.001$.

Conclusion: Sonography to rule out appendicitis in the pediatric patient is in general most successful when performed by experienced sonographers with adequate time to perform the scan. Triaging patients to those sonographers who have displayed optimal perceptual ability of the normal appendix may help optimize patient care and hospital resources. Having experienced sonographers available after hours would allow for optimal care in the setting of 'query' appendicitis.

Keywords: Appendicitis, Sonographer experience, Pediatric, Perception skills, Radiology residents

Background

Recognition of diagnostic error and more specifically perception error remains a significant challenge in radiologic practice with the overall prevalence appearing unchanged from the first estimates by Garland in 1949 [1–4]. The process of image interpretation is based on individual complex psychophysiological and cognitive activities not readily observable and subject to a wide variety of error types [5–7]. Studies investigating cognitive and systemic factors contributing to diagnostic error have mostly been focused on assessment of missed breast or lung nodules. Perception in sonography is fundamentally different than the other modalities where images are

*Correspondence: jyang@qmed.ca
[2] Queen's School of Medicine, Queen's University, 80 Barrie Street, Kingston, ON K7L 3N6, Canada
Full list of author information is available at the end of the article

produced in a formatted nature and then later evaluated by the observer (passive perception). Ultrasound is performed in a less standardized way, requiring the most appropriate acoustic window to evaluate the region of concern. Image production requires the operator's perceptual skills while acquiring the images (active perception). The objective of this study was to determine if an inherent perception skill along with sonographer experience, knowledge base or scan time was associated with an imager's ability to perceive the normal pediatric appendix.

Materials and methods

Study population

This was a retrospective review of all pediatric patients (< 18 years) sent to the imaging department from the emergency room (ER) of two affiliated academic tertiary care hospitals over a 1-year time span to rule out appendicitis. This centre is a general tertiary care hospital with an embedded pediatric department. A further 1-year review limited to the cases performed by residents was undertaken to acquire more numbers. The sonographic study was performed by one of 15 general sonographers within the diagnostic imaging department or by one of 8 on-call radiology residents. The patients with positive findings for appendicitis or any other identifiable pathology with subsequent treatment were excluded from the database. Patients with a sonogram depicting a normal appendix with subsequent discharge from ER and normal follow-up were included in the study, as were those with an appendix not visualized on sonography with subsequent normal follow-up imaging (CT) and/or discharge from hospital with resolution of symptoms on follow-up. Cases in which there was a discrepancy in the sonographers or residents impression with the attending radiologist were also excluded.

Ultrasound equipment utilized

Scans were performed on Logic 9 Scanner (GE Medical Systems, Milwaukee, WI), employing a linear 6–15 MHz or convex 1–6 MHz transducer probe. The exams were targeted to the right lower quadrant and performed in a manner consistent with the typical techniques used including graded compression. The initials of the sonographer were used to identify the scanner and data findings extracted from the technical or resident note. The time taken to perform the scan was determined by the time noted on the first obtained image and the last obtained image.

Statistical analysis

A priori sample size calculations were not done, as this was a convenience sample of all eligible pediatric patients referred to imaging over a 1-year period. Data were collected in an Excel file and imported into IBM SPSS (version 25.0 for Windows, Armonk, New York, 2018) for statistical analysis. Data were initially analyzed descriptively, including frequencies and percentages for categorical data and means and standard deviations for continuous data. The Shapiro–Wilk test was used to assess the normality of the underlying distribution of continuous data. Comparisons of the groups with a normal or non-visualized appendix were made using Chi-square tests for categorical data and independent samples *t*-tests or Mann–Whitney U for continuous data. A multivariable logistic regression model was developed to assess the relative contributions of the variables that had a moderate association ($p < 0.15$) in univariate analysis, while also controlling for patient sex.

Results

The study group included a total of 127 pediatric patients who were sent to the imaging department over a 1-year time span with a clinical suspicion of acute appendicitis. Of these, 60 (47%) had a normal appendix (6 mm caliber or less with no adjacent inflammatory changes) visualized on sonography and 67 (53%) patients underwent sonography with the appendix not visualized. The population consisted of 76 female and 51 male patients. Table 1 outlines the association between scanner experience, amount of time spent scanning and resident level of training with the ability to perceive the normal appendix on sonography.

Table 1 Description of sample and univariate results

Characteristics	Normal appendix $N=60$	Appendix not visualized $N=67$	*p* value
Patient sex			
Male *n* (%)	27 (45.0)	24 (35.8)	0.292
Female *n* (%)	33 (55.0)	43 (64.2)	0.113
Patient age (mean ± SD)	12.5 ± 3.5	11.2 ± 4.7	0.001
US time in minutes (mean ± SD)	29.1 ± 15.5	20.4 ± 12.6	< 0.001
Experience in years (median, 25th and 75 percentile)	15 (9, 15)	8 (3, 14)	
Expertise			
Technician *n* (%)	54 (91.5)	35 (53.8)	< 0.001
Junior residents ≤ 3 *n* (%)	3 (5.1)	20 (30.8)	
Senior residents 4+ *n* (%)	2 (3.4)	10 (15.4)	

Numbers do not always add up to overall totals due to small amounts of missing data

p values are based on the Chi-square test (sex), independent samples *t*-test (patient age as continuous, US time in minutes) and the Mann–Whitney U (experience in years)

The sonographers who were unable to perceive the normal appendix had significantly less experience (median 8 years) than those who did visualize the normal appendix (median 15 years), $p<0.001$. The minutes spent performing the scan was significantly shorter for those where the appendix was not visualized (mean 20.4 ± 12.6 min) as compared to the time spent when able to perceive a normal appendix (mean 29.1 ± 15.5), $p=0.001$. These two variables were significantly and positively correlated; those with more scanning experience took more time to do the assessment ($r=0.310$, $p=0.001$).

Multivariable logistic regression (Table 2) demonstrated that increased minutes spent scanning was significantly associated with greater odds of perceiving the normal appendix (OR 1.04, 95% CI 1.01, 1.07, $p=0.012$). Increased sonographer experience was also significantly associated with greater odds of seeing the appendix (OR 1.07, 95% CI 1.02, 1.13, $p=0.012$). A patient of older age and male sex was also associated with greater odds, but failed to reach statistical significance ($p=0.43$ and $p=0.099$, respectively).

When comparing junior (PGY2/3) to senior radiology residents (PGY4/5), the junior residents were somewhat less successful in identifying the normal appendix (3/23 or 13.0% as compared to 2/10 or 16.7%); however, this was not statistically significant ($p=0.771$) in this small subset of 35 observations.

Independent of experience, there was a marked difference among the 15 sonographers in their ability to perceive the normal appendix. However, the large number of low-frequency cells in the descriptive table made the tests of significance invalid. Table 3 illustrates a comparison among the 4 sonographers with the highest success in perceiving the normal appendix, to the remainder of the sonographers and the residents in the study. The top 4 were significantly more likely to visualize the appendix (88.0%) than all of the other combined (20.8%, $p<0.001$), and also had considerably more years of experience (median 15 versus 8 years). Sonographers in general were more likely to see a normal appendix (60.7%) than the residents (14.0%, $p=0.001$).

Table 2 Multivariable logistic regression model (0 = not seen, 1 = visualized)

Model for pediatrics (age < 18)	Odds ratio (95% confidence interval)	*p* value
Age in years	1.04 (0.94, 1.15)	0.430
Patient sex (0 = male (ref), 1 = female)	0.50 (0.22, 1.14)	0.099
US time in minutes	1.04 (1.01, 1.07)	0.012
Experience in years	1.07 (1.02, 1.13)	0.012

Cox and Snell R-square = 0.17; overall model Chi-square = 22.0, $p<0.001$

Discussion

Diagnostic/perception error has been defined as a diagnosis that is missed, delayed or wrong as determined by a subsequent definitive test or finding. The lack of perception of a normal finding may also constitute a diagnostic error when clinically relevant. Initial work by Garland in 1949, who estimated an average radiology perception error rate of up to 30%, has led to extensive study in human perception and factors in perception error which, for the most part, remain poorly understood [4, 7, 8]. Increasing workloads, cognitive biases, systemic factors such as lighting, along with rising quality expectations are potential yet minor factors that contribute to perception error, often the result of mental or visual fatigue [1, 3, 5]. Attempts to improve error by work hour alterations, improved environmental setting such as decreased interruptions and changes in luminescence of monitors have had limited success [5].

Errors in imaging have been classified into two broad categories comprising errors in perception versus interpretive errors. Perception error accounts for 60–80% of radiologists errors in clinical practice. The majority lacks any identifiable cause [5, 9]. The persistence of investigative studies depicting the degree of perceptual error among imagers worldwide despite the level of training or experience and spanning multiple modalities would suggest that errors related to carelessness, negligence or underperformance of some kind are not the typical cause. Rather, there appears to be an inherent misperception or under perception associated with the complex process of image interpretation perhaps below the threshold of conscious awareness [5]. More recent studies have further defined perceptual error into three basic types. These include (1) scanning error—a failure to fixate on the

Table 3 Comparison of top 4 sonographers to all others

	Top 4 sonographers, $N=50$	All others, $N=77$	*p* value
US result appendix normal, *n* (%)	44 (88.0)	16 (20.8)	< 0.001
Appendix not visualized, *n* (%)	6 (12.0)	61 (79.2)	
Years of experience, median (25th, 75th percentile)	15 (9, 15)	8 (3, 14)	< 0.001

The *p* value is based on the Pearson Chi-square test and the Mann–Whitney U

adequate region; (2) recognition error—a fixation on the region but for inadequate time and (3) decision-making error—fixation on the appropriate region for adequate time, but an unexplained lack of recognition of pathology [3]. We believe that a lack of perception of a normal finding during the scanning process, rather than the usual lack of recognition on a set of provided images, that will alter patient care and management should be included in this third type.

Previous studies have shown the value of sonographer experience in patient diagnosis [10–12]. Our study hopes to also illustrate the role of an inherent perceptual skill that some sonographers display that can affect patient care. Missed and misinterpreted diagnosis in sonography are often too easily attributed to technical factors such as body habitus or overlying bowel gas. While these factors may limit an examination, the sonographer's ability to adequately perceive anatomic fascial planes in the region of concern will often determine the ultimate clinical value of the study. Intuitively, one would expect that increased experience (years of training) in scanning or increase in knowledge base (as one would expect the senior residents to have gained more imaging knowledge than the juniors) would correlate with an improved ability to perceive the normal appendix. We found this to be the case, as our junior residents demonstrated a lower ability to identify the normal appendix as compared to their more senior colleagues. Although in general, sonographers with more years of experience correlated with an increase in perceiving the normal appendix, within the group of experienced sonographers there was a wide discrepancy in frequency of perception of a normal appendix suggesting there may be an inherent individual perceptual skill. Just as some radiologists are able to more quickly spot the lung nodule on chest radiographs or the individual who is able to perceive "Waldo" more easily than others, we suggest that there are sonographers that find the normal appendix more easily than others [13].

Utilizing the "query" appendicitis ER population illustrates the potential clinical effect of this difference in sonographer perceptual skill. Demonstration of a normal appendix on sonography can, for the most part, eliminate this potentially dangerous disease process from the physician's list of concern, potentially saving the patient from further studies such as CT/MR and expediting patient care through the emergency department. Interestingly, if all the patients sent to the imaging department to rule out appendicitis could have been triaged to the four sonographers with the greatest success in perceiving the normal appendix, an additional 50 patients would have had their appendix visualized, and the overall percentage of cases where the appendix was not seen would drop from 52 to 12%. As such, it may be of benefit for less experienced sonographers to accompany sonographers who are more experienced to gain experience and technical skills in visualizing the appendix. Alternatively, this discrepancy in sonographer perceptual skill may suggest that triaging query appendicitis cases to a set of sonographers more adept than others may result in higher efficiency and a decrease in unnecessary further testing for the patient.

The study has multiple limitations which need to be acknowledged. We are a relative small center which resulted in variable and sometimes insufficient number of cases for adequate assessment of each sonographer and an overall small sample volume. The body mass index (BMI) was not utilized, which may affect the ability to see the appendix. As the patients were referred to the department without direction to a specific sonographer it was felt that over time the differences in BMI would likely equalize out among the scanners. Further limitations were a potential bias related to the sonographer choosing not to perform a 'query' appendicitis case deferring to a sonographer with more confidence if possible. In addition, the ability of the staff radiologists to perceive the normal appendix was not assessed. Given, we are at an academic center, the majority of the ER cases sent to the department were initially performed by the trained sonographers who then present the case to the radiology resident on service. The cases may not be reviewed initially by the staff unless a concern or question is raised by the resident. Additionally, the cases are often performed after hours with the resident on-call or available sonographer. It is possible that availability of staff radiologists may have improved detection of the normal appendix. Lastly, a further limitation was utilizing the initial sonography image recorded on the PACS images as the start of the exam as this may not take into account the full time the sonographer took to perform a "scout" scan before acquiring images.

Conclusion

Similar to previous studies involving mammography and chest imaging modalities, perception/diagnostic error in sonographic image acquisition and interpretation should be recognized. The lack of perception of a normal appendix has the potential to adversely affect patient care and resource allocation. Further research endeavors to better understand, train and test for individual differences in perception ability and the complex cognitive processes involved in image interpretation are needed. Triaging of patients and their related imaging to those sonographers who have displayed the optimal perceptual ability for the suspected disease process may help optimize patient care and hospital resources. Sonography of pediatric patients is most successful when performed by experienced sonographers with adequate allotted time for the study with a history of successful perception of the normal appendix. Having experienced sonographers available after hours would allow for optimal care in the setting of 'query' appendicitis.

Abbreviations
ER: emergency room; PGY: postgraduate year.

Acknowledgements
Not applicable.

Authors' contributions
DC and DS were responsible for developing the idea for this project and the steps required for data collection, and obtaining research ethics approval. JY, PP, ES, and MK were involved with data analysis and significant writing of the manuscript, and subsequent editing. WH was responsible for data analysis and drafting of the statistical models and results. All authors played a significant role in contribution towards the final manuscript draft and have approved of this submission. All authors read and approved the final manuscript.

Author details
[1] Department of Radiology, Kingston Health Sciences Centre, Queen's University, 76 Stuart Street, Kingston, ON K7L 2V7, Canada. [2] Queen's School of Medicine, Queen's University, 80 Barrie Street, Kingston, ON K7L 3N6, Canada. [3] WJ Henderson Centre for Patient Oriented Research, Queen's University, 76 Stuart Street, Kingston, ON K7L 2V7, Canada. [4] Department of Surgery, Kingston Health Sciences Centre, Queen's University, 76 Stuart Street, Kingston, ON K7L 2V7, Canada.

References
1. Lee CS, Nagy PG, Weaver SJ, Newman-Toker DE (2013) Cognitive and system factors contributing to diagnostic errors in radiology. AJR Am J Roentgenol 201:611–617
2. Krupinski EA (2000) The importance of perception research in medical imaging. Radiat Med 18:329–334
3. Pow RE, Mello-Thoms C, Brennan P (2016) Evaluation of the effect of double reporting on test accuracy in screening and diagnostic imaging studies: a review of the evidence. J Med Imaging Radiat Oncol 60:306–314
4. Garland LH (1949) On the scientific evaluation of diagnostic procedures. Radiology 52:309–328
5. Bruno MA, Walker EA, Abujudeh HH (2015) Understanding and confronting our mistakes: the epidemiology of error in radiology and strategies for error reduction. Radiographics 35:1668–1676
6. Provenzale JM, Kranz PG (2011) Understanding errors in diagnostic radiology: proposal of a classification scheme and application to emergency radiology. Emerg Radiol 18:403–408
7. Tourassi G, Voisin S, Paquit V, Krupinski E (2013) Investigating the link between radiologists' gaze, diagnostic decision, and image content. J Am Med Inform Assoc 20:1067–1075
8. Cochrane AL, Garland LH (1952) Observer error in the interpretation of chest films; an international investigation. Lancet 2:505–509
9. Pitman AG (2006) Perceptual error and the culture of open disclosure in Australian radiology. Australas Radiol 50:206–211
10. Lee JH, Jeong YK, Park KB, Park JK, Jeong AK, Hwang JC (2005) Operator-dependent techniques for graded compression sonography to detect the appendix and diagnose acute appendicitis. Am J Roentgenol 184(1):91–97
11. Tegnander E, Eik-Nes SH (2006) The examiner's ultrasound experience has a significant impact on the detection rate of congenital heart defects at the second-trimester fetal examination. Ultrasound Obstet Gynecol 28(1):8–14
12. O'Connor PJ, Rankine J, Gibbon WW, Richardson A, Winter F, Miller JH (2005) Interobserver variation in sonography of the painful shoulder. J Clin Ultrasound 33:53–56
13. Waite S, Grigorian A, Alexander RG, Macknik SL, Carrasco M, Jeeger DJ, Martinez-Conde S (2019) Analysis of perceptual expertise in radiology—current knowledge and a new perspective. Front Hum Neurosci 13:213

26

Transesophageal echocardiography (TEE) in cardiac arrest: results of a hands-on training for a simplified TEE protocol

Peiman Nazerian[1*], Giuliano De Stefano[1], Giovanni Albano[1], Vera Gaspari[1], Sergio Bevilacqua[2], Valter Campagnolo[2], Pierluigi Stefàno[3] and Stefano Grifoni[1]

Abstract

Background: Integration of transesophageal echocardiography (TEE) with Focused Cardiac Ultrasound (FoCUS) can impact decision-making, assist in the diagnosis of reversible etiologies and help guiding resuscitation of patients with cardiac arrest.

Objective: To evaluate the ability of emergency physicians (EPs) to obtain and maintain skills in performing resusTEE after a course with clinical training in the cardiac surgery theatre.

Methods: Ten EPs without previous TEE experience underwent a resusTEE course, based on a 2-h workshop and an 8-h hands-on training. The training was performed in a cardiac surgery theatre tutored by cardiovascular anesthesiologists. The six taught views were mid-esophageal four-chamber (ME4CH), mid-esophageal long axis (MELAX), mid-esophageal two-chamber (ME2CH), mid-esophageal bicaval view (MEbicaval), transgastric short axis (TGSAX) and aorta view (AOview). The EPs were evaluated by a cardiovascular anesthesiologist at the end of the course as well as after 12 weeks according to a standardized evaluation method. Once the course was completed, resusTEE exams, performed by EPs in Emergency Department (ED), were monitored for a 12-week period.

Results: The average assessment of the ten EPs by the tutors was higher than 4 points out of 5, both at the end of the course and after 12 weeks. Probe insertion, acquisition and interpretation of the different views scored on average more than 4 points out of 5 except for TGSAX that showed worsening after 12 weeks. Trainees performed twelve resusTEE exams in ED in patients with out-of-hospital cardiac arrest (OHCA) over 12 weeks after the course. EPs used only four out of six taught views in clinical practice, in the following order of frequency: ME4CH, AOview, MEbicaval and MELAX.

Conclusions: EPs, after a course with clinical training in the cardiac surgery theatre, can successfully acquire and maintain the skills needed to perform resusTEE. However, among the six views learned in the course, EPs used only four of them (ME4CH, MEbicaval, MELAX and AOview).

Keywords: Transesophageal echocardiography, Cardiocirculatory arrest, Emergency medicine, Emergency department, Resuscitation, Ultrasound, Training course

Background

Emergency physicians (EPs) routinely use Focused Cardiac Ultrasound (FoCUS) in the management of cardiac arrest. The European Resuscitation Council guidelines suggest integrating FoCUS into the advanced life support algorithm for the identification of potentially reversible

*Correspondence: pnazerian@hotmail.com
[1] Department of Emergency Medicine, Careggi University Hospital, Largo Brambilla 3, 50134 Florence, Firenze, Italy
Full list of author information is available at the end of the article

causes of cardiac arrest, pseudo-pulseless electrical activity (PEA), and to help the decision to interrupt cardiopulmonary resuscitation (CPR) [1]. However, an important limitation of FoCUS is the technical difficulty to obtain adequate cardiac windows in the few seconds available during the scheduled pauses in compressions performed for rhythm check. Common reasons for the poor acoustic windows obtained in cardiac arrest patients are insufflation of air into the stomach during pulmonary ventilation, and the presence of defibrillator pads, automated compression devices, and other monitoring equipment [2]. The aforementioned limitations of FoCUS could be overcome by adding other ultrasound views with transesophageal echocardiography (TEE) [3].

TEE offers several advantages in critical care because of the excellent acoustic window, due to the position of the TEE probe in the esophagus or stomach, very close to the heart [4, 5]. Additionally, TEE provides a better identification of aortic dissection [6] and can be used to guide cannulation for extracorporeal life support (ECLS) [7]. Furthermore, it can be performed during CPR without interrupting chest compressions, offering continuous support to improve CPR quality and to decide when to discontinue resuscitation [3, 8–10].

Although, only small, single-center observational studies have been published on the use of focus TEE in the ED [3, 11]. The American College of Emergency Physicians recommends the utilization of a simplified protocol of TEE (resuscitative TEE, resusTEE) including only few of the twenty-eight views needed for a comprehensive TEE examination [12, 13]. The best simplified institutional protocol of resus TEE and the methods of training needed for EPs to learn the technique should be defined before implementing the use of TEE in the ED.

TEE is rarely used in ED and it is performed in emergency situations, when teaching is often impossible; for these reasons, practical skills need to be learned outside ED. High-fidelity simulators have an important and well-known role in the learning of new skills and are currently used also for resusTEE training. Arntfield et al. evaluated the ability of EPs to acquire and maintain the skills required for performing TEE at 6 weeks after a course based on simulations [14]. However, TEE simulators have elevated costs and are available only in a few EDs. Clinical training performed in a "controlled" environment such as the cardiac surgery theatre could be an alternative option that still needs to be evaluated. In our institution, we have no simulator available for training. Therefore, we decided to implement resusTEE by training EPs in the cardiac surgery theatre.

The primary objective of this study was to evaluate the ability of EPs to acquire and maintain the skills to perform six views of resusTEE after a 10-h course based on a clinical training. As additional endpoint, we evaluated which views were used in clinical practice in ED, during the period of implementation of the technique.

Methods

ResusTEE course and protocol

The study was approved by the Regional Ethical Committee.

ResusTEE course was attended by ten EPs (six specialists and four residents) with at least 1 year of experience in FoCUS. The course was composed of 2 hours of formal lectures and 8 hours of a hands-on clinical training. The lectures included the review of basic TEE principles, indications and contraindications for TEE, demonstration of probe insertion and the technique needed to acquire six views of a simplified TEE protocol and to identify, through video loops, anatomic structures as well as the most common pathologic findings.

The clinical training was performed in three cardiac surgery operating rooms with cardiovascular anesthesiologists, certified as tutors in adult transesophageal echocardiography by the European Association of Cardiovascular Imaging. Each operating room was equipped with an ultrasound system provided with a 7.0-MHz TEE probe: SONOS 5500 (Phillips Medical Systems, Bothell, WA), iE33 (Philips, Andover, MA) and EPIQ 7(Philips, Andover, MA).

The tutor guided the trainees to acquire the manual and interpretive skills needed for the insertion of the probe, acquisition, and interpretation of six different TEE views. The trainees inserted the probe in patients scheduled for elective cardiac surgery, already intubated, under general anesthesia. TEE is routinely performed in such patients for monitoring purposes and to check the result of surgery. Therefore, patients were not subjected to any additional risk due to the teaching procedure and, since the same TEE views were used also for clinical purposes, the training did not interfere with the surgery.

ResusTEE protocol was composed of six sequential views: mid-esophageal four-chamber (ME4CH) (Fig. 1a–Additional file 1: video 1a), mid-esophageal long axis (MELAX) (Fig. 1b–Additional file 2: video 1b), mid-esophageal two-chamber (ME2CH) (Fig. 1c–Additional file 3: video 1c), mid-esophageal bicaval view (MEbicaval) (Fig. 1d–Additional file 4: video 1d), transgastric short axis (TGSAX) (Fig. 1e–Additional file 5: video 1e) and aorta view (AOview) (Fig. 1f–Additional file 6: video 1f) (Additional file). This protocol differed from the one proposed by the American College of Emergency Physicians because of the addition of three views (ME2CH, MEbicaval and AOview) [12] and from the protocol proposed by the University of Pennsylvania due to the addition of two views (ME2CH and AOview) [15].

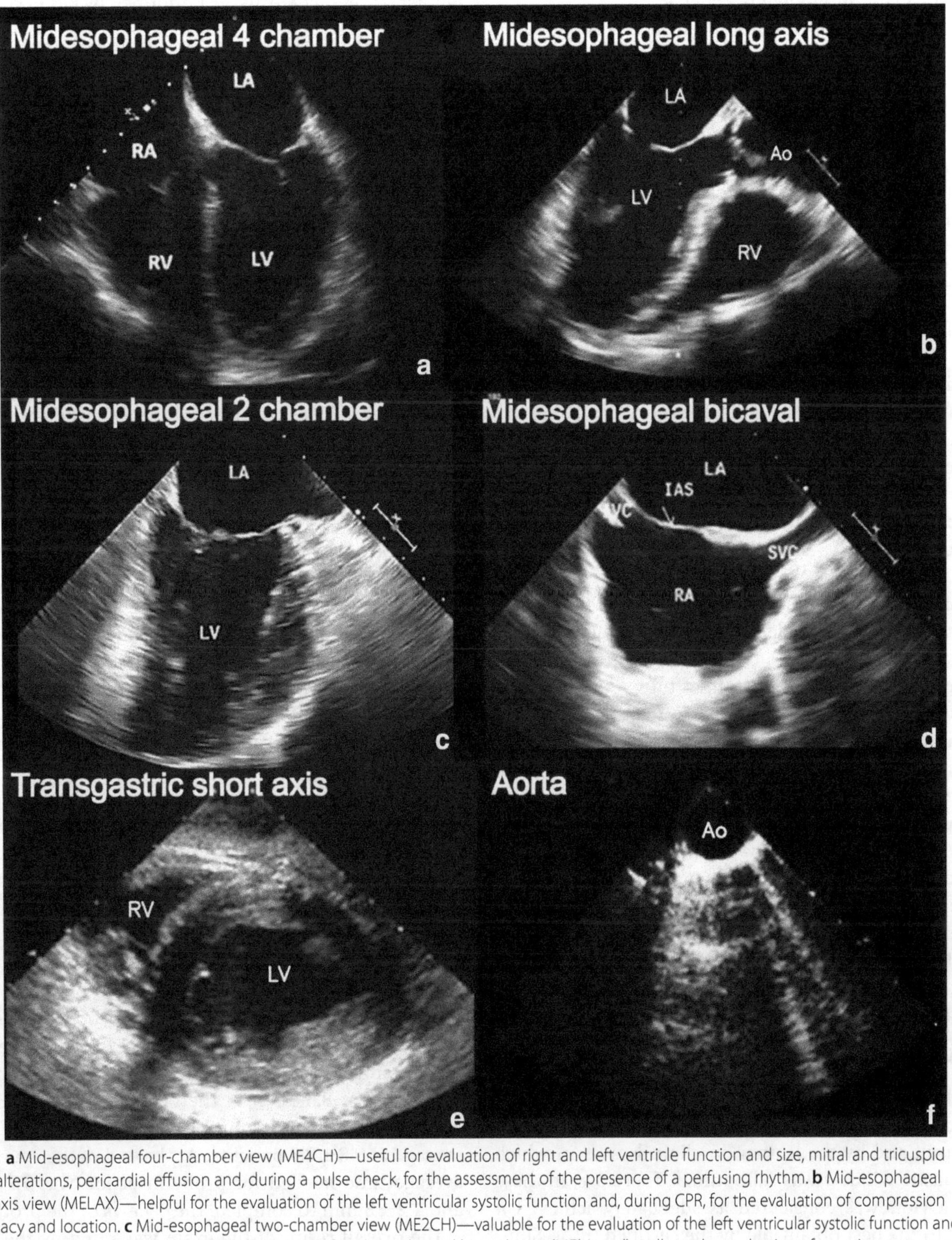

Fig. 1 **a** Mid-esophageal four-chamber view (ME4CH)—useful for evaluation of right and left ventricle function and size, mitral and tricuspid valve alterations, pericardial effusion and, during a pulse check, for the assessment of the presence of a perfusing rhythm. **b** Mid-esophageal long-axis view (MELAX)—helpful for the evaluation of the left ventricular systolic function and, during CPR, for the evaluation of compression adequacy and location. **c** Mid-esophageal two-chamber view (ME2CH)—valuable for the evaluation of the left ventricular systolic function and the regional motion of the anterior and inferior wall. **d** Mid-esophageal bicaval view (MEbicaval)—allows the evaluation of superior vena cava thrombus, catheters or venous cannula position (as for ECLS) and respiratory dimensions variations that can be related to volume status and fluid responsiveness. **e** Transgastric short-axis view (TGSAX)—provides information about pericardial effusion, left ventricle systolic function and regional wall motion abnormalities. **f** Aorta view (AOview)—useful for guiding vessel cannulation for ECLS and for the identification of aortic dissection/aneurysm involving the aortic arch and the descending thoracic aorta. *Ao* aorta, *IAS* interatrial septum, *IVC* inferior vena cava, *LA* left atrium, *LV* left ventricle, *RA* right atrium, *RV* right ventricle, *SVC* superior vena cava

Skill assessment throughout the course

During the practical training, the trainees were monitored and the effective hours in which they handled the probe, the number of exams performed, and the type and number of inspected pathological findings were registered. Furthermore, at the end of the training period, an observer medical student registered the time needed to insert the probe and to acquire the six views of the protocol. One of the two anesthesiologists rated the skills of the trainees. The same assessment was repeated after 2 h of hands-on retraining, 12 weeks after the completion of the course, to evaluate skills retention over time.

The skill assessment consisted of a practical exam, by which the technique of probe insertion, acquisition and interpretation of the six different views (ME4CH, ME2CH, MELAX, MEbicaval, TGSAX, AOview) were evaluated and rated separately. The tutors used a rating system (from 1 to 5) as follows: 1 = inadequate, 2 = insufficient, 3 = sufficient, 4 = good and 5 = excellent.

The insertion of the probe was assessed considering the quickness time required for insertion and taking into account the possible need for help from the tutor, according to the following scale: 1 = insertion failed; 2 = insertion achieved only with substantial tutor's intervention; 3 = insertion achieved in > 2 min; 4 = insertion achieved in > 1 and ≤ 2 min; 5 = insertion achieved in ≤ 1 min. The learner's ability to acquire each of the 6 views was also assessed on the basis of a similar evaluation scale previously published taking into account quickness the time required to obtain the view and the amount of help needed by the learner to reach the target [16]. This scale has been adapted on the basis of the aforementioned 5 skill levels according to the following scheme: 1 = image acquisition failed; 2 = image achieved only after substantial tutor's help; 3 = image achieved slowly but with small tutor instruction; 4 = image achieved slowly but without any tutor instruction; 5 = image obtained quickly and fluidly as part of a complete examination without any help from the tutor. To attribute the score, the tutor also took into account the objective difficulties encountered both by himself and by the learner, in clinical cases in which the acoustic window was suboptimal. Therefore, in these cases, a view was considered as adequately achieved if similar to the best obtainable by the certified tutor. Similarly, criteria to consider an adequately interpreted view (rating ≥ 3) were the confidence in the correct identification of all the anatomic structures and the completeness in the discussion of all the potential pathological conditions that could be identified by each view. In this regard, the tutor assigned a score ranking from 1 to 5 according to his personal experience and at his discretion.

Implementation of resusTEE performed by EPs in clinical practice

For 12 weeks, after the end of the course, we monitored the effective application of resusTEE performed by all the trainees in ED. Each one of the EPs trained in the course was involved in resuscitation in case of out-of-hospital cardiac arrest (OHCA) and the decision to perform a resusTEE in addition to FoCUS was decided by the resuscitation team leader. The FoCUS was already part of the standard management of OHCA in our ED and was always performed according to the European Resuscitation Council guidelines [1]. ResusTEE was performed by EPs, with the supervision of a cardiologist or an anesthesiologist, part of the resuscitation team, after patients' intubation, using a dedicated ultrasound machine (Vivid S5 ultrasound multiprobe machine provided with a GE 6Tc-RS TEE Probe, GE Healthcare, Wauwatosa, WI, USA), available in the shock room 24 h a day, 7 days a week. The time from the patient's arrival in the shock room to the successful probe insertion, the time needed to complete the TEE exam and the different views performed by EPs were recorded by a medical student. The resuscitation team leader completed a standardized form after having finished the clinical management. The form reported if resusTEE had led to a modification of the diagnosis made by FoCUS, when it suggested a shift of the site of chest compression during CPR, when it was used to guide vessel cannulations as well as for the interruption of CPR.

The results were presented as a percentage for dichotomous variables, as mean ± standard deviation for normally distributed variables. The analysis was conducted using Excel 15.30 (Office, Microsoft, United States of America).

Results

The ten trainees had 8.3 ± 6.2 years of experience in FoCUS, but none had any previous TEE experience.

All trainees participated in all the courses and each trainee spent 8.5 ± 3 h in the operating room, 6.8 ± 3 h effectively handling the probe and performed TEE in an average of 9.8 ± 2.9 patients. At the end of the course, the average time needed for probe insertion was 75 ± 42 s, and 4.2 ± 3 min to complete the 6 views of the protocol.

The overall result of the exam was rated by the tutors as "good to excellent" both at the end of the course (mean rating 4.8 ± 0.4) and after 12 weeks (mean rating 4.8 ± 0.6). The evaluation of the skill for the insertion of the probe, the acquisition and interpretation of the six views was rated by the tutors as "good to excellent" except for the transgastric short axis, that showed worsening of the acquisition ability after 12 weeks (Table 1).

Table 1 Probe insertion, acquisition, and interpretation of resusTEE views at the end of the course and after 12 weeks rated by tutors

Tutor's assessment	End of the course Mean ± SD	After 12 weeks Mean ± SD	Difference mean ± SD
Probe insertion	4.8 ± 0.4	4.7 ± 0.4	0.1 ± 0
Views acquisition			
Mid-esophageal four-chamber	4.8 ± 0.4	4.8 ± 0.6	0 ± 0.2
Mid-esophageal two-chamber	4.8 ± 0.4	4.9 ± 0.3	0.1 ± 0.1
Mid-esophageal long axis	4.8 ± 0.4	4.9 ± 0.3	0.1 ± 0.1
Mid-esophageal Bicaval view	4.7 ± 0,4	4.8 ± 0.6	0.1 ± 0.2
Aorta and aortic arch views	4.8 ± 0.4	4.8 ± 0.6	0 ± 0.2
Transgastric short axis	4.5 ± 0.7	3.7 ± 1.2	-0.8 ± 0.5
Color doppler images	4.8 ± 0.4	5	0.2 ± 0.4
Views interpretation			
Mid-esophageal four-chamber	4.8 ± 0.4	4.8 ± 0.6	0 ± 0.2
Mid-esophageal two-chamber	4.8 ± 0.4	4.9 ± 0.3	0.1 ± 0.1
Mid-esophageal long axis	4.8 ± 0.4	4.9 ± 0.3	0.1 ± 0.1
Mid-esophageal Bicaval view	4.8 ± 0.4	4.8 ± 0.6	0 ± 0.2
Aorta and aortic arch views	4.8 ± 0.4	4.8 ± 0.6	0 ± 0.2
Transgastric short axis	4.7 ± 0.4	4.2 ± 1.3	− 0.5 ± 0.9
Overall	4.8 ± 0.4	4.8 ± 0.6	0 ± 0.2

SD standard deviation

Table 2 ResusTEE operative findings during the hands-on training

ResusTEE operative findings	Frequency (number of occurrences)	Mean for each trainee ± SD
Reduced global left ventricular function	66	6.6 ± 4.8
Regional wall motion abnormalities	64	6.4 ± 4.9
Guidance of insertion of catheters	64	6.4 ± 4.9
Absence of cardiac motion	44	4.4 ± 3.2
Right ventricular dysfunction	26	2.6 ± 1.8
Pericardial effusion/tamponade	24	2.4 ± 1.7

Table 2 summarizes the number of different operative findings evaluated by trainees during the course in the cardiac surgery theatre.

During the 12 weeks following the completion of the course, the ten trainees performed resusTEE in ED on twelve OHCA, intubated patients (1.2 ± 1.1 for each trainee). ResusTEE exams were performed on ten patients during RCP, while on the other two patients the exams were performed after the return of spontaneous circulation. In one patient with major thoracic trauma, although the probe was inserted, it was not possible to obtain any adequate view. Median time from the patient's arrival in the shock room to the probe insertion was 14.4 ± 13.18 min and the time needed to complete resusTEE exam was 4.2 ± 1.4 min. The most used views in order of occurrence were ME4CH, AOview, MEbicaval and MELAX while ME2CH and TGSAX views were not used.

In nine patients (81%), resusTEE confirmed the diagnosis obtained by FoCUS (5 cases of acute coronary syndrome, 1 case of pulmonary embolism, 1 case of septic shock, 2 cases of undetermined cardiac arrest); while in 2 cases (19%), it led to changes in diagnosis and management: one case of acute aortic dissection previously diagnosed as acute coronary syndrome (Additional file 7: video 2) and one case of cardiac tamponade unidentified by FoCUS, because of a poor acoustic window. Furthermore, resusTEE was of pivotal importance during resuscitation in 4 cases, in which it indicated to shift the selected site of compression for cardiac massage over the left ventricle, showing appropriate opening of the mitral and aortic valves. Additionally, it guided vascular cannulation for ECLS in six patients (Additional file 8: video 3) and led to the interruption of CPR in other 4 cases.

Discussion

Our study showed that EPs who attended a 2-h lectures and an 8-h hands-on clinical training in a cardiac surgery theatre can successfully acquire the skills needed to learn a simplified TEE protocol, and that these skills can be maintained after 12 weeks. A previous study on simulation training had showed similar results at the end of the course and after a shorter period (6 weeks) [14]. The perioperative environment is ideal to practice probe insertion and image acquisition because the patient is intubated under general anesthesia, and undergoes a long operation such as cardiac surgery. This is the reason why the time spent by the trainees effectively handing the probe was long in this study. Besides, trainees faced many different pathologic conditions and rapid changes in hemodynamics during the different phases of the cardiac surgical intervention. A potential disadvantage of this approach is the risk of mechanical injury from probe insertion and manipulation, given the employ of real patients for the training of clinicians who had no prior experience with this device, although we did not report any injury to patients during the training under the supervision of expert cardiovascular anesthesiologists. Another limitation is the lack of possibility of facing situations of cardiac arrest and CPR in the operating room, even if the trainees frequently observed the absence of cardiac motion. While resusTEE training based on simulators has already proved to be an optimal method, this study showed that clinical training could be a feasible alternative when simulators are not available [14, 15].

In the 12-week period after the course, the trainees performed resusTEE exams on few patients, corresponding to 22% of OHCA patients managed in the same period in ED. An excessively long median time from patient's arrival in the shock room to the probe insertion was recorded. A further implementation in the practice of resusTEE is, therefore, mandatory. Since participants can maintain their abilities 12 weeks post-course but with some deterioration in their skills, and given the few opportunities to practice resusTEE in their clinical practice, it could be advisable to offer a continuous training with a 2-h retraining in the operating theatre every 12 weeks.

The trainees showed good performances in the acquisition and interpretation of all of the six suggested views, except for TGSAX view, for which a decrease of performance after 12 weeks was recorded. This view was not used in clinical practice in ED. Different factors could explain this finding: first of all, a technical reason, because TGSAX requires more complex movements to be obtained, and because the acquisition of the image may be prevented by anatomic factors, such as gastrectasia and hiatal hernia. Besides, some information such as evaluation of systolic function, wall motion abnormalities and presence of pericardial effusion can be derived from other easier views. However, we have to consider that TGSAX is an ideal view for anatomic monitoring when conducting resuscitation. It is less subject to cranio-caudal displacement, given the gastric location and it is the only view that characterizes all of the six major wall segments and allows even the inexperienced user to best evaluate wall motion and global LV function. Lastly, the TGSAX is the only view that teaches the value of the transgastric position and ante-flexion, thereby preparing the participants for the motor skills required to obtain additional views. Therefore, we believe that the importance of this view needs to be reinforced and more effort should be dedicated to its learning throughout the course.

The other view that was not used in clinical practice was ME2CH, despite being easily obtained. The reasons for the non-utilization of this view by the trainees are not technical, as for TGSAX, but only related to the few additive information achieved by this view during OHCA. Unlike TGSAX view, ME2CH was not included in the previous protocols and, thus, could be omitted from the protocol [12, 14, 15].

AOview was taught in our course, although not included in the previous resusTEE protocols [12, 14, 15]. In our study, this view was not only outstandingly acquired and interpreted during the course by trainees, but it was also frequently used in clinical practice in ED. This view was useful for guiding vessel cannulation for ECLS and as an additive view to MELAX for the diagnosis of acute aortic dissection. However, we must highlight that AOview was often used for guiding cannulations as our ED is a "hub" center for ECLS. This view would probably be less important and less commonly used in EDs without ECLS facilities.

Given the limited data (only a few cases performed on real patients), a further period of observation is mandatory to assess the inclusiveness of the AOview view in the protocol and its effective utility in emergency situations.

This study, as already reported by others [10], showed that EPs can easily learn resusTEE and that resusTEE is useful to make the correct diagnosis, take the decision to interrupt CPR, and be a guidance for vessel cannulation for ECLS. However, it is still unknown if resusTEE can modify the outcomes of critical patients.

Limitations

All the participants were experts in FoCUS; therefore, it is not known if similar results can be obtained by EPs who have lower or no experience in FoCUS.

Practical training was carried out in one of the major Italian cardiac surgery centers with 3 operating theatres working simultaneously. This exposed trainees to many different cases, and this situation is uncommon in smaller centers.

Lastly, the utilization of resusTEE in clinical ED practice was monitored for a relatively short period of time and immediately after the end of the course, therefore no definitive conclusions can be drawn about which views should be included or excluded in a final and acknowledged simplified protocol; furthermore, the ten trainees performed on average just one study and their performances could only be assessed once.

Conclusions

EPs can successfully learn and maintain the skills which are required for the use of a simplified resusTEE protocol through a 10-h theoretical–practical course, performed in a cardiac surgery theatre. While high-fidelity simulation is the ideal modality for the training of novices in TEE, clinical training in the operating theater can be a feasible alternative if simulators are not available. Among views incorporated in the previous resusTEE protocols,

TGSAX was not used in clinical practice; therefore, its importance needs to be reinforced during the course.

Supplementary information

Additional file 1: Video 1a. Mid-esophageal four-chamber view (ME4CH).

Additional file 2: Video 1b. Mid-esophageal long-axis view (MELAX).

Additional file 3: Video 1c. Mid-esophageal two-chamber view (ME2CH).

Additional file 4: Video 1d. Mid-esophageal bicaval view (MEbicaval).

Additional file 5: Video 1e. Transgastric short-axis view (TGSAX).

Additional file 6: Video 1f. Aorta view (AOview).

Additional file 7: Video 2. Acute aortic dissection.

Additional file 8: Video 3. Cannulation of vessels for ECLS.

Additional file 9: Standard technique used to obtain the six views of the simplified TEE protocol.

Abbreviations

TEE: Transesophageal echocardiography; FoCUS: Focused cardiac ultrasound; OHCA: Out-of-hospital cardiac arrest; ResusTEE: Resuscitative TEE; EP: Emergency physician; ED: Emergency department; ECLS: Extracorporeal life support; PEA: Pulseless electrical activity; CPR: Cardiopulmonary resuscitation; SD: Standard deviation.

Acknowledgements

Study group: Eleonora de Villa, Mirco Donati, Cosimo Caviglioli, Piero Ticali, Antonio Gaspardini, Arianna Gandini, Giuseppe Giannazzo. The authors thank Isabel Sciberras and Sara Mucaj for the collaboration in writing the manuscript. On behalf of Winfocus and US SIMEU study group.

Authors' contributions

PN is the guarantor of the manuscript. PN contributed to the conception and design of the study, acquisition of the data, analysis and interpretation the data, drafting of the manuscript and editing it for important intellectual and scientific content; served as the principal author; edited the revision and approved the final draft. GDS, GA, SB, VC contributed to the conception and design of the study, acquisition of the data, analysis and interpretation the data, drafting of the manuscript and editing it for important intellectual and scientific content; VG contributed to acquisition of the data; edited the revision and approved the final draft. PS and SG contributed to analysis and interpretation of the data; approved the final draft. All authors read and approved the final manuscript.

Author details

[1] Department of Emergency Medicine, Careggi University Hospital, Largo Brambilla 3, 50134 Florence, Firenze, Italy. [2] Department of Anaesthesiology, Careggi University Hospital, Florence, Italy. [3] Department of Cardiac Surgery, Careggi University Hospital, Florence, Italy.

References

1. Soar J, Nolan JP, Böttiger BW, Perkins GD, Lott C, Carli P et al (2015) European Resuscitation Council guidelines for resuscitation 2015. Section 3. Adult advanced life support. Resuscitation 95:100–147
2. Cook CH, Praba AC, Beery PR, Martin LC (2002) Transthoracic echocardiography is not cost-effective in critically ill surgical patients. J Trauma 52(2):280–284
3. Arntfield R, Pace J, Hewak M, Thompson D (2016) Focused transesophageal echocardiography by emergency physicians is feasible and clinically influential: observational results from a novel ultrasound program. J Emerg Med 50(2):286–294
4. Mayo PH, Narasimhan M, Koenig S (2015) Critical care transesophageal echocardiography. Chest 148(5):1323–1332
5. Vignon P, Mentec H, Terre S, Gastinne H, Gueret P, Lemaire F (1994) Diagnostic accuracy and therapeutic impact of transthoracic and transesophageal echocardiography in mechanically ventilated patients in the ICU. Chest 106:1829–1834
6. Nienaber CA, von Kodolitsch Y, Nicolas V, Siglow V, Piepho A, Brockhoff C et al (1993) The diagnosis of thoracic aortic dissection by noninvasive imaging procedures. N Engl J Med 328:1–9
7. Fair J, Tonna J, Ockerse P, Galovic B, Youngquist S, McKellar SH et al (2016) Emergency physician–performed transesophageal echocardiography for extracorporeal life support vascular cannula placement. Am J Emerg Med 34(8):1637–1639
8. van der Wouw PA, Koster RW, Delemarre BJ, de Vos R, LampeSchoenmaeckers AJ, Lie KI (1997) Diagnostic accuracy of transesophageal echocardiography during cardiopulmonary resuscitation. J Am Coll Cardiol 30(3):780–783
9. Levitov A, Frankel HL, Blaivas M, Kirkpatrick AW, Su E, Evans D et al (2016) Guidelines for the appropriate use of bedside general and cardiac ultrasonography in the evaluation of critically ill patients–Part II: cardiac ultrasonography. Crit Care Med 44(6):1206–1227
10. Teran F, Dean AJ, Centeno C, Panebianco NL, Zeidan AJ, Chan W (2019) Evaluation of out-of-hospital cardiac arrest using transesophageal echocardiography in the emergency department. Resuscitation 137:140–147
11. Blaivas M (2008) Transesophageal echocardiography during cardiopulmonary arrest in the emergency department. Resuscitation 78:135–140
12. Guidelines for the use of transesophageal echocardiography (TEE) in the ED for cardiac arrest (2017) Ann Emerg Med 70:442–445
13. Hahn RT, Abraham T, Adams MS, Bruce CJ, Glas KE, Lang RM et al (2013) Guidelines for performing a comprehensive transesophageal echocardiographic examination: recommendations from the American Society of Echocardiography and the Society of Cardiovascular Anesthesiologists. J Am Soc Echocardiogr 26:921–964
14. Arntfield R, Pace J, McLeod S, Granton J, Hegazy A, Lingard L (2015) Focused transesophageal echocardiography for emergency physicians—description and results from simulation training of a structured four-view examination. Crit Ultrasound J 7(1):1–7
15. TeranF, Zeidan A. Implementation of a resuscitative TEE Program in the ED-ICU Interface. (2017) https://www.acep.org/how-we-serve/sections/critical-care-medicine/news/March-2018/implementation-of-a-resuscitative-tee-program-in-the-ed-icu-interface
16. Damp J, Anthony R, Davidson MA, Mendes L (2013) Effects of transesophageal echocardiography simulator training on learning and performance in cardiovascular medicine fellows. J Am Soc of Echocardiogr 26(12):1450–1456

27

Ultrasound measurement of optic nerve sheath diameter pre- and post-lumbar puncture

Christopher K. Schott[1,2*], Mohammad I. Hirzallah[3], Rock Heyman[4], Daniel N. Lesky[5], Emily B. Brant[3] and Clifton W. Callaway[6]

Abstract

Background: To test the hypothesis that optic nerve sheath diameter (ONSD) correlates with real-time changes in intracranial pressure, we performed ultrasound measurements of the ONSD in ambulatory patients undergoing elective lumbar puncture (LP). We conducted a prospective cohort study, including adult patients undergoing LP in a non-emergent setting. We measured ONSD perpendicular to the optic nerve at 3 mm behind the globe in both eyes in the traverse and sagittal planes, with the patient supine. The primary outcome was change in ONSD from pre-LP to post-LP. We calculated association of opening and closing LP pressures with changes in the pre- and post-LP ONSD measurements.

Results: The mean patient age was 49.0 years (SD = 37–61, range 19–67) with 21 females (72.4%) and 26 (89.7%) white American (not Hispanic or Latino). The average opening pressure and closing pressures were 20.4 cm and 13.5 cm with a difference of 6.9 cm, (95% CI 3.9–10.0 cm). Pressures between the participants with baseline ONSD measurement > 5 mm (average opening pressure = 21.3 cm) to those < 5 mm (20.2 cm) differed by 1.1 cm (95% CI − 5.7 to 8.0). Linear regression revealed no association between the sagittal, transverse, average, and change in ONSD measurements with the observed LP opening pressure, change in LP pressure, or volume of cerebral spinal fluid (CSF) drained.

Conclusions: In this study of ambulatory patients undergoing rapid decreases in ICP via elective LP, we detected no acute changes in ultrasonographic measurement of the ONSD.

Keywords: Optic nerve sheath diameter, Intracranial pressure, Ultrasound

Background

Optic nerve sheath diameter (ONSD) measurement by ultrasonography is a promising method to detect elevated intracranial pressure (ICP) [1, 2] and is gaining popularity as a beside assessment of ICP in critically ill patients [3]. This may be of particular benefit to undifferentiated patients presenting to the emergency department with concerns for elevated ICP and where Point-of-care ultrasound (POCUS) has a significant role in patient care.

Increased intracranial pressure transmits directly along the optic nerve and leads to papilledema [4, 5]. Several studies found that increase in ONSD correlates with increase in ICP [6–9]. Meta-analyses and systematic reviews support use of ONSD as a non-invasive ICP assessment modality [10]. However, different studies report variable inter-rater agreement and wide confidence intervals in measurements, suggesting caution-pending larger and more comprehensive studies [3, 11, 12].

In some studies, ICP and ONSD change simultaneously. These include when CSF drainage is used to reduce ICP [6, 13, 14], when ICP rises during endotracheal suctioning [15] and when intrathecal infusion tests increase ICP and are followed by intrathecal crystalloid injections

*Correspondence: Christopher.Schott@va.gov; schottck@upmc.edu
[1] VA Pittsburgh Health Care Systems * Critical Care Service Line (124U), University Drive, Pittsburgh, PA 15240, USA
Full list of author information is available at the end of the article

that decrease ICP [16]. However, a cohort of subarachnoid hemorrhage patients showed that ONSD values did not normalize after normalization of ICP [17] and a study of relapse-free multiple sclerosis patients showed that the ONSD was smaller than normal controls [18].

This variability in ONSD changes by pathology and chronicity suggests that studies specific to acute ICP changes may not be generalizable to patients with chronic ICP elevation in outpatient settings. In this study, we investigated the effect of routine CSF drainage performed in the outpatient setting on ONSD.

Methods

Our primary research question was to determine if the optic nerve sheath diameter demonstrates a measurable change via ultrasound assessment in real time for patients undergoing elective lumbar punctures correlated with changes in intracranial pressure. This study was approved by the University of Pittsburgh institutional review board (PRO14040248). Study investigators obtained written informed consent from all patients (or guardians of participants) in the study prior to enrollment.

We conducted a prospective cohort convenience study. The participants were patients of a collaborating neurologist at the University of Pittsburgh Medical Center who were scheduled to receive diagnostic lumbar puncture. These patients represented a unique sample for assessing the dynamics of acute ICP changes. All measurements took place during scheduled out-patient lumbar puncture clinics at the office of this neurologist. Study team members had specific training on how to perform ONSD measurements with POCUS. The PI (CS) has extensive training in POCUS, particularly in regard to ONSD measurements. He directly taught and supervised the other team members (comprised an EM POCUS fellow, EM residents and a medical student research assistant) for hands-on training across several sessions as well as their initial patient enrollments to ensure accuracy of technique and measurements. Subsequent, unsupervised scans were reviewed for accuracy of the saved measurements.

We included adult patients, ages 18–89, undergoing a non-emergent, scheduled lumbar puncture for diagnostic indications. We excluded pregnant women, and patients with prosthetic eyes, cataracts, glaucoma, or recent eye trauma or surgery. Patient who received their LP sitting up were excluded as CSF pressure measurement in the sitting position is not known to be reliable.

We calculated sample size based on prior studies of the relationship between ONSD and ICP in human subjects. ONSD measurement has a median inter-observer variation of $\pm$0.2–0.3 mm [19]. In an intrathecal infusion test conducted in human subjects that induced raised ICP in subjects, the ONSD-to-ICP ratio varied from 0.019 to 0.071 mm/cm [16]. Choosing conservative values of an ONSD-to-ICP ratio of 0.025 mm/cm, and an ICP change of 10 cm, we calculated that we would need to enroll 17 patients with elevated ICP. With the addition of a 35% buffer for dropout (i.e., inability to complete LP or done while sitting up), this yielded an anticipated enrollment of 23 patients. However, as the investigators were blinded to these data, all consecutive patients meeting inclusion criteria had these measurements obtained. We planned to enroll consecutive patients until at least 17 patients with elevated ICP had been included. Anticipating that 20% of the patients will have high intracranial pressure (> 25 cm), we determined that the anticipated number to include would be 115.

After screening, enrolling and obtaining written informed consent, the study investigators performed ultrasound (US) measurements of the participants' ONSD. All study team members were competent in the use of US to acquire these views and accurately obtain the ONSD measurements. The investigators used a GE vivid i ultrasound machine with an 8–16 MHz high-frequency linear probe (GE Healthcare, Chicago, IL, USA). ONSD measurements were obtained with the patient supine to correspond with opening pressure measurements of patients in the lateral decubitus position. Each subject received four pre-LP US ONSD measurements: both eyes were evaluated in the traverse and sagittal planes. Consistent with previously published studies, the width of the ONSD was measured at 3 mm behind the globe, in the axis perpendicular to the optic nerve, with the patient supine [20]. These images were saved as digital files, de-identified from any patient information, locally to the US device itself for subsequent quality assurance review of the images and accuracy of measurement by the senior members of the research team. At this time, the patient was taken for their scheduled LP.

The second set of measurements was performed after the patients' LP. The research team member, blinded from the patients pre- and post-LP pressures and amount of cerebral spinal fluid (CSF) removed, performed repeat measurements from the both of the participant's ONSD in transverse and sagittal plane. These images were also saved locally to the device. After the images were saved, the neurologist performing the LP provided the participant's opening pressure, closing pressure and amount of CSF he removed. These results were entered into our database as well as the ONSD measurements pre- and post-LP. Opening pressure > 25 cm was used to categorize patients as having increased ICP. However, we included all patients to assess the changes in ONSD pre- and post-LP in those both with and without elevated ICP in order to better understand the elasticity on the ONSD in vivo.

Patient data were de-identified and blinded to the research team members performing the ONSD measurements. However, demographic information of the patients was collected, including indication for LP (i.e., presently ongoing or resolved symptoms) and other existing co-morbidities.

We used descriptive statistics to characterize the study subjects. We calculated average ONSD for each eye as the arithmetic mean of sagittal and transverse measurements. For each eye, we compared sagittal and transverse and average ONSD before and after LP using two-tailed paired t test. We calculated change in ONSD at each eye and axis from pre-LP to post-LP. We also examined LP opening pressure in the subset of subjects with abnormal ONSD (>5 mm). We used linear regression to measure association of sagittal, transverse, average, and change in ONSD with LP opening pressure, change in LP pressure, and volume of CSF drained. We considered p values < 0.05 to be significant. We used STATA 14.2 for all analyses (STATA Corp., College Park, Tx).

Data Availability: Anonymized data not published within this article will be made available by request from any qualified investigator.

Results

Between February 2015 and December 2017, we screened 113 patients. Thirty-two were enrolled with 29 completing all ONSD ultrasound and LP measurements (Fig. 1). We ended the study early due to slower than anticipated enrollment, which made the project no longer feasible.

The average patient age was 49.0 years (SD = 37–61, range 19–67 years of age) with 21 females (72.4%) and 26 (89.7%) white American (not Hispanic or Latino) with the remainder as Black or African American (Table 1). Twenty (69.0%) of the patients were scanned by investigator CS, 6 (20.7%) by DL, 2 (6.9%) by EB and 1 (3.4%) by MS. There was a mean of 68 min (SD = 48–88 min) between pre- and post-lumbar puncture ONSD measurements.

The skewness and kurtosis test of normality confirmed that continuous variables did not differ from normal except for LP opening pressure. Therefore, mean (SD) is used for most variables. The only continuous variable that deviated from normal distribution was LP opening pressure, where we report as median (IQR). For all participants, the median opening pressure was 19 cm (IQR 16–24) with average closing pressure of 13.5 cm with a

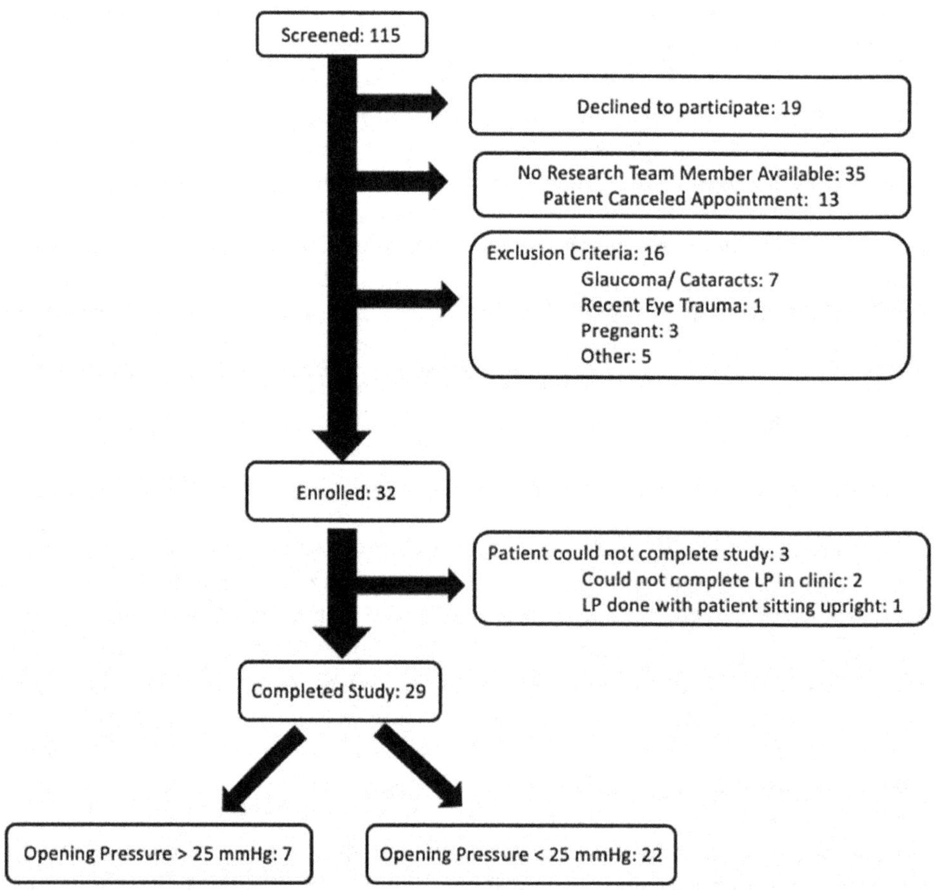

Fig. 1 Patient enrollment flow chart. *LP* lumbar puncture

Table 1 Patient demographics

Characteristic	No (%)	Co-morbidities	No
Sex		Parkinson's	1
Male	8 (27.59%)	Hypertension	5
Female	21 (72.41%)	Narcolepsy	1
Age	Avg = 49.03 (range 19–67)	Cervical stenosis	1
Race		Multiple sclerosis	2
White	26 (89.66)	Transverse myelitis	1
African America	3 (10.34%)	Depression/anxiety	2
		CAD	2
		Diabetes	5
Symptoms at present	No	Hyperlipidemia	2
Extremity paresthesias	6	Arthritis	1
Headache	3	Iron deficiency	1
Blurred vision	5	Lupus	1
Dizzy	3	Rheumatoid arthritis	1
Weakness (generalized)	4	Sjogren's syndrome	1
Nausea	2	Reynaud's	1
Back pain	1	Bipolar	3
		Pseudotumor cerebri	1
		Pre-eclampsia (history of)	1
		Psoriasis	1
		Hypothyroidism	1
		Prostate cancer	1
		Thyroid cancer	1

difference of 6.9 cm (95% CI 3.9–10.0 cm). There was no statistically significant difference in opening pressures between the participants who had an ONSD measurement > 5 mm (average opening pressure = 21.3 cm) to those < 5 mm (20.2 cm) with a difference of 1.1 cm ($p = 0.7395$, 95% CI = −8.0–5.7). The volume of CSF removal was normally distributed, with a mean of 13.4 cc's (SD 4.2).

We observed an increase of 0.3 mm in the left eye sagittal plane ONSD ($p = 0.0318$, 95% CI 0.03–0.6) as well as in the averaged left transverse and sagittal planes (delta = 0.3 mm, $p = 0.0027$, 95% CI = 0.1–0.5), but we did not observe any other reliable changes from pre- to post- lumbar puncture ONSD measurements (Table 2). We separately examined the 7 patients who had elevated ICP on opening pressure measurement (25 cm or greater; Table 3). Again, we observed an *increase* in the ONSD measurement for the left eye transverse plane (average increase of 0.8 mm, $p = 0.0451$, 95% CI = 0.03–1.1) and the averaged left eye measurements (average increase of 0.63 mm, $p = 0.0293$, 95% CI = 0.09–1.2), but no other changes from pre- to post-lumbar puncture ONSD measurements (Fig. 2; Tables 4, 5).

In linear regression models, there were no independent associations between the sagittal, transverse, average, and change in ONSD measurements with the observed LP opening pressure, change in LP pressure, and volume of CSF drained. Comparison of

Table 2 Comparison of participant optic nerve sheath diameter, by plane of measurement, pre-lumbar puncture compared to post-lumbar puncture for all participants

	Average diameter (PRE)	Average diameter (POST)	Delta	*p*	95% CI
Left eye Transverse	5.09	4.8	0.29	0.0566	−0.0088 to 0.5959
Left eye sagittal	5.02	4.72	0.3	0.0318	0.028 to 0.572
Left eye (averaged ONSD)	5.06	4.76	0.297	0.0037	0.1039 to 0.4896
Right eye transverse	4.84	4.86	−0.02	0.8873	−0.3451 to 0.2999
Right eye sagittal	5.04	4.82	0.223	0.0747	−0.0237 to 0.4703
Right eye (averaged ONSD)	4.92	4.84	0.867	0.5042	−0.1754 to 0.3488

Table 3 Comparison of participant optic nerve sheath diameter, by plane of measurement, pre-lumbar puncture compared to post-lumbar puncture, for participants with elevated intracranial pressure (opening pressure > 25 cm)

	Average diameter (PRE)	Average diameter (POST)	Delta	*p*	95% CI
Left eye Transverse	5.228571	4.4	0.8285714	0.0452	0.0245 to 1.2626
Left eye sagittal	5.257143	4.814286	0.442857	0.2336	−0.3754 to 1.2612
Left eye (averaged ONSD)	5.242857	4.607143	0.6357142	0.0293	0.0894 to 1.1820
Right eye transverse	4.785714	4.8	−0.0142856	0.9696	−0.8939 to 0.8654
Right eye sagittal	5.4	5.016667	0.3833	0.2701	−0.4115 to 1.1782
Right eye (averaged ONSD)	5.008333	4.891667	0.1166666	0.7165	−0.6635 to 0.8968

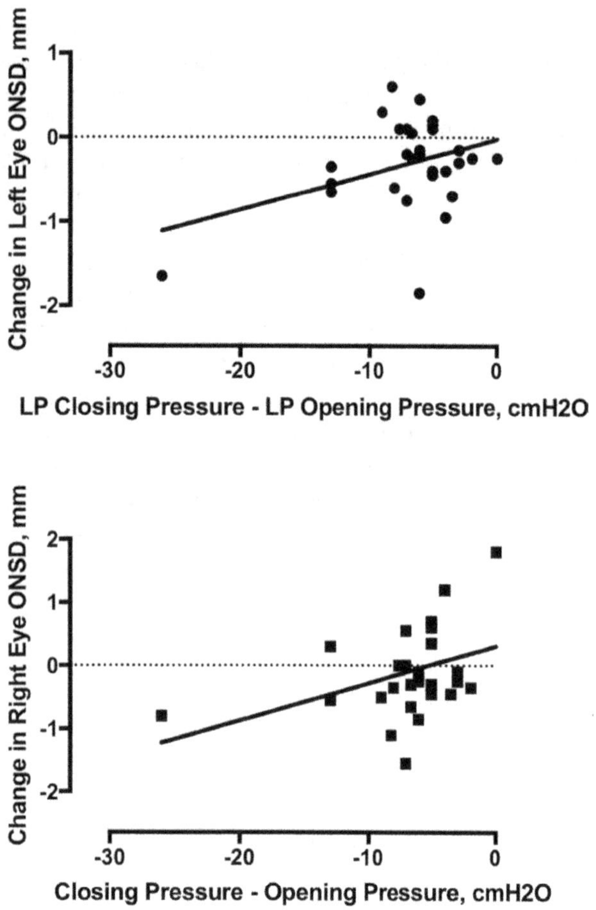

Fig. 2 Linear regression analysis of change in between opening and closing pressures (in cmH_2) compared against the change in optic nerve sheath diameter (mm), averaged between transverse and sagittal plan measurements, for the left and right eyes, respectively

measurements in the 2 planes (transverse vs sagittal) at the same time period (pre- or post-lumbar puncture) demonstrates moderate to good levels of agreement (0.65–0.88; Table 6). However, there is a greater variation between eyes (left vs right) for measurements in the same plane and period of time (range = 0.33–0.84; Table 7).

Discussion

This study provides evidence that the use of ONSD measurement via ultrasound (2D/B mode imaging with measurement of the ONSD 3 mm posterior to the globe in supine patients) does not correlate with real-time changes in ICP (as measured in cm of H_20) in ambulatory patients undergoing an elective lumbar puncture. Linear regression revealed no association between the sagittal, transverse, average, and change in ONSD measurements with the observed LP opening pressure, change in LP pressure, or volume of CSF drained, except for an *increase* in the ONSD measurement for the left eye transverse plane (average increase of 0.8 mm, $p = 0.0451$, 95% CI = 0.03–1.1) and the averaged left eye measurements (average increase of 0.63 mm, $p = 0.0293$, 95% CI = 0.09–1.2).

Our results suggest that clinically significant changes in ONSD measurements via ocular ultrasound may not be seen among ambulatory patients. Only ONSD in the left transverse and left averaged (transverse and sagittal) planes changed before and after LP. The direction of this change was actually an increase in the ONSD, contrary to our hypothesis. Moreover, the magnitude of this change (0.3 mm) is not clinically significant, being much less than the standard deviation of observed ONSD measurements and potentially less than inter-rater and intra-rater variation in measurement. These findings were no different when we separated out the patients with proven elevated ICP.

There was moderate to good correlation between the measured planes (transverse vs sagittal) for the ONSD at the same periods of time (pre-LP vs post-LP). However, there was a wide range of agreement in measurements between left and right eyes (range of agreement 0.33–0.84). This finding suggests an agreement in the ONSD measurement between planes of the same eye, but wider range of agreements between eyes (i.e., asymmetric ONSD among this patient population). This could be due to the underlying etiology of the ONSD enlargement, as many of the patients were presenting for neurologic complaints with workups for multiple sclerosis.

Table 4 Linear regression analysis of ONSD measurements to opening pressure

Measurement	Correlation coefficient	*p*	R^2	95% CI
Left eye transverse (Pre)	0.12	0.924	0.0003	− 2.502532 to 2.749281
Left eye sagittal (Pre)	0.28	0.801	0.0024	− 1.967434 to 2.524459
Left eye (averaged ONSD, pre)	0.24	0.848	0.0014	− 2.336629 to 2.82292
Right eye transverse (pre)	0.23	0.863	0.0011	− 2.442073 to 2.894984
Right eye sagittal (pre)	1.27	0.38	0.0286	− 1.652574 to 4.194005
Right eye (averaged ONSD, post)	0.797	0.589	0.011	− 2.194456 to 3.789119

Table 5 Linear regression analysis of ONSD measurements to volume of CSF removal

Measurement	Correlation coefficient	p	R^2	95% CI
Right eye delta (transverse)	−1.07	0.225	0.0502	−2.824557 to .693879
Right eye delta sagittal	−1.66	0.167	0.0669	−4.057 to 0.7390722
Right eye delta (averaged)	−1.64	0.146	0.0738	−3.893995 to 0.6095693
Left eye delta (transverse)	1.18	0.209	0.0538	−0.696745 to 3.04977
Left eye delta (sagittal)	0.96	0.358	0.0292	−1.145068 to 3.072341
Left eye delta (averaged)	2.41	0.098	0.0915	−0.4728556 to 5.283155

Table 6 Agreement of measurements between planes (transverse and sagittal) for each eye, pre- and post-lumbar puncture

Measurement plane 1	Measurement plane 2	Cronbach's alpha
L pre-transverse	L pre-sagittal	0.7629
R pre-transverse	R pre-sagittal	0.7485
L post-transverse	L post-sagittal	0.6456
R post-transverse	R post-sagittal	0.8825

Table 7 Agreement of measurements between eyes (right vs left) for each plane, pre- and post-lumbar puncture

Measurement Plane 1	Measurement plane 2	Cronbach's alpha
Left eye pre, transverse	Right eye pre, transverse	0.3297
Left eye pre, sagittal	Right eye pre, sagittal	0.4405
Left eye post, transverse	Right eye post, transverse	0.8399
Left eye post, sagittal	Right eye post, sagittal	0.6885

Therefore, one explanation may be that the enlargement in a unilateral eye could be due to inflammation (e.g., optic neuritis), as opposed to increased intracranial pressure, and may not demonstrate changes with intracranial pressures. No ONSD measurement in either plane, eye or time period (pre-LP or post-LP) demonstrated a significant relationship with opening intracranial pressure or amount of CSF removed.

A recent publication by Wang et al. reported a higher correlation between ONSD and changes in lumbar puncture ($r=0.724$, 95% CI 0.470–0.876; $p<0.001$) among patients admitted for suspected elevated ICP [21]. However, their reported statistical correlation may be limited in clinical application. Their results show that a patient with a 20-cm drop in ICP may have a measured ONSD change of as little as 0.5 mm on bedside ultrasound. This raises the question of whether a potential observed change of 0.5 mm is clinically useful or detectable, particularly with previously published inter-rater variability of 0.2–0.3 mm [19]. Furthermore, the validity of these results has been questions, as noted in a letter to the editor addressing this particular publication [22]. Therefore, though studies like this and others support a statistical correlation between changes in ICP and ONSD measurements, it is important to keep in mind potential the clinical limitations and applicability of this measurement when attempting to apply to patient care.

A recent systematic review and meta-analysis of 71 studies, inclusive of adult and pediatric populations, report pooled sensitivity, specificity, positive likelihood ratio, and negative likelihood ratio of ONSD measurements to be 97% (95% CI 92–99%), 86% (CI 74–93%), 6.93 (CI 3.55–13.54), and 0.04 (CI 0.02–0.10), respectively [10]. However, in contrast to our study, the included papers used in their meta-analysis predominantly come from a patient population with known intracranial pathology (18 with traumatic brain injury, 26 without and 27 mixed). This is in contrast to our study, examining ambulatory patients without known elevations in ICP. We may not have observed as noticeable results with potential etiologies for enlarged ONSD measurements from etiologies other than elevation in ICP. The contrast in patient populations suggests that this method to assess for elevation in ICP via ONSD may not be generalizable to all patient populations.

Limitations

The study has several limitations. First, the study was stopped early secondary to slow enrollment. Patients did not consent to participate in the study at a rate we felt was feasible for continued data collection. Though we did not reach our anticipated target enrollment, there were enough patients to detect some differences between left eye (transverse, averaged transverse and sagittal) ONSD measures pre- and post-LP, and to provide point estimates for the changes in ONSD. The study is also limited in that we used a convenience sample population of ambulatory patients undergoing scheduled lumbar punctures. The majority of this population were white females, potentially limiting generalizability. Moreover, this patient population may have had changes in ONSD from other etiologies, such as inflammation from underlying neurologic condition, opposed to elevated intracranial pressures. Since we used a convenience sample of patients during their scheduled LP, we were only able to record pre- to post-LP within the timeframe of their office visit. We cannot exclude potential changes in ONSD that occur longer after LP.

Conclusions

Our study suggests that there are limitations to the use and application of ONSD ultrasound measurements in ambulatory patients, in contrast to prior studies in critically ill patients [1–3, 7–9, 11, 23] In this study, we were not able to consistently detect changes in the ONSD across each eye or multiple planes of view. Observed changes in single eyes were too small in magnitude to trust for clinical decision making. We did not observe any correlation between ONSD measurements by ultrasound and opening pressures, change in pressure or amount of CSF removed, either in all patients or in the group of patients with elevated ICP. In addition, we did not find a relationship between enlarged ONSD and ICP.

While point-of-care ultrasound has many applications for bedside assessments and clinical decision making, this study suggests caution in using ultrasound measurements of the ONSD in ambulatory patients.

Abbreviations

ONSD: Optic nerve sheath diameter; LP: Lumbar puncture; CSF: Cerebral spinal fluid; ICP: Intracranial pressure; POCUS: Point-of-care ultrasound.

Acknowledgements

The authors and study investigators would like to thanks the University of Pittsburgh Department of Emergency Medicine Applied Physiology Laboratory for loaning the ultrasound machine used in this study.

The opinions expressed in this paper do not reflect those of the Veteran's Healthcare administration.

Statistical analysis

Conducted by Clifton W. Callaway, MD, PhD[f], Department of Emergency Medicine, University of Pittsburgh and University of Pittsburgh Medical Center (UPMC).

Authors' contributions

CKS designed and conceptualized the study; analyzed the data; drafted the manuscript for intellectual content. MIH analyzed the data; drafted the manuscript for intellectual content. RH served major role in the acquisition of data. DNL designed and conceptualized the study; major role in the acquisition of data. EBB served major role in the acquisition of data. CWC analyzed the data and performed statistical analysis. All authors read and approved the final manuscript.

Author details

[1] VA Pittsburgh Health Care Systems * Critical Care Service Line (124U), University Drive, Pittsburgh, PA 15240, USA. [2] Department of Critical Care Medicine and Emergency Medicine, University of Pittsburgh, and University of Pittsburgh Medical Center (UPMC), 3550 Terrace Street Scaife Hall, Suite 600, Pittsburgh, PA 15213, USA. [3] University of Pittsburgh Multidisciplinary Critical Care Training Program, 3550 Terrace Street Scaife Hall, Suite 600, Pittsburgh, PA 15213, USA. [4] Department of Neurology, University of Pittsburgh, and University of Pittsburgh Medical Center (UPMC), 300 Halket Street, Suite 4500, Pittsburgh, PA, USA 15213. [5] School of Medicine 401 Scaife Hall, University of Pittsburgh, 3550 Terrace Street, Pittsburgh, PA 15261, USA. [6] Department of Emergency Medicine, University of Pittsburgh, and University of Pittsburgh, Medical Center (UPMC), 3600 Forbes at Meyran Avenue Forbes Tower, Suite 10028, Pittsburgh, PA 15213, USA.

References

1. Gangemi M, Cennamo G, Maiuri F, D'Andrea F (1987) Echographic measurement of the optic nerve in patients with intracranial hypertension. Neurochirurgia (Stuttg). 30(2):53–55. https://doi.org/10.1055/s-2008-1053656
2. Galetta S, Byrne SF, Smith JL (1989) Echographic correlation of optic nerve sheath size and cerebrospinal fluid pressure. J Clin Neuroophthalmol. 9(2):79–82
3. Robba C, Santori G, Czosnyka M et al (2018) Optic nerve sheath diameter measured sonographically as non-invasive estimator of intracranial pressure: a systematic review and meta-analysis. Intensive Care Med 44(8):1284–1294. https://doi.org/10.1007/s00134-018-5305-7
4. De Moraes CG (2013) Anatomy of the visual pathways. J Glaucoma 22(Suppl 5):S2–7. https://doi.org/10.1097/ijg.0b013e3182934978
5. Selhorst JB, Chen Y (2009) The optic nerve. Semin Neurol 29(1):29–35. https://doi.org/10.1055/s-0028-1124020
6. Moretti R, Pizzi B, Cassini F, Vivaldi N (2009) Reliability of optic nerve ultrasound for the evaluation of patients with spontaneous intracranial hemorrhage. Neurocrit Care 11(3):406–410. https://doi.org/10.1007/s12028-009-9250-8
7. Liu D, Li Z, Zhang X et al (2017) Assessment of intracranial pressure with ultrasonographic retrobulbar optic nerve sheath diameter measurement. BMC Neurol. 17(1):188. https://doi.org/10.1186/s12883-017-0964-5
8. Jeon JP, Lee SU, Kim S-E et al (2017) Correlation of optic nerve sheath diameter with directly measured intracranial pressure in Korean adults using bedside ultrasonography. PLoS ONE 12(9):e0183170. https://doi.org/10.1371/journal.pone.0183170
9. Raffiz M, Abdullah JM (2017) Optic nerve sheath diameter measurement: a means of detecting raised ICP in adult traumatic and non-traumatic neurosurgical patients. Am J Emerg Med 35(1):150–153. https://doi.org/10.1016/j.ajem.2016.09.044
10. Koziarz A, Sne N, Kegel F et al (2019) Bedside optic nerve ultrasonography for diagnosing increased intracranial pressure. Ann Intern Med 3:1. https://doi.org/10.7326/m19-0812
11. Dubourg J, Javouhey E, Geeraerts T, Messerer M, Kassai B (2011) Ultrasonography of optic nerve sheath diameter for detection of raised intracranial pressure: a systematic review and meta-analysis. Intensive Care Med 37(7):1059–1068. https://doi.org/10.1007/s00134-011-2224-2
12. Ohle R, McIsaac SM, Woo MY, Perry JJ (2015) Sonography of the optic nerve sheath diameter for detection of raised intracranial pressure compared to computed tomography: a systematic review and meta-analysis. J Ultrasound Med 34(7):1285–1294. https://doi.org/10.7863/ultra.34.7.1285
13. Williams P (2017) Optic nerve sheath diameter as a bedside assessment for elevated intracranial pressure. Case Reports Crit Care. 2017:3978934. https://doi.org/10.1155/2017/3978934
14. Hassen GW, Al-Juboori M, Koppel B, Akfirat G, Kalantari H (2018) Real time optic nerve sheath diameter measurement during lumbar puncture. Am J Emerg Med 36(4):736.e1–736.e3. https://doi.org/10.1016/j.ajem.2018.01.037
15. Maissan IM, Dirven PJAC, Haitsma IK, Hoeks SE, Gommers D, Stolker RJ (2015) Ultrasonographic measured optic nerve sheath diameter as an accurate and quick monitor for changes in intracranial pressure. J Neurosurg 123(September):1–5. https://doi.org/10.3171/2014.10.JNS141197
16. Hansen HC, Helmke K (1997) Validation of the optic nerve sheath response to changing cerebrospinal fluid pressure: ultrasound findings during intrathecal infusion tests. J Neurosurg 87(1):34–40. https://doi.org/10.3171/jns.1997.87.1.0034
17. Bäuerle J, Niesen WD, Egger K, Buttler KJ, Reinhard M (2016) Enlarged optic nerve sheath in aneurysmal subarachnoid hemorrhage despite

normal intracranial pressure. J Neuroimaging 26(2):194–196. https://doi.org/10.1111/jon.12287
18. De Masi R, Orlando S, Conte A et al (2016) Transbulbar B-mode sonography in multiple sclerosis: clinical and biological relevance. Ultrasound Med Biol 42(12):3037–3042. https://doi.org/10.1016/j.ultrasmedbio.2016.07.018
19. Ballantyne S, O'Neill G, Hamilton R, Hollman A (2002) Observer variation in the sonographic measurement of optic nerve sheath diameter in normal adults. Eur J Ultrasound. 15(3):145–149. https://doi.org/10.1016/S0929-8266(02)00036-8
20. Soldatos T, Chatzimichail K, Papathanasiou M, Gouliamos A (2009) Optic nerve sonography: a new window for the non-invasive evaluation of intracranial pressure in brain injury. Emerg Med J. 26(9):630–634. https://doi.org/10.1136/emj.2008.058453
21. Wang L, Chen L, Chen Y et al (2018) Correlation between noninvasive ultrasonography and dynamically monitored intracranial pressure. JAMA Ophthalmol. 136(3):250–256. https://doi.org/10.1001/jamaophthalmol.2017.6560
22. Hoffman RS (2018) Measuring optic nerve sheath diameter as a proxy for intracranial pressure. JAMA Ophthalmol. 136(3):1309. https://doi.org/10.1159/000366451
23. Moretti R, Pizzi B (2011) Ultrasonography of the optic nerve in neurocritically ill patients. Acta Anaesthesiol Scand 55(6):644–652. https://doi.org/10.1111/j.1399-6576.2011.02432.x

Optic nerve sheath diameter sonography during the acute stage of intracerebral hemorrhage: a potential role in monitoring neurocritical patients

M. Bender[1*], S. Lakicevic[1], N. Pravdic[1], S. Schreiber[2] and B. Malojcic[3]

Abstract

Background: Optic nerve sheath diameter (ONSD) sonography has been proposed as a reliable bedside tool for the detection of increased intracranial pressure (ICP). ONSD reacts almost simultaneously to oscillations in ICP. The aim of this study was to investigate the ONSD dynamics in the acute stage of intracerebral hemorrhage (ICH) and to compare ONSD dynamics to the clinical outcome.

Methods: We enrolled 35 acute ICH patients and 20 healthy volunteers in this prospective study. At the admission, all patients underwent brain CT scan and ONSD sonography. We repeated the ONSD on the second and the third day in all patients while CT scan was repeated if a patient condition deteriorated. The changes in serial ONSD measurements were termed as stable or unstable ONSD trend. ONSD trend was considered as unstable if variations of average ONSD were above 5%. The outcome of the patient was assessed with the Modified Rankin Scale (mRS) and Glasgow Outcome Scale (GOS).

Results: In healthy volunteers serial ONSD recordings for 3 days revealed a stable trend in 100%. However, in the study group, 23 patients had unstable and 12 had stable ONSD trend during the acute stage of ICH. The patients with unstable ONSD trend were more likely to have worse outcomes (p value 0.003).

Conclusion: In patients with ICH, the acute-phase ONSD dynamics can help in predicting the clinical outcome.

Keywords: Optic nerve sheath diameter, Intracranial hemorrhage, Ultrasound, Outcome

Introduction

ONSD has been proposed as a reliable, non-invasive bedside tool for the detection of raised ICP. Increased ICP, transmitted through the subarachnoid space, causes ONSD enlargement, which can easily be detected using ultrasound (US) [1, 2]. This was first demonstrated by Hansen and Helmke in an experimental study on cadaveric specimens with the greatest degree of distension occurring at 3 mm behind the optic globe, whereupon this location has become a standard measurement point [3]. Since then, ONSD has been well studied in experimental and clinical settings, in healthy populations as well as in patients with elevated ICP of different etiologies. Quite a few studies have compared ONSD sonography to invasive ICP measurements and most of them proven a good correlation. Furthermore, they demonstrated that the ONSD reflects an immediate change in ICP and changes almost concurrently with rapid ICP variations [2, 4]. However, the optimal ONSD cutoff point for detection of increased ICP has not been well established, the range of proposed values varies from 4.8 to 5.9 mm [5–9]. Available data regarding normal ONSD are also inconclusive, with a wide inter-individual range

*Correspondence: marijabender@yahoo.com
[1] Department of Neurology, University Hospital Mostar, Bijeli Brijeg bb, 88 000 Mostar, Bosnia and Herzegovina
Full list of author information is available at the end of the article

of ONSD in the general healthy population [10–13]. Even though ONSD sonography is not as accurate as invasive ICP monitoring, many studies have demonstrated that ONSD reflects an immediate change in ICP, hence, serial ONSD recordings might be useful in monitoring the patients with elevated ICP when invasive monitoring is not possible or is not recommended. Accepting limitations of the method, we investigated the dynamics or relative ONSD changes rather than the absolute ONSD changes in the acute phase of spontaneous, non-traumatic ICH and we evaluated its association with clinical course and outcome.

Methods

Study population

This prospective observational study was carried out in University Hospital Mostar, over a period of 15 months from January 2018 to March 2019. The study was approved by the Ethics Committee of the hospital in accordance with the guidelines of the Declaration of Helsinki [14]. All participants provided written informed consent, for the unconscious patients, the informed consent was obtained by a proxy. All patients presenting to our hospital, no more than 6 h after the symptom onset, with a diagnosis of supratentorial non-traumatic ICH were enrolled in the study. Exclusion and inclusion criteria are listed in Table 1. A control group ($n=20$) consisted of healthy volunteers, without a known intracranial or ocular pathology. The patients and the control group were not paired.

Measurements—study protocol

The study protocol included at least two brain CT scan. First CT scan was done at the admission and second during the follow-up phase during the hospitalization. The brain CT scan was evaluated by an investigator blinded to other results, including ONSD measurements and clinical status. At the level of the third ventricle, midline shift was measured [15] and the ICH volume was assessed using a widely recognized ABCD/2 method [16]. Clinical status was evaluated daily using the National Institute of Health Stroke Scale (NIHSS) and Glasgow Coma Scale (GCS) performed simultaneously to ONSD measurement [17]. Intracerebral Hemorrhage (ICH) Score was also performed at the admission and the outcome of the patient was assessed when the patients were discharged from the hospital, using the mRS and the GOS [18, 19].

Ultrasound examination

Ocular sonography was performed at admission, on the second and the third day, by an investigator with previous experience in sonography measurements of the ONSD in more than 100 patients. Sonography was performed using a GE Logiq P6 scanner (General Electrics Medical Systems, Milwaukee, WI, USA) with a 13–10 MHz linear transducer. The patients were examined in Semi-Fowler's position. They were asked to try to suppress eye movements. If the patient was unconscious and not able to fix on primary gaze, a slight adjustment of angulation was required. The insonation program was set to "small parts" or "superficial" with an insonation depth set to 5–8 cm and with optimally adjusted gain to obtain good contrast between the structures. The mechanical index was set to 0.2. ONSD was measured 3 mm behind the globe. Video of every ultrasound was recorded and analyzed later by a single-blinded investigator. Each measurement was performed three times and the mean value was calculated afterward. Changes in serial ONSD measurements were termed as stable or unstable ONSD trend. We considered that the patient has an unstable ONSD trend if the variations (increase or decrease) of average ONSD (left or right) were above 5% (Fig. 1) [20].

Statistical analysis

Categorical variables were presented as frequencies and percentages, and numerical variables were presented as medians either with interquartile range or confidence intervals. The differences between categorical groups were tested using Chi-squared, while the differences between numerical values were tested using the Mann–Whitney *U* test.

Table 1 Inclusion and exclusion criteria

Inclusion criteria	Supratentorial non-traumatic ICH confirmed by brain CT
	Admission to the hospital within 6 h after symptom onset
	≥ 18 years of age
	Brain neuroimaging (CT) within 6 h after symptom onset
Exclusion criteria	Ocular trauma or a disease involving the optic nerve
	Inability to preform US measurement within 1 h from brain CT

ICH intracerebral hemorrhage, *CT* computed tomography, *US* ultrasound

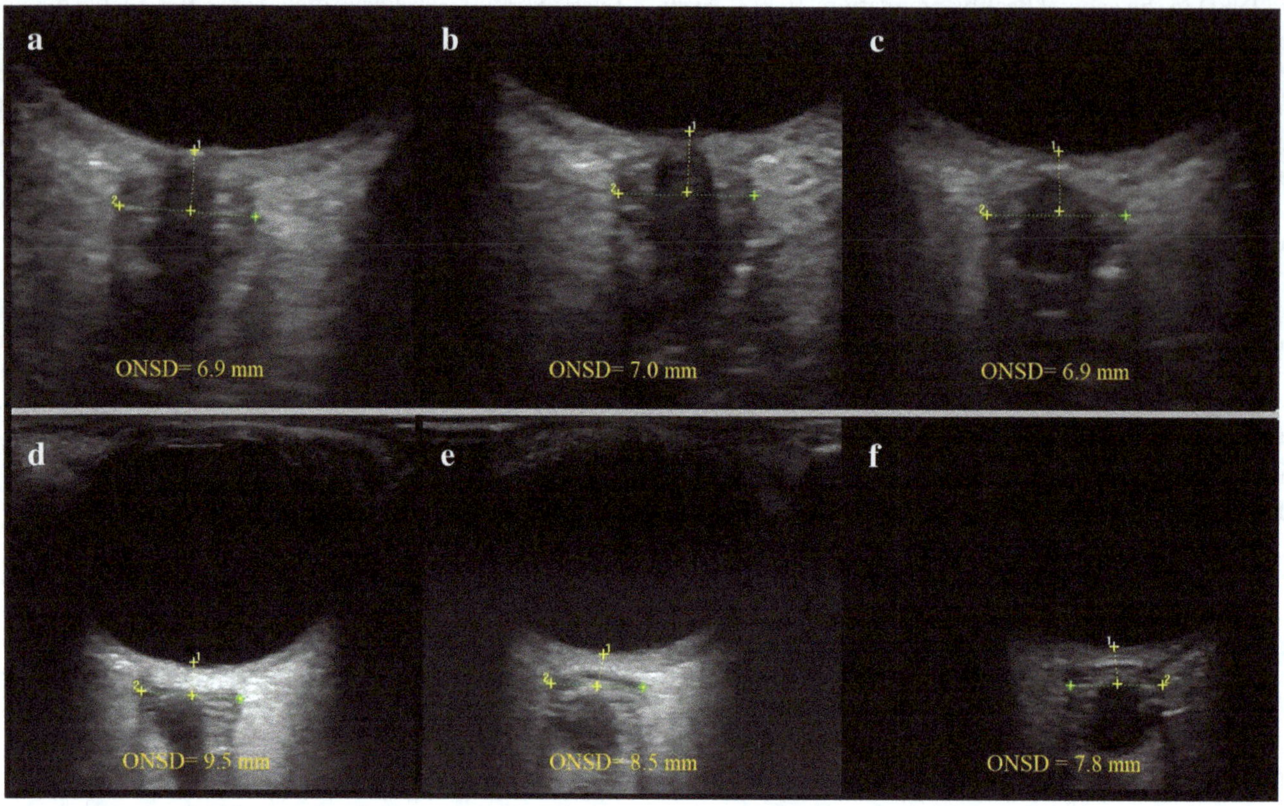

Fig. 1 An example of different ONSD trends during the acute stage of ICH. ONSD ultrasound in a patient with ICH performed at admission (**a**), on the second (**b**), and the third day (**c**), representing the stable ONSD trend and example of unstable ONSD trend in another patient (**d**–**f**) (*ONSD* optic nerve sheath diameter)

Results

During the study period, 35 patients met the inclusion criteria. Clinical and demographic data are shown in Table 2. The patient group and the control group did not significantly differ in terms of gender ($\chi^2=0.012$, $P=1.00$). However, groups differed significantly in age ($\chi^2=55.0$, $P<0.001$). Patients were significantly older. Median binocular ONSD values in patients with acute ICH were significantly higher from those in the control group ($\chi^2=55.0$, $P=0.041$). The median intra-observer variation was ± 0.1 mm (ICC$=0.99$, $P<0.001$, 95% CI 0.99–1.00). In healthy volunteers, serial ONSD recordings revealed a stable trend in 100%. However, in the study group, 23 patients had unstable and 12 had stable ONSD trend during the acute stage of ICH. Serial ONSD sonography recordings during the acute stage of ICH are shown in Table 3. The patients in the unstable ONSD group trend were more likely to have higher ICH scores, ICH volume, mRS, and lower GCS and GOS. On the other hand, no correlation was demonstrated between ONSD trend and midline shift, localization of ICH, NIHSS, and ONSD at admission (Table 4). There were no

Table 2 Demographic and clinical data in study and control groups

	Acute ICH ($n=35$)	Healthy volunteers ($n=20$)	*P*-value*
Age [median (IQR)] (years)	74 (66–79)	30.5 (27–36)	<0.001
Male sex [n (%)]	24 (69.0)	14 (70.0)	1.00
NIHSS score at admission [median (IQR)]	13 (9–18)		
GCS at admission [median (IQR)]	12 (11–15)		
ONSD [median (IQR)] (mm)	7.1 (6.6–7.5)	6.2 (6.0–6.7)	0.041
ICH volume (cm^3) [median (IQR)]	2 (1–3)		

GCS Glasgow Coma Scale, *ICH* intracerebral hemorrhage, *NIHSS* National Institute of Health Stroke Scale, *ONSD* optic nerve sheath diameter, *IQR* interquartile range

*Mann–Whitney continuous data test Chi-square for categorical data

Table 3 ONSD serial recordings during the acute stage of ICH

Patient (n), age (years), sex	Time since admission (days)	ONSD (mm)			ONSD trend	ICH volume (cm^3); midline shift (mm)	GCS	NIHSS	ICH score	MrS; GOS
		Right	Left	Average						
1	0	7.03	7.10	7.06	Unstable (ascending)	31; 8	6	30	4	6; 1
91, F	1	7.10	7.30	7.20			6	30		
	2	7.70	7.76	7.73			6	30		
2	0	5.56	5.33	5.44	Unstable (ascending)	43; 6	6	28	3	6; 1
58, F	1	5.83	6.10	5.96			6	28		
	2	6.06	5.80	5.93			6	28		
3	0	6.73	6.03	6.38	Stable	94; 9	15	13	1	6; 1
76, M	1	6.46	5.96	6.21			15	12		
	2	6.73	5.93	6.33			15	12		
4	0	7.60	7.20	7.40	Stable	11; 4	15	12	1	4; 4
83, M	1	7.23	7.26	7.22			15	12		
	2	7.30	7.23	7.25			15	10		
5	0	8.16	7.85	8.05	Stable	25; 2	15	6	0	2; 5
61, M	1	8.20	7.75	7.98			15	6		
	2	7.93	7.80	7.86			15	5		
6	0	7.10	6.93	7.01	Stable	69; 7.3	8	31	3	6; 1
79, F	1	6.96	6.90	6.93			9	31		
	2	7.00	6.86	6.93			9	31		
7	0	6.76	6.66	6.71	Stable	37; 6	15	13	2	4; 3
59, F	1	6.66	6.56	6.61			15	11		
	2	6.63	6.63	6.63			15	11		
8	0	7.10	6.96	7.03	Stable	10; 6	15	7	1	4; 4
65, M	1	7.07	6.80	6.94			15	6		
	2	7.00	6.70	6.85			15	6		
9	0	7.70	7.63	7.66	Stable	10; 0	15	11	0	4; 3
62, M	1	7.90	7.60	7.75			15	10		
	2	7.63	7.50	7.56			15	10		
10	0	7.50	7.60	7.55	Unstable (oscillating)	71; 8	4	31	4	6; 1
71, M	2 h*	7.40	6.55	6.80			3	31		
	1	7.90	6.50	7.20			3	31		
	2	6.55	6.55	6.55			3	31		
11	0	6.50	6.85	6.68	Unstable (descending)	49; 8	12	12	4	6; 1
82, M	1	6.6	6.90	6.55			12	12		
	2	6.0	6.66	6.43			12	12		
	3	5.65	6.50	6.08			12	12		
12	0	8.56	8.10	8.33	Unstable (descending)	13; 7	11	11	2	4; 3
77, F	1	7.86	8.10	7.98			11	11		
	2	8.20	7.66	7.93			12	11		
13	0	6.50	6.55	6.52	Unstable (descending)	13; 7	12	7	3	5; 3
88, F	1	6.56	6.55	6.54			12	7		
	2	6.45	5.75	6.10			13	7		
14	0	6.96	7.40	7.18	Unstable (descending)	8; 0	15	4	1	1; 5
72, M	1	7.25	7.16	7.20			15	4		
	2	6.10	6.75	6.45			15	3		
15	0	7.13	7.20	7.16	Unstable (ascending)	34; 9	12	15	3	5; 3
67, F	1	7.26	7.80	7.53			12	15		
	2	7.23	7.56	7.41			12	15		

Table 3 (continued)

Patient (n), age (years), sex	Time since admission (days)	ONSD (mm)			ONSD trend	ICH volume (cm³); midline shift (mm)	GCS	NIHSS	ICH score	MrS; GOS
		Right	Left	Average						
16 71, M	0	7.60	7.40	7.50	Unstable (ascending)	78; 5	11	11	3	6; 1
	1	7.73	8.13	7.93			11	12		
	2	7.46	7.80	7.63			11	12		
17 55, M	0	6.96	7.23	7.10	Unstable (descending)	76; 11	12	13	3	6; 1
	2 h*	6.06	6.50	6.28			3	30		
	1	6.36	6.36	6.36			3	30		
	2	6.26	6.70	6.46			3	30		
18 72, F	0	6.00	7.10	6.55	Unstable (ascending)	31; 0	15	3	1	2; 4
	1	6.93	7.60	6.98			15	3		
	2	7.40	7.65	7.52			15	3		
19 74, M	0	6.96	7.50	7.23	Unstable (descending)	66; 14	10	16	3	6; 1
	1	7.10	7.60	7.35			11	16		
	2	6.66	6.63	6.64			11	15		
	3	6.73	7.10	6.91						
20 67, M	0	7.20	7.46	7.33	Unstable (oscillating)	30; 5	12	17	3	6; 1
	1	7.70	8.20	7.95			12	17		
	2	7.20	7.73	7.26			12	17		
	3	7.60	7.60	7.60						
	4	6.96	7.65	7.30						
	5	6.96	7.50	7.22						
21 76, M	0	7.26	8.23	7.75	Unstable (descending)	31; 0	11	9	2	2; 4
	1	7.30	7.90	7.60			15	4		
	2	7.30	7.66	7.48			15	1		
22 74, M	0	6.30	6.43	6.36	Unstable (descending)	62; 7	12	19	3	6; 1
	1	6.26	6.60	6.43			12	19		
	2	7.23	6.86	7.05			12	19		
23 66, M	0	6.66	6.56	6.61	Unstable (descending)	33; 6	12	18	3	6; 1
	1	6.30	6.16	6.23			12	18		
	2	6.35	6.05	6.27			12	18		
24 63, M	0	6.36	6.20	6.28	Stable	1; 0	15	5	0	1; 5
	1	6.40	6.16	6.28			15	4		
	2	6.36	6.10	6.23			15	4		
25 80, F	0	7.10	6.90	7.00	Unstable (ascending)	50; 9	7	29	4	6; 1
	1	7.63	7.53	7.58			7	29		
	2	7.60	7.53	7.56			7	30		
26 61, M	0	6.63	6.96	6.79	Unstable (descending)	5.8; 0	15	10	0	4; 3
	1	6.06	6.45	6.25			15	10		
	2	5.6	6.53	6.08			15	8		
27 83, F	0	6.60	6.56	6.58	Stable	7; 7	15	17	1	4; 3
	1	6.66	6.46	6.56			15	17		
	2	6.80	6.70	6.80			15	17		
28 77, M	0	7.86	7.20	7.53	Unstable (oscillating)	8.3; 0	15	12	0	5; 3
	1	8.16	6.66	7.41			15	12		
	2	8.35	7.03	7.69			15	12		

Table 3 (continued)

Patient (n), age (years), sex	Time since admission (days)	ONSD (mm)			ONSD trend	ICH volume (cm^3); midline shift (mm)	GCS	NIHSS	ICH score	MrS; GOS
		Right	Left	Average						
29 67, M	0	9.16	9.70	9.43	Unstable (descending)	97; 13	5	31	4	6; 1
	1	8.86	9.66	9.26			4	31		
	2	8.2	9.33	8.79			4	31		
	3	8.30	8.66	8.48			4	31		
	4	8.00	8.00	8.00			4	31		
30 78, M	0	7.46	8.25	7.85	Stable	1; 0	15	5	0	2; 5
	1	7.36	8.30	7.83			15	5		
	2	7.46	8.36	7.91			15	5		
31 79, M	0	7.10	7.00	7.05	Stable	4; 0	15	6	0	1; 5
	1	7.00	7.00	7.00			15	6		
	2	7.10	7.10	7.10			15	6		
32 82, M	0	7.46	7.40	7.43	Unstable (oscillating)	30; 8	12	15	4	6; 1
	1	8.16	8.06	8.11			12	16		
	2	7.96	7.56	7.76			12	16		
33 76, F	0	7.13	7.33	7.23	Unstable (descending)	75; 14	4	31	4	6; 1
	1	7.16	6.53	6.84			4	31		
	2	7.05	6.66	6.85			4	31		
34 87, M	0	6.66	6.60	6.63	Stable	31; 6	15	11	2	2; 4
	1	6.66	6.60	6.63			15	11		
	2	6.90	6.90	6.90			15	11		
35 71, M	0	6.80	7.55	7.18	Unstable (oscillating)	40; 5	14	13	2	6; 1
	1	7.46	7.26	7.36			14	13		
	2	7.50	6.66	7.08			14	13		

ICH intracerebral hemorrhage, *ONSD* optic nerve sheath diameter, *M* male, *F* female

* Placement of intraventricular catheter

Table 4 Comparison between patients with stable and unstable ONSD trend

	Median (95% CI)		
	Stable ONSD trend	Unstable ONSD trend	*P*-value*
Number	12	23	
ONSD admission	7.0 (6.6–7.6)	7.2 (6.9–7.4)	0.532
mRS	4.0 (2.0–4.0)	6.0 (5.0–6.0)	0.003
GOS	4.0 (3.0–5.0)	1.0 (1.0–3.0)	0.002
ICH score	1.0 (0.0–1.9)	3.0 (2.4–3.7)	<0.001
GCS	15.0 (15.0–15.0)	12.0 (10.4–12.0)	<0.001
NIHSS	11.0 (6.0–13.0)	15.0 (11.4–18.7)	0.073
ICH volume (cm^3)	10.5 (4.5–35.9)	34.0 (30.3–57.8)	0.029
Midline shift (mm)	5.0 (0.0–6.8)	7.0 (5.0–8.0)	0.079

ONSD optic nerve sheath diameter, *mRS* Modified Rankin Scale, *GCS* Glasgow Coma Scale, *ICH* intracerebral hemorrhage, *NIHSS* National Institute of Health Stroke Scale, *GOS* Glasgow Outcome Scale

*Mann–Whitney continuous data test Chi-square for categorical data

differences between left and right ONSD in the healthy volunteers, but 11 patients had one ONSD significantly larger (> 5%) than the other and in 8 of 11 cases larger ONSD was on the same side as the ICH.

Discussion

To the best of our knowledge, this work for the first time provides information about the dynamics of ONSD measured by means of ultrasound in the acute stage of ICH. We demonstrated that in some ICH patients ONSD values change significantly during the acute stage, whether they rise or fall, and those patients are more likely to have worse functional outcomes when compared to ICH patients with stable acute-phase ONSD values.

ONSD sonography seems to be a reliable surrogate of ICP, with high intra- and interobserver reliability [11, 21, 22] and good correlation between US and MRI measurements of the ONSD [23]. However, most of the published studies rely on a single ONSD measurement or the absolute values of ONSD for ICP diagnosis, rather than on serial recordings and relative changes that might be more useful.

Previous studies have demonstrated that ONSD changes concurrently with rapid ICP variations. Consequently, we could detect changes in ICP by detecting changes in ONSD values. This makes serial ONSD sonography a good non-invasive alternative for ICP assessment in neurocritical patients in whom invasive monitoring is not available or not indicated.

Only a few studies have investigated the utility of serial ONSD measurements. Toscano et al. performed daily ONSD measurements in 21 sedated neurocritical patients who eventually developed brain death (BD) and observed that ONSD values were increasing over time with the widest values occurring just after the BD. The increase of the ONSD was constantly correlated with elevated values of ICP [24]. Thotakura confirmed the utility of serial ONSD measurements in 40 patients with TBI who were in a conservative management program at the time of admission. All the patients with the descending trend had a good outcome and required no surgery, on the other hand, out of four patients who died, three were in ascending trend and the other in static trend [20]. Daily ONSD monitoring has proven to be useful in monitoring pediatric patients during diabetic ketoacidosis management as well as in monitoring patients with MCA infarction who are at risk of developing malignant MCA syndrome [25, 26]. Skoloudik et al. investigated the utility of ONSD sonography during the acute stage of ICH. They emphasize that relative enlargement of the ONSD is a more sensitive indicator of raised ICP than the absolute ONSD value [27]. Naldi et al. also investigated ONSD in patients with ICH and have shown that the second assessment of ONSD measurements may be useful in identifying patients with the persistency of elevated ICP [28]. Both studies have indicated the need for more research in this field.

Furthermore, we demonstrated that ONSD reacts almost simultaneously to oscillations in ICP. Two patients underwent placement of external ventricular drain (EDV) and ONSD descending trend appeared right after. The average left and right ONSD at admission for patient 10 and patient 17 (Table 3) were 7.55 mm and 7.10 mm, respectively. Only a few minutes after the placement of EDV, sonography of ONSD was done again, this time showing a significant decline in ONSD values, on 6.80 mm for patient 10 and 6.28 mm for patient 17. This could be one more proof that ONSD reacts to ICP changes in real-time, especially because ONSD significantly decreased immediately after the placement of EDV.

The values of ONSD in a healthy subject in this study were higher than has usually been found previously (median 6.2 mm; 95% CI 6.1–6.7). This could be due to multiple reasons including ethnic diversity and genetic difference as well as measuring the technique of ultrasound and expertise of the observer.

This study has some limitations. The lack of ICP data makes it impossible to correlate ONSD values with the actual ICP. Although the sample size in the study was sufficient for adequate statistical analysis, the number of participants was relatively small and future studies with a larger number of patients are needed to strengthen our results. One of the limitations was that there was no uniform time of control neuroimaging. Control brain CT was not necessarily done during the first 2 days which is the period in which we monitored ONSD. Consequently, a comparison of the ONSD dynamics with the dynamics of intracranial status would not be valid. Control CT scan was available for 32 patients (3 died before follow-up brain CT). 10 patients had significant worsening of intracranial status in terms of increased ICH volume, perifocal edema, or progression of midline shift, and 9 of these 10 patients had an unstable ONSD trend (3 oscillating, 3 ascending and 3 descending trends).

Furthermore, the ONSD trend was marked as stable or unstable, but in the unstable ONSD group, there were patients with clear ascending, descending, and oscillating trends (alternating increase or decrease value) (Table 3). The sample size was not sufficient enough for adequate statistical analysis among these subgroups of the unstable trend. Mean mRS for oscillating, ascending, and a descending trend was 5.8, 5.2, and 4.8, respectively. Mean GOS values for these subgroups of ONSD unstable trend also differ similarly: 1.4 for oscillating, 1.8 for ascending, and 2.1 for descending trend. The patients with oscillating ONSD trends were most likely to have a worse outcomes, followed by ascending and then a descending trend.

Although the acute phase ONSD dynamics can help in predicting the clinical outcome in ICH patients, this study does not address whether ONSD trend improves prognostication over already known variables.

Conclusion

The role of daily ONSD sonography in the acute stage of ICH has not yet been investigated. According to our results, the assessment of acute-phase ONSD dynamics can help predicting the outcome in ICH patients and serial ONSD assessment may be a useful noninvasive tool for the detection of ICP changes in neurocritical patients without invasive monitoring.

Abbreviations

EDV: External ventricular drain; NIHSS: National Institute of Health Stroke Scale; GCS: Glasgow Coma Scale; ONSD: Optic nerve sheath diameter; ICP: Intracranial pressure; ICH: Intracerebral hemorrhage; mRS: Modified Rankin Scale; GOS: Glasgow Outcome Scale; CT: Computer tomography; US: Ultrasound.

Acknowledgements
None.

Authors' contributions
MB and BM designed the study. MB prepared the manuscript draft with important intellectual input from SS and BM. MB, SL, and NP conducted the study including patient recruitment, data collection, and data analysis. All authors contributed to manuscript revision. All authors read and approved the final manuscript.

Author details
[1] Department of Neurology, University Hospital Mostar, Bijeli Brijeg bb, 88 000 Mostar, Bosnia and Herzegovina. [2] Department of Neurology, Asklepios Kliniken, Brandenburg, Germany. [3] Department of Neurology, University Hospital Center Zagreb, Zagreb, Croatia.

References

1. Ohle R, McIsaac SM, Woo MY, Perry JJ (2015) Sonography of the optic nerve sheath diameter for detection of raised intracranial pressure compared to computed tomography: a systematic review and meta-analysis. J Ultrasound Med 34:1285–1294
2. Dubourg J, Javouhey E, Geeraerts T, Messerer M, Kassai B (2011) Ultrasonography of optic nerve sheath diameter for detection of raised intracranial pressure: a systematic review and meta-analysis. Intensive Care Med 37:1059–1068
3. Hansen HC, Helmke K (1996) The subarachnoid space surrounding the optic nerves. An ultrasound study of the optic nerve sheath. Surg Radiol Anat 18:323–328
4. Soldatos T, Chatzimichail K, Papathanasiou M, Gouliamos A (2009) Optic nerve sonography: a new window for the non-invasive evaluation of intracranial pressure in brain injury. Emerg Med J 26:630–634
5. Maissan IM, Dirven PJ, Haitsma IK, Hoeks SE, Gommers D, Stolker RJ (2015) Ultrasonographic measured optic nerve sheath diameter as an accurate and quick monitor for changes in intracranial pressure. J Neurosurg 123:743–747
6. Kimberly HH, Shah S, Marill K, Noble V (2008) Correlation of optic nerve sheath diameter with direct measurement of intracranial pressure. Acad Emerg Med 15:201–204
7. Geeraerts T, Newcombe VF, Coles JP, Abate MG, Perkes IE, Hutchinson PJ et al (2008) Use of T2-weighted magnetic resonance imaging of the optic nerve sheath to detect raised intracranial pressure. Crit Care 12:R114
8. Lochner P, Fassbender K, Knodel S, Andrejewski A, Lesmeister M, Wagenpfeil G et al (2019) B-mode transorbital ultrasonography for the diagnosis of idiopathic intracranial hypertension: a systematic review and meta-analysis. Ultraschall Med 40:247–252
9. Bauerle J, Nedelmann M (2011) Sonographic assessment of the optic nerve sheath in idiopathic intracranial hypertension. J Neurol 258:2014–2019
10. Chen H, Ding GS, Zhao YC, Yu RG, Zhou JX (2015) Ultrasound measurement of optic nerve diameter and optic nerve sheath diameter in healthy Chinese adults. BMC Neurol 15:106
11. Bauerle J, Lochner P, Kaps M, Nedelmann M (2012) Intra- and interobserver reliability of sonographic assessment of the optic nerve sheath diameter in healthy adults. J Neuroimaging 22:42–45
12. Soldatos T, Karakitsos D, Chatzimichail K, Papathanasiou M, Gouliamos A, Karabinis A (2008) Optic nerve sonography in the diagnostic evaluation of adult brain injury. Crit Care 12:R67
13. Romagnuolo L, Tayal V, Tomaszewski C, Saunders T, Norton HJ (2005) Optic nerve sheath diameter does not change with patient position. Am J Emerg Med 23:686–688
14. Stockhausen K (2000) The Declaration of Helsinki: revising ethical research guidelines for the 21st century. Med J Aust 172:252–253
15. Hara M, Kadowaki C, Shiogai T, Takeuchi K (1998) Correlation between intracranial pressure (ICP) and changes in CT images of cerebral hemorrhage. Neurol Res 20:225–230
16. Kothari RU, Brott T, Broderick JP, Barsan WG, Sauerbeck LR, Zuccarello M et al (1996) The ABCs of measuring intracerebral hemorrhage volumes. Stroke 27:1304–1305
17. Young FB, Weir CJ, Lees KR, Committee GITS, Investigators (2005) Comparison of the National Institutes of Health Stroke Scale with disability outcome measures in acute stroke trials. Stroke 36:2187–2192
18. Hemphill JC 3rd, Farrant M, Neill TA Jr (2009) Prospective validation of the ICH score for 12-month functional outcome. Neurology 73:1088–1094
19. Broderick JP, Adeoye O, Elm J (2017) Evolution of the modified Rankin scale and its use in future stroke trials. Stroke 48:2007–2012
20. Thotakura AK, Marabathina NR, Danaboyina AR, Mareddy RR (2017) Role of serial ultrasonic optic nerve sheath diameter monitoring in head injury. Neurochirurgie 63:444–448
21. Ballantyne SA, O'Neill G, Hamilton R, Hollman AS (2002) Observer variation in the sonographic measurement of optic nerve sheath diameter in normal adults. Eur J Ultrasound 15:145–149
22. Cimilli Ozturk T, Demir H, Yorulmaz R, Ozdemir S, Isat G, Ecmel OO (2015) Assessment of intra-interobserver reliability of the sonographic optic nerve sheath diameter measurement. Kaohsiung J Med Sci 31:432–436
23. Steinborn M, Fiegler J, Ruedisser K, Hapfelmeier A, Denne C, Macdonald E et al (2012) Measurement of the optic nerve sheath diameter in children: comparison between transbulbar sonography and magnetic resonance imaging. Ultraschall Med 33:569–573
24. Toscano M, Spadetta G, Pulitano P, Rocco M, Di Piero V, Mecarelli O et al (2017) Optic nerve sheath diameter ultrasound evaluation in intensive care unit: possible role and clinical aspects in neurological critical patients' daily monitoring. Biomed Res Int 2017:1621428
25. Albert AF, Kirkman MA (2017) Clinical and radiological predictors of malignant middle cerebral artery infarction development and outcomes. J Stroke Cerebrovasc Dis 26:2671–2679
26. Hansen G, Vallance JK, Beer DL, Clark I, Sellers EAC (2016) Serial optic nerve sheath diameter ultrasonography during pediatric diabetic ketoacidosis management: a pilot study. J Diabetes Complicat 30:1600–1602
27. Skoloudik D, Herzig R, Fadrna T, Bar M, Hradilek P, Roubec M et al (2011) Distal enlargement of the optic nerve sheath in the hyperacute stage of intracerebral haemorrhage. Br J Ophthalmol 95:217–221
28. Naldi A, Pivetta E, Coppo L, Cantello R, Comi C, Stecco A et al (2019) Ultrasonography monitoring of optic nerve sheath diameter and retinal vessels in patients with cerebral hemorrhage. J Neuroimaging 29:394–399

Permissions

All chapters in this book were first published by Springer; hereby published with permission under the Creative Commons Attribution License or equivalent. Every chapter published in this book has been scrutinized by our experts. Their significance has been extensively debated. The topics covered herein carry significant findings which will fuel the growth of the discipline. They may even be implemented as practical applications or may be referred to as a beginning point for another development.

The contributors of this book come from diverse backgrounds, making this book a truly international effort. This book will bring forth new frontiers with its revolutionizing research information and detailed analysis of the nascent developments around the world.

We would like to thank all the contributing authors for lending their expertise to make the book truly unique. They have played a crucial role in the development of this book. Without their invaluable contributions this book wouldn't have been possible. They have made vital efforts to compile up to date information on the varied aspects of this subject to make this book a valuable addition to the collection of many professionals and students.

This book was conceptualized with the vision of imparting up-to-date information and advanced data in this field. To ensure the same, a matchless editorial board was set up. Every individual on the board went through rigorous rounds of assessment to prove their worth. After which they invested a large part of their time researching and compiling the most relevant data for our readers.

The editorial board has been involved in producing this book since its inception. They have spent rigorous hours researching and exploring the diverse topics which have resulted in the successful publishing of this book. They have passed on their knowledge of decades through this book. To expedite this challenging task, the publisher supported the team at every step. A small team of assistant editors was also appointed to further simplify the editing procedure and attain best results for the readers.

Apart from the editorial board, the designing team has also invested a significant amount of their time in understanding the subject and creating the most relevant covers. They scrutinized every image to scout for the most suitable representation of the subject and create an appropriate cover for the book.

The publishing team has been an ardent support to the editorial, designing and production team. Their endless efforts to recruit the best for this project, has resulted in the accomplishment of this book. They are a veteran in the field of academics and their pool of knowledge is as vast as their experience in printing. Their expertise and guidance has proved useful at every step. Their uncompromising quality standards have made this book an exceptional effort. Their encouragement from time to time has been an inspiration for everyone.

The publisher and the editorial board hope that this book will prove to be a valuable piece of knowledge for researchers, students, practitioners and scholars across the globe.

List of Contributors

Pablo Blanco
Intensive Care Unit, Hospital Dr. Emilio Ferreyra, 4801, 59 St., 7630 Necochea, Argentina
Intensive Care Unit, Clínica Cruz Azul, 2651, 60 St., 7630 Necochea, Argentina

Giovanni Volpicelli
Emergency Medicine, San Luigi Gonzaga University Hospital, 10043 Turin, Italy

Babar Fiza, Michael Tang and Michael Maile
Department of Anesthesiology, University of Michigan Hospitals, 1500 East Medical Center Drive, Ann Arbor, MI 48109-5861, USA

Brian Lentz
Department of Emergency Medicine, Highland Hospital-Alameda Health System, 1411 E. 31st Street, QIC 22123, Oakland, CA 94602, USA

Tiffany Fong, Randall Rhyne and Nicholas Risko
Department of Emergency Medicine, Johns Hopkins University School of Medicine, 1800 Orleans St, Baltimore, MD 21287, USA

Marta Alfageme, Jorge González Plaza, Santiago Méndez, Juan A. Gómez Patiño, María L. Collado, Rocío González Costero and Agustín García Suárez
Department of Interventional Radiology, Hospital Universitario Puerta de Hierro, Majadahonda, España

José M. Abadal
Department of Interventional Radiology, Hospital Universitario Severo Ochoa, Leganés, España

Teresa Fontanilla
Department of Radiology, Hospital Universitario Puerta de Hierro, Majadahonda, España

Christian D. Yic, Leandro Moraes, Marcos E. Lasso and Alberto Biestro
Department of Critical Care Medicine, Hospital de Clínicas, Montevideo, Uruguay

Sergio I. Paz and Julio C. Pontet
Department of Critical Care Medicine, Hospital Pasteur, Montevideo, Uruguay

Gabriel Prada
Department of Critical Care Medicine, Mayo Clinic, Jacksonville, USA

David Rene Rodriguez Lima
Emergency Medicine and Critical and Intensive Care Medicine, Hospital Universitario Mayor Méderi-Universidad del Rosario, Bogotá, Colombia

Andrés Felipe Yepes, Claudia Inés Birchenall Jiménez and Mario Andrés Mercado Díaz
Critical and Intensive Care Medicine, Hospital Universitario Mayor Méderi-Universidad del Rosario, Bogotá, Colombia

Ever Julián Duran and Ever Leonardo Rojas Díaz
Resident, Critical and Intensive Care Medicine, Hospital Universitario Mayor Méderi-Universidad del Rosario, Bogotá, Colombia

Darío Isaías Pinilla Rojas
Anesthesiology and Critical and Intensive Care Medicine, Hospital Universitario Mayor Méderi-Universidad del Rosario, Bogotá, Colombia

Yury Forlán Bustos Martínez
Emergency Medicine Department of Ultrasound and Simulation, Universidad del Rosario, Bogotá, Colombia

M. J. Blans and F. H. Bosch
Department of Intensive Care, Rijnstate Hospital, 6800 TA Arnhem, The Netherlands

J. G. van der Hoeven
Department of Intensive Care, Radboud University Medical Center, 6500 HB Nijmegen, The Netherlands

Pablo Rodriguez, Igor Sviridenko, Sylvia Noveri and Ana Soca
Intensive Care Unit, Hospital Pasteur, Administración de Servicios de Salud del Estado, Montevideo, Uruguay

Christian Yic, Diego Méndez and Mario Cancela
Intensive Care Unit, Asociación Española Primera de Socorros Mutuos, Montevideo, Uruguay

José L. Díaz-Gómez
Department of Critical Care Medicine, Mayo Clinic, Jacksonville, USA

Julio Pontet
Intensive Care Unit, Hospital Pasteur, Administración de Servicios de Salud del Estado, Montevideo, Uruguay
Intensive Care Unit, Asociación Española Primera de Socorros Mutuos, Montevideo, Uruguay
Larravide 2458, Montevideo, Uruguay

Gert Jan Scheffer
Radboud Institute for Health Sciences, Department of Anesthesiology, Pain, and Palliative Medicine, Radboud university medical center, Geert Grooteplein-Zuid 10, 6525 GA Nijmegen, The Netherlands

Rein Ketelaars, Geert-Jan van Geffen and Nico Hoogerwerf
Radboud Institute for Health Sciences, Department of Anesthesiology, Pain, and Palliative Medicine, Radboud university medical center, Geert Grooteplein-Zuid 10, 6525 GA Nijmegen, The Netherlands
Radboud Institute for Health Sciences, Helicopter Emergency Medical Service Lifeliner 3, Radboud university medical center, Geert Grooteplein-Zuid 10, 6525 GA Nijmegen, The Netherlands

Gabby Reijnders
Department of Intensive Care, Catharina Hospital, Michelangelolaan 2, 5623 EJ Eindhoven, The Netherlands

E. Rancinger
The Research Section, Department of Surgery (A), Odense University Hospital, Baagoes Allé 15, 5700 Svendborg, Denmark

M. Riishede
The Research Section, Department of Surgery (A), Odense University Hospital, Baagoes Allé 15, 5700 Svendborg, Denmark
Department of Clinical Research, University of Southern Denmark, SDU, Odense, Denmark
Department of Internal Medicine & Emergency Medicine (M/FAM), Odense University Hospital, Svendborg, Denmark

G. Baatrup
The Research Section, Department of Surgery (A), Odense University Hospital, Baagoes Allé 15, 5700 Svendborg, Denmark
Department of Clinical Research, University of Southern Denmark, SDU, Odense, Denmark

C. B. Laursen
Department of Clinical Research, University of Southern Denmark, SDU, Odense, Denmark
Department of Respiratory Medicine, Odense University Hospital, Odense, Denmark

L. S. Teglbjærg
Department of Internal Medicine & Emergency Medicine (M/FAM), Odense University Hospital, Svendborg, Denmark

P. B. Pedersen
Department of Clinical Research, University of Southern Denmark, SDU, Odense, Denmark
Department of Internal Medicine & Emergency Medicine (M/FAM), Odense University Hospital, Svendborg, Denmark

S. M. Luef
Department of Respiratory Medicine, Odense University Hospital, Odense, Denmark

J. H. Clausen
Department of Cardiology, Hospital of Southern Jutland, Aabenraa, Denmark

O. Graumann
Department of Clinical Research, University of Southern Denmark, SDU, Odense, Denmark
Department of Radiology, Odense University Hospital, Odense, Denmark

A. T. Lassen
Department of Clinical Research, University of Southern Denmark, SDU, Odense, Denmark
Department of Emergency Medicine, Odense University Hospital, Odense, Denmark

Tyler Beals
Beth Israel Deaconess Medical Center, 1 Deaconess Rd, Rosenberg 2, Boston, MA 02215, USA

Kay Odashima, Lawrence E. Haines, Antonios Likourezos, Jefferson Drapkin and Eitan Dickman
Maimonides Medical Center, Brooklyn, NY, USA

Antonio Anile and Giacomo Castiglione
Intensive Care Unit, Ospedale Vittorio Emanuele, AOU Policlinico-Vittorio Emanuele, Catania, Italy

Silvia Ferrario
Section of Nephrology, Department of Clinical and Experimental Medicine, Policlinico Universitario, University of Catania, Catania, Italy

Lorena Campanello and Maria Antonietta Orban
School of Anaesthesia and Intensive Care, University Hospital "G. Rodolico", University of Catania, Catania, Italy

Emily L. Wilson
Pulmonary Division, Intermountain Medical Center, Salt Lake City, UT, USA

Ezekiel Egan
University of Utah School of Medicine, Salt Lake City, UT, USA

Michael J. Lanspa, Colin K. Grissom and Samuel M. Brown
Pulmonary Division, Intermountain Medical Center, Salt Lake City, UT, USA
Pulmonary Division, University of Utah School of Medicine, Salt Lake City, UT, USA
Critical Care Echocardiography Service, Intermountain Medical Center, Salt Lake City, UT, USA

Elliotte L. Hirshberg
Pulmonary Division, Intermountain Medical Center, Salt Lake City, UT, USA
Pulmonary Division, University of Utah School of Medicine, Salt Lake City, UT, USA
Critical Care Echocardiography Service, Intermountain Medical Center, Salt Lake City, UT, USA
Department of Pediatrics, University of Utah School of Medicine, Salt Lake City, UT, USA

Rebecca Burk
Pulmonary Division, Intermountain Medical Center, Salt Lake City, UT, USA
Critical Care Echocardiography Service, Intermountain Medical Center, Salt Lake City, UT, USA

Sarah J. Beesley
Pulmonary Division, Intermountain Medical Center, Salt Lake City, UT, USA
Pulmonary Division, University of Utah School of Medicine, Salt Lake City, UT, USA
Shock Trauma Intensive Care Unit, 5121 South Cottonwood Street, Murray, UT 84107, USA

Christian Villavicencio, Julen Leache, Iban Oliva, Alejandro Rodriguez and María Bodí
Critical Care Department, Joan XXIII-University Hospital, Mallafre Guasch 4, 43007 Tarragona, Spain

Judith Marin
Critical Care Department, Hospital del Mar-Research Group in Critical Illness (GREPAC), Institut Hospital del Mar d'investigacions Mèdiques (IMIM), Barcelona, Spain

Nilam J. Soni
Division of Pulmonary & Critical Care Medicine, University of Texas Health San Antonio, San Antonio, TX, USA
Division of General & Hospital Medicine, University of Texas Health San Antonio, San Antonio, TX, USA
Section of Hospital Medicine, South Texas Veterans Health Care System, San Antonio, TX, USA

Mohamed Amine Msolli, Adel Sekma, Maryem Ben Marzouk, Khaoula Bel Haj Ali, Nasri Bzeouich, Kamel Laaouiti, Mohamed Habib Grissa, Kaouthar Beltaief, Wahid Bouida, Hamdi Boubaker and Semir Nouira
Emergency Department, Fattouma Bourguiba University Hospital, 5000 Monastir, Tunisia
Research Laboratory LR12SP18, University of Monastir, 5019 Monastir, Tunisia

Wael Chaabane, Lotfi Boukadida and Riadh Boukef
Emergency Department, Sahloul University Hospital, 4011 Sousse, Tunisia
Research Laboratory LR12SP18, University of Monastir, 5019 Monastir, Tunisia

Imen Gannoun and Imen Trabelssi
Research Laboratory LR12SP18, University of Monastir, 5019 Monastir, Tunisia

Zohra Dridi
Cardiology Department, Fattouma Bourguiba University Hospital, 5000 Monastir, Tunisia

Asma Belguith
Department of Preventive Medicine, Fattouma Bourguiba University Hospital, 5000 Monastir, Tunisia

Mehdi Methamem
Emergency Department, Farhat Hached University Hospital, 4031 Sousse, Tunisia

Tom Terboven, Ivette Betka, Tim Viergutz, Georg Leonhard and Michael Schöler
Department of Anaesthesiology and Intensive Care Medicine, University Medical Center Mannheim, Theodor-Kutzer-Ufer 1-3, 68167 Mannheim, Germany

Christel Weiss
Department of Medical Statistics, University Medical Center Mannheim, Theodor-Kutzer-Ufer 1-3, 68167 Mannheim, Germany

Marcus Rudolph
Department of Anaesthesiology and Intensive Care Medicine, University Medical Center Mannheim, Theodor-Kutzer-Ufer 1-3, 68167 Mannheim, Germany
DRF Stiftung Luftrettung gemeinnützige AG, Filderstadt, Germany

Anurag Dalai, Leanne Langford and Haron Obaid
Department of Radiology, College of Medicine, University of Saskatchewan, 103 Hospital Drive, Saskatoon, SK S7N 0W8, Canada

Cole Beavis
Department of Orthopedic Surgery, College of Medicine, University of Saskatchewan, Saskatoon, Canada

Naima Kilhamn
Department of Perioperative Medicine and Intensive Care, Karolinska University Hospital, Solna, 171 76 Stockholm, Sweden

Mårten Renberg, Claire Rimes-Stigare, Max Bell and Daniel Hertzberg
Department of Perioperative Medicine and Intensive Care, Karolinska University Hospital, Solna, 171 76 Stockholm, Sweden
Department of Physiology and Pharmacology, Karolinska Institutet, Stockholm, Sweden

Olof Jonmarker
Department of Radiology, Karolinska University Hospital, Huddinge, Stockholm, Sweden

Osman Adi, Azma Haryaty Ahmad and Chan Pei Fong
Resuscitation & Emergency Critical Care Unit, Department of Emergency and Trauma, Raja Permaisuri Bainun Hospital, Jalan Raja Ashman (Jalan Hospital), 30400 Ipoh, Perak, Malaysia

Asri Ranga
Department of Cardiology, Hospital Serdang, Serdang, Selangor, Malaysia

Nova Panebianco
Division of Emergency Ultrasound, Department of Emergency Medicine, Hospital of the University of Pennsylvania, 3400 Spruce St, Philadelphia, PA 19104, USA

Ilaria Pulzato
Dipartimento di Medicina interna e Specialità mediche, Di.M.I. Università degli Studi di Geniva, Viale Benedetto XV, 10, 16132 Genoa, GE, Italy

Enrico Boero
Dipartimento di scienze Chirurgiche, Università degli Studi di Torino, Turin, Italy

Elona Shaipi and Luciano Cardinale
SCDU Radiodiagnostica e Medicina Nucleare, Azienda Ospedaliero-Universitaria S.Luigi Gonzaga, Regione Gonzole 10, 10043 Orbassano, TO, Italy

Daria Antipova, Leila Eadie and Philip Wilson
Centre for Rural Health, University of Aberdeen, Old Perth Road, Inverness IV2 3JH, UK

Ashish Stephen Macaden
Department of Stroke and Rehabilitation Medicine, Raigmore Hospital, NHS Highland, Inverness IV2 3UJ, UK

Denise Castro, Prasan Patel, Eric Sauerbrei and Don Soboleski
Department of Radiology, Kingston Health Sciences Centre, Queen's University, 76 Stuart Street, Kingston, ON K7L 2V7, Canada

Joseph Yang
Queen's School of Medicine, Queen's University, 80 Barrie Street, Kingston, ON K7L 3N6, Canada

Wilma Hopman
WJ Henderson Centre for Patient Oriented Research, Queen's University, 76 Stuart Street, Kingston, ON K7L 2V7, Canada

Mila Kolar
Department of Surgery, Kingston Health Sciences Centre, Queen's University, 76 Stuart Street, Kingston, ON K7L 2V7, Canada

Peiman Nazerian, Giuliano De Stefano, Giovanni Albano, Vera Gaspari and Stefano Grifoni
Department of Emergency Medicine, Careggi University Hospital, Largo Brambilla 3, 50134 Florence, Firenze, Italy

Sergio Bevilacqua and Valter Campagnolo
Department of Anaesthesiology, Careggi University Hospital, Florence, Italy

Pierluigi Stefàno
Department of Cardiac Surgery, Careggi University Hospital, Florence, Italy

Christopher K. Schott
VA Pittsburgh Health Care Systems Critical Care Service Line (124U), University Drive, Pittsburgh, PA 15240, USA
Department of Critical Care Medicine and Emergency Medicine, University of Pittsburgh, and University of Pittsburgh Medical Center (UPMC), 3550 Terrace Street Scaife Hall, Suite 600, Pittsburgh, PA 15213, USA

Emily B. Brant and Mohammad I. Hirzallah
University of Pittsburgh Multidisciplinary Critical Care Training Program, 3550 Terrace Street Scaife Hall, Suite 600, Pittsburgh, PA 15213, USA

Rock Heyman
Department of Neurology, University of Pittsburgh, and University of Pittsburgh Medical Center (UPMC), 300 Halket Street, Suite 4500, Pittsburgh, PA, USA 15213

Daniel N. Lesky
School of Medicine 401 Scaife Hall, University of Pittsburgh, 3550 Terrace Street, Pittsburgh, PA 15261, USA

Clifton W. Callaway
Department of Emergency Medicine, University of Pittsburgh, and University of Pittsburgh, Medical Center (UPMC), 3600 Forbes at Meyran Avenue Forbes Tower, Suite 10028, Pittsburgh, PA 15213, USA

M. Bender, S. Lakicevic and N. Pravdic
Department of Neurology, University Hospital Mostar, Bijeli Brijeg bb, 88 000 Mostar, Bosnia and Herzegovina

S. Schreiber
Department of Neurology, Asklepios Kliniken, Brandenburg, Germany

B. Malojcic
Department of Neurology, University Hospital Center Zagreb, Zagreb, Croatia

Index

www.ingramcontent.com/pod-product-compliance
Lightning Source LLC
LaVergne TN
LVHW082222200926
848484LV00008B/2287